THE PROSTATE BOOK

DR. PETER T. SCARDINO, M.D.

and

JUDITH KELMAN

MICHAEL JOSEPH
an imprint of
PENGUIN BOOKS

MICHAEL JOSEPH

Published by the Penguin Group
Penguin Books Ltd, 80 Strand, London WC2R 0RL, England
Penguin Group (USA) Inc., 375 Hudson Street, New York, New York 10014, USA
Penguin Group (Canada), 10 Alcorn Avenue, Toronto, Ontario, Canada m4v 3b2
(a division of Pearson Penguin Canada Inc.)
Penguin Ireland, 25 St Stephen's Green, Dublin 2, Ireland (a division of Penguin Books Ltd)
Penguin Group (Australia), 250 Camberwell Road,
Camberwell, Victoria 3124, Australia (a division of Pearson Australia Group Pty Ltd)
Penguin Books India Pvt Ltd, 11 Community Centre,
Panchsheel Park, New Delhi – 110 017, India
Penguin Group (NZ), cnr Airborne and Rosedale Roads, Albany,
Auckland 1310, New Zealand (a division of Pearson New Zealand Ltd)
Penguin Books (South Africa) (Pty) Ltd, 24 Sturdee Avenue,
Rosebank 2196, South Africa

Penguin Books Ltd, Registered Offices: 80 Strand, London WC2R 0RL, England

www.penguin.com

First published in the United States of America by The Penguin Group 2005
First published in Great Britain by Michael Joseph 2005
1

Copyright © Peter T. Scardino and Judith Kelman, 2005

The moral right of the authors has been asserted

Neither the author or the publishers is engaged in rendering professional advice or services to the individual reader.
The ideas, procedures and suggestions in this book are not intended as a substitute for consulting a physician. All matters
regarding health require medical supervision. Neither the authors or the publisher shall be liable or responsible for any loss,
injury, or damage allegedly advising from any information or suggestion in this book. The opinions expressed in this book
represent the personal views of the author and not of the publisher. While the authors have made every effort to provide
accurate telephone numbers and Internet addresses at the time of publication, neither the authors or the publisher
assumes any responsibility for errors, or for changes that occur after publication.

Printed in Great Britain by Clays Ltd, St Ives plc

A CIP catalogue record for this book is available from the British Library

ISBN 0–718–14694–8

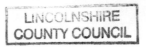

In memory of Dr. Peter L. Scardino, a fine urologist, a charming gentleman, and a generous father. And to Cecilia and Lillian, who hold the future in their lovely little hands.

To George Edelstein, who always wished to be a healer, and was.

To David Golde, M.D., 1941–2004, a man of unusual insight, a brilliant physician, and a wise leader.

And to all the patients and their families whose courage has been a constant source of wonder and whose insightful questions led to this book.

ACKNOWLEDGMENTS

This book is not intended to be one doctor's point of view. To provide comprehensive, up-to-date information, we sought the help of top medical experts, scientists working in cutting-edge research, nurses, and many patients and their loved ones who have experienced these problems themselves. The authors wish to thank the following for their thoughtful and most generous input.

Memorial Sloan-Kettering urologists Drs. James Eastham and Bertrand Guillonneau provided countless insights from their vast experience in caring for patients with prostate cancer.

Dr. Howard Scher leads the team of superb medical oncologists who have pioneered the treatment of prostate cancer with drugs. He and Dr. Michael Morris provided valuable perspectives on advanced prostate cancer.

Drs. Zvi Fuks, Michael Zelefsky, and Steve Leibel, pioneers in the development of modern radiation oncology, read the chapters related to radiation therapy and its complications and offered many helpful suggestions.

Dr. Victor Reuter contributed his insights as one of the country's leading prostate pathologists. Dr. Hedvig Hricak, an outstanding radiologist who virtually invented MRI of the prostate, reviewed all the sections on diagnostic imaging.

Dr. Michael Kattan, a wizard of medical informatics, offered many insights on decision making and those invaluable predictive tools: nomograms.

Dr. Carlos Cordon-Cardo, a pioneer in studying and battling cancer at a molecular level, lent his extraordinary, cutting-edge insights. Dr. Hans Lilja, who discovered "free" PSA, helped us to define and explain the importance of PSA in prostate cancer and other prostatic diseases.

Psychiatrist Dr. Andrew Roth lent his expertise on the emotional and psychiatric problems of prostate-cancer patients and their partners. Gastroenterologist Dr. Moshe Shike provided valuable advice about the treatment of intestinal complications of radiation therapy for prostate cancer. Dr. Karyn Eilber contributed to the sections on the diagnosis and treatment of urinary problems, and Dr. John Mulhall assisted with the sections on the sexual complications of prostate diseases and their treatments. Dr. Barrie Casselith graciously reviewed the manuscript and offered the latest, scientifically grounded information about alternative and complementary medicine. Karrie Zampini, CSW, ACSW, who developed the country's first post-treatment resource program for cancer survivors, lent her unique perspective on the needs of patients and their loved ones.

Thanks to a most extraordinary nurse practitioner, Mary Schoen, N.P., and to Tara Stevenson, R.N., for their valuable observations and practical suggestions.

We are grateful to Dr. E. Darracott Vaughan of the Weill Medical College of Cornell University for his insights about BPH in particular and for his many other helpful comments. Thanks to Dr. Anthony Schaeffer of Northwestern University, one of the country's leading experts on prostatitis, for offering his up-to-date views.

Many of the staff at Memorial Sloan-Kettering provided valuable support. Special thanks to Hope Lafferty for her organizational skills and to David Kuo for the skill and intelligence he brought to our information system and for his countless effective responses to our distress signals at all hours when our laptops crashed or the network went down. Thanks also to Kim Gibbons, Barbara Kristaponis, Ophelia Chu, and many others.

We're indebted to Sidney Kimmel, Jim Robinson, Sandy Warner, Paul Marks, Bob Wittes, and Harold Varmus. Without them the Prostate Cancer Program at Memorial Sloan-Kettering would not exist. And special thanks to Jan Calloway, Mickey Tarnopol, Michael Milken, David Koch, Joe Allbritton, Grant Gregory, and many others who have so generously supported the program.

Kudos to Mary Higgins Clark and John Conheeney for hosting the most elegant writers' retreat imaginable. We are grateful to David Storrs, Virgil Simons, Steve Gragg, Ken Borow, Salvatore and Connie Natale, David Elsasser, Richard Barlow, Gregg Wiita, both Ed Grossmans, Steve Joseph, Jamie Janoff, Randolph Duke, Mel Lerman, Karl Seib, and Ivan Wolff for all the thoughtful discussions and valuable input. Thanks also to Liz Polizzi, for a job so thoughtfully and well done.

It's been a privilege to work with top-notch literary agent Peter Lampack, and with all the good people in the Penguin Group, especially Susan Petersen Kennedy, David Shanks, Megan Newman, and Marilyn Ducksworth.

CONTENTS

Part Three

∎

PROSTATE CANCER

INTRODUCTION

I n 1971, the U.S. government declared war on cancer, and for men with prostate cancer, there is excellent news from the front! We now have tests that can detect this common cancer so early in its course that most patients can be cured with surgery or radiation therapy. Modern techniques have lowered the risk of troubling side effects from these treatments, improving quality as well as length of life. Recent landmark studies have proven for the first time that chemotherapy prolongs survival for men with advanced prostate cancer. The mortality rate from this disease has declined more than 25 percent in the past decade. And we now have exciting evidence that it may be possible to prevent prostate cancer with a simple pill!

Decades of intense research efforts are also paying off in the diagnosis and treatment of other prostate diseases. New medical therapies for benign prostate hyperplasia (prostate enlargement) shrink the gland and reduce the need for surgery. Finally, we've begun to understand the cause of prostatitis (inflammation or infection in the gland) and how to cure it.

Still, despite all the progress we've made, men facing these diseases continue to grapple with troubling questions. If you have prostate cancer, how dangerous is it? Do you need to be treated now, or can you wait and monitor the disease, hoping the cancer will not progress? If you need treatment, is surgery or radiation the better choice? What about laparoscopic surgery, with or without robotics, instead of the traditional open procedure? If you opt for radiation, should you have seed implants, external beam therapy, or a combination of the two? Do you need hormone therapy, and if the answer is yes, which drugs should you take and when should you start? What about alternative and complementary medicine? Should you consider experimental therapies or a clinical trial? The vast array of diagnostic tests and treatment alternatives leaves many men frustrated and confused.

If you have urinary problems because of an enlarged prostate, should you take medicine or have surgery? If medicine is the answer, is one drug enough, or do you need two? If surgery is the best option for you, should the tissue be removed by laser? Is hyperthermia (heating the prostate) as effective as TURP (removal of excess tissue through a scope)? Which treatment is safer? Which is more likely to solve the problem permanently? Should you start taking a powerful antibiotic at the first symptoms of prostatitis, or is there a better approach? Prostate diseases are highly variable and enormously complex. Until trouble strikes, most men know little about their prostate gland. Knowledge in the field is constantly evolving. Persistent myths and misconceptions abound, not only among the general public but among doctors as well. To find the right answers, you may have to navigate some very tricky terrain.

Over the years, I've met with thousands of men in my office face-to-face and tried to arm them with sound, up-to-date, comprehensive, and comprehensible information about their medical issues and options. In these pages, I hope to make the same information available to all men confronting serious prostate problems and to their loved ones. Understanding what you're up against and how to respond can make all the difference. As baseball great Joe Torre said of his own experience with prostate cancer, "When you get the information, the fear just sort of melts away."

To equip you with the knowledge you'll need to make wise choices, this book is organized into three parts. Part One deals with the normal prostate, where it is located, what it does, and how it relates to urinary, bowel, and sexual function. Since many prostate problems are closely associated with aging, we'll go on to explore what typically happens to sexual and urinary function as men age and what you can do to increase your odds of aging successfully. Part Two focuses on prostate problems other than cancer—prostatitis and BPH (prostate enlargement)—that cause so much grief for so many men. We'll look at strategies for dealing with these strikingly common prostate ailments, and we'll also examine how these conditions can confound our ability to diagnose prostate cancer and how they might affect your treatment options if you develop a malignancy in the gland. Part Three takes an in-depth look at prostate cancer: what it is, how it develops and progresses, and what can be done about it. I'll introduce you to state-of-the-art predictive tools called nomograms that have helped many patients and physicians to make sound treatment choices. In these pages, you'll find the facts you need to resolve the major issues: Is treatment necessary now? If so, which approach makes the most sense? Which is more important—the type or the quality of treatment? How can you ensure that you'll get the best available care and the best possible outcome?

Being diagnosed with a prostate disease is no picnic. But today we have the necessary information and tools to provide real options and enable men to make informed decisions. Not long ago, things looked very different indeed.

I first heard about prostate cancer as a teenager, when one of my father's close friends, I'll call him Dan O'Conner, developed the disease. Mr. O'Conner was a strapping, vibrant man in his fifties, a highly successful businessman with an amazing intellect and a terrific sense of humor. He was always great fun to be around, always armed with a fascinating story—someone who seemed to me larger than life.

My father was both Mr. O'Conner's friend and his urologist. I'll never forget the day Dad came home from the office in an uncharacteristically somber mood. When I asked what was wrong, he told me that he had just had to tell a dear friend that he had prostate cancer. Mr. O'Conner was an extrovert in the best sense of the word, always open about the critical events of his life. His daughter was in my high school class, and she had her father's way of being honest and direct, so her dad's illness was no secret.

Several weeks later, my father operated to remove Mr. O'Conner's prostate gland. To my young mind, that surely meant that he would be fine, back to his old self again as soon as the effects of the surgery wore off. For a while this proved true, but some years later the cancer recurred. While it responded initially to further treatment, over the next few years his condition deteriorated. Even though Mr. O'Conner remained outwardly cheerful, it was clear that he was sinking. He was weakened by bone pain and the narcotic medication needed to control it. He had difficulty walking. I could tell from the bleak look on my father's face when it was Mr. O'Conner on the phone, asking for advice about another in the endless string of medical crises. Back in those days, there was little my dad could do beyond being there for his friend, listening with empathy and trying to keep him as comfortable as possible.

When Mr. O'Conner died, my friends and family went to his funeral. By then I was in my last year of medical school. I had begun to learn about cancer in general, but the medical school curriculum in those days included almost nothing about prostate cancer. During the funeral service and for weeks afterward, I kept thinking that there had to be some way to battle this disease more effectively. My father's outlook was not encouraging. Though prostate cancer was far more common than most people realized, medical science had made little progress toward detecting it early or figuring out better ways to treat it and save men's lives.

As I went through my own specialty training at the Massachusetts General Hospital, the National Cancer Institute, and UCLA, I became increasingly determined to focus on prostate cancer: to understand it better and to try to develop or apply new treatments. Like my father, my professors unanimously discouraged that choice. Prostate cancer was far too complex, they argued. The disease typically grew and spread so slowly that confirming whether a particular treatment worked or not took longer than the duration of most doctors' careers! Inexplicably, some men with this disease lived for decades without treatment, yet most cancers had already spread to distant sites (metastasized), as Dan O'Conner's had, by the time they were detected. While hormone therapy brought dramatic relief of painful metastases to bone, the remission typically lasted for only a few years and the cancer always recurred.

Treating advanced prostate cancer with the chemotherapy that was then available was like rearranging the deck chairs on the *Titanic,* for all the difference it made.

Fortunately, my dad and my teachers were wrong. The slowly expanding research in prostate cancer in the 1970s began to pay off in the 1980s, and the outlook for men with prostate cancer improved dramatically. By the late 1980s, a simple blood test for prostate-specific antigen (PSA), a protein made in the prostate that leaks into the blood when the prostate is disrupted by disease, revolutionized the diagnosis of prostate cancer. For the first time, most prostate cancers could be detected at an early, curable stage. Using ultrasound imaging, we could see the internal structure and measure the size of the prostate, but a major breakthrough came with the development of ultrasound-guided needle biopsy of the prostate. A biopsy of the gland became a safe, simple office procedure— last year over 800,000 were performed in the United States—so doctors could easily diagnose whether a patient had cancer or not. Advances in surgery placed the radical prostatetectomy (complete removal of the prostate) on firm anatomical grounds, improving the chances for cure and reducing the onerous side effects. Both brachytherapy (seed implants) and external beam radiation therapy were refined to increase the dose of radiation delivered precisely to the prostate, minimizing damage to surrounding structures and decreasing the risk of urinary, sexual, and bowel complications. Drugs to promote penile erections or to relax an irritated bladder, and devices and procedures to control urinary incontinence, give us highly effective means to deal with the side effects of treatment that sometimes occur.

Nevertheless, many doctors continue to have an incomplete understanding of prostate diseases, and even seasoned experts can disagree. When Ralph S., a 62-year-old financial planner, learned that he had prostate cancer, he used his well-honed research skills to track down top-notch professionals to consult. The first urologist he saw recommended surgery as the best way to get rid of the cancer. Ralph expected a second opinion to confirm this, but the next urologist was firmly in favor of seed implants. After all, he said, seeds were much less invasive and would require no time lost from work. Hoping to break the tie, Ralph went to see yet another specialist, this time a medical oncologist, who disagreed with the first two doctors and weighed in strongly on the side of external beam radiation. Ralph's reward, for all his scrupulous efforts, was utter confusion. How could three capable doctors with fine reputations have such strikingly different ideas about what he should do? Were they analyzing and interpreting the data differently? Or were there simply three equally effective alternatives from which he could choose? If that were the case, how on Earth was he supposed to make such a daunting decision when, weeks before, he barely knew where his prostate was?

To make a wise choice, you need to understand exactly what you're up against, the risks and benefits of each treatment alternative, and—perhaps most critically—yourself. It's crucial to assess your personal values and concerns. What are the key issues driving your decision? Might some unrealistic expectations or unnecessary concerns be standing in your way?

Take the case of Frank R. When I saw him recently, he was in a panic over the news that his prostate biopsy was positive for cancer. His uncle had suffered with unspecified "prostate troubles" when Frank was a child, with memorably disastrous consequences. Now, Frank was convinced that he would wind up as his uncle had: in diapers, sexually disabled, isolated, lonely, and depressed. He told me he thought his wisest course would be to forget about treatment and retire immediately, so that he could spend what little good time he had left with his wife, children, and friends.

Frank's diagnostic results painted a completely different picture. He was 69 years old, and his biopsy had turned up only one minuscule area of low-risk cancer. In my mind, the central question was whether Frank needed treatment at all. Given the typical slow course of such an early cancer, a reasonable alternative was to monitor him closely, postponing treatment unless and until there were warning signs that the cancer was beginning to grow. There was a good chance that he would live out the rest of his natural life with no problems from his prostate cancer whatsoever.

Frank's situation is far from unique. With prostate cancer, the gulf between reality and expectation can be enormous. Finding accurate, reliable information to narrow that breach is not easy. Advice from other men who have experienced prostate cancer may be misleading, outmoded, or entirely irrelevant to you. If you seek enlightenment from the Internet, you'll find plenty of wishful thinking, blind supposition, and raw bias overwhelming the few nuggets of sound, scientific advice. To make wise choices and cope well with this disease, you have to understand exactly what you're up against. To that end, this book reflects the generous input of leading specialists working to conquer prostate diseases, including medical oncologists, radiation therapists, radiologists, pathologists, research scientists, biostatisticians, nurses, and mental health practitioners, as well as other urologists from around the country who specialize in prostate cancer, infections in the gland, BPH, infertility, erectile dysfunction, and incontinence. In addition, many of our patients and their partners have graciously contributed their valuable insights, illustrative anecdotes, and practical advice. To keep you apprised of new developments as they emerge, I will offer regular updates on my Web site (www.drscardino.com or www.theprostatebook.com).

As you read, keep in mind that you can and will get through this. Millions of men have weathered serious problems with their prostates successfully. Today, the vast majority of patients are spared the urinary problems and sexual decline that were once seen as virtually inevitable. Given good modern care, they are able to put the disease behind them and get on with their lives.

Getting the word out is crucial. Ironically, though most men have scanty knowledge about their prostates, nearly everyone has heard that prostate diseases and their treatments can impair or alter a man's most intimate personal functions. Preferring not to think about such things, some young, healthy men avoid simple screening with the digital rectal exam and the PSA test, even though regular testing would virtually guarantee that any cancer they developed would be discovered at an early, curable stage. Out of fear of side effects, some men forgo lifesaving treatment, even though the side effects of modern treatment are not inevitable, are often transient, and are almost always correctable when they occur. Some men refuse treatment even though the disease itself, if left to progress, can cause serious side effects of its own.

Thankfully, many prominent men have come forward in recent years to discuss their experiences with prostate diseases frankly and to encourage others to become more vigilant, better informed, and more proactive about their own health. Leading political figures Rudy Giuliani, Colin Powell, and John Kerry; General Norman Schwarzkopf; media mogul Rupert Murdoch; Intel CEO Andy Grove; baseball legend Joe Torre; leading educator Cornel West; and entertainment greats Robert De Niro, Jerry Lewis, Mandy Patinkin, and Harry Belafonte represent the new forthright face and increasingly optimistic voice of male prostate health. Their message and examples are clear, inspiring, and true: Prostate diseases can be confronted, treated, and overcome.

I'm grateful to these remarkable individuals and to all the men with prostate cancer I've been privileged to know over the years, especially my family friend, Dan O'Conner. Witnessing his struggle against this disease all those years ago gave me the will to join in the fight against prostate cancer. I know Dan would be delighted by how things have changed for men with this disease and what huge strides we've made toward winning the battle.

Dr. Peter T. Scardino
October 2004

Part One

THE PROSTATE
AND THE
NORMAL MALE

1

■

The Prostate

READ THIS CHAPTER TO LEARN:

- Where does the prostate lie, how is it constructed, and what does it do?
- What can go wrong with this troublemaking gland, and why do these problems develop so frequently?

What is the prostate? Where is it? What does it do? Can you live without it? Or perhaps more to the point if you're plagued by prostate problems: Is there any way that you and this gland can peacefully coexist?

Few men are able to answer any, let alone all, of these fundamental questions. Until trouble strikes, the prevailing attitude holds that this small, obscure gland is probably best ignored. If you're a typical man, you were aware that the prostate exists; you knew that it can cause all manner of unpleasantness; and, quite frankly, you preferred not to think about it.

But now you have no choice. If you or someone you love has been diagnosed with prostate cancer or another serious prostate disease, you need to understand precisely what you're up against in order to determine which response makes sense.

WHAT IS THE PROSTATE?

The **prostate** is a gland, the term used to describe fluid-producing organs. Salivary glands, predictably, manufacture saliva, which aids in digestion. The prostate churns out part of the seminal fluid, which protects and nourishes sperm as they navigate the female reproductive tract.

Terminology related to the prostate and its function can seem deliberately geared to maximize confusion. In a prime example, the plum-shaped prostate "gland" is made up of many fluid-producing sacs that are also called "glands" (just as many hairs on a person's head are collectively referred to as "hair"). Another name for these microscopic glands, though it may not strike you as particularly user-friendly, is acini.

In addition to abundant microscopic glands, the prostate contains a network of internal piping (ducts) and supporting muscle and fibrous cells (stroma). When ejaculation occurs, the muscular stroma contracts like a pumping fist, deploying the seminal fluid out through the penis, along with the sperm it is charged to preserve and defend.

NOTE: People writing about the prostate commonly describe the gland as resembling a walnut. While the general size and shape are somewhat similar, the analogy evokes a hard shell and dry, solid contents, which in no way resemble the healthy human prostate. A small plum, with its spongy, fluid-filled interior and soft skin, is far closer to the way a typical prostate appears after puberty. With the benign enlargement (BPH) or prostate cancer that so often accompanies advancing age, a larger and sometimes more irregular plum would serve as a reasonable surrogate image.

WHAT DOES THE PROSTATE DO?

In young boys, the prostate gland is minuscule. It lies dormant until puberty, when, stimulated by a surge of male hormones, the gland grows and begins its lifelong task of churning out seminal fluid (**semen**). The seminal vesicles (attached just above the prostate) and the Cowper's glands (along the urethra just below the prostate) also add to the seminal fluid that is released during ejaculation. Within the prostate, fluid manufacturing occurs in the **epithelial cells** that line the microscopic glands and ducts.

Seminal fluid contains a complex stew of proteins and minerals specially designed to preserve and protect sperm as they make their way along the female reproductive tract. A critical component, contributed by the prostate, is a protein called **prostate-specific antigen (PSA)**. While finding a high level of PSA on the blood screening test for prostate cancer can be a harbinger of trouble, PSA in the seminal fluid is perfectly normal. In fact, PSA plays the essential role of liquefying coagulated semen so the sperm are free to journey toward an egg.

WHERE IS THE PROSTATE LOCATED?

Deep in the pelvis, below the urinary bladder, the prostate encircles the urethra, the conduit that allows both urine and semen to pass through the penis to the outside. The prostate lies directly behind the pubic bone and in front of the rectum, which is why the rear surface of the gland can be felt by a doctor during a **digital rectal exam (DRE)**.

In the 1966 sci-fi film classic *Fantastic Voyage,* an intrepid rescue team is drastically miniaturized and deployed through the circulatory system of a brilliant government scientist to track down and eradicate a life-threatening blood clot in an artery. Had Command Central sent these germ-sized heroes southward to tackle a troubling condition in Professor Benes's prostate gland instead, getting there would have been the least of their troubles. The crew's greater challenge by far would have been finding a way to treat Benes's prostate problem without damaging his urinary, bowel, or sexual functions.

While some major organs—such as the kidneys, liver, and lungs—live in relative isolation akin to a private home on a quiet suburban street, the prostate sits smack at the hub of a frenzied anatomical intersection. Here, structures responsible for sexual, urinary, and bowel function operate in

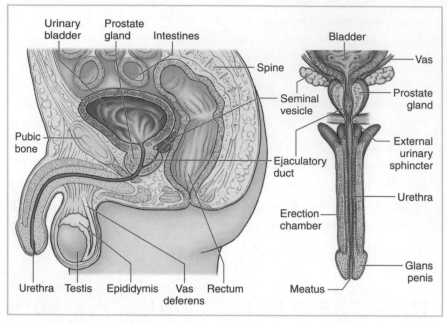

The prostate and neighboring organs. Cutaway views from the side (in left-hand drawing) and from the front (in right-hand drawing).

perilously close proximity to one another. Like an accident at the frantic juncture of a major highway, a minor glitch in any one of these structures can precipitate a chain of destructive events. One driver stops short, and the trailing vehicles pile up in a mile-long fender bender. One lane is consumed by construction, and smoothly flowing traffic slows to a frustrating trickle. The prostate expands with benign enlargement or becomes inflamed or develops a malignant tumor, and suddenly a man collides head-on with the frightening specters of erectile dysfunction, urinary incontinence, or loss of bowel control—whether from the disease itself or from the treatment.

Mere millimeters separate the rear of the prostate from the rectal wall, so the rectum lies directly in the line of fire of a radiation beam targeted at a cancerous prostate. Running in the neurovascular bundle just beside the prostate and rectum are the exquisitely delicate **cavernous (erectile) nerves**, which are essential for penile erections. These nerves can be easily damaged by imprecise attempts to treat prostate cancer, whether with

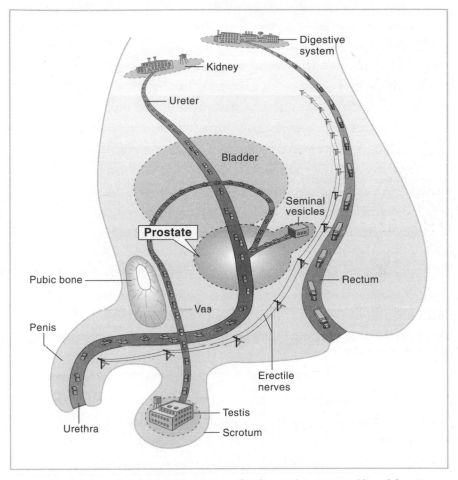

The prostate is located at the busy intersection of male sexual, urinary, and bowel functions.

surgery, radiation, or **cryotherapy** (freezing). Since the urethra runs from the bladder directly through the prostate, BPH (benign enlargement of the gland) or a large cancer can slow the urinary stream and eventually block its flow completely. In front of the prostate looms the pubic bone, which can add to the challenge faced by a surgeon trying to remove the gland or by a radiation therapist doing seed implants.

The bladder and delicate **ureters** (tubes that channel urine from the kidneys) perch directly above the prostate, and the penis extends out from below. These organs can be injured if radiation for prostate cancer is not targeted with scrupulous care. If the bladder, urethra, or ureters are hit by damaging rays, **inflammation** or bleeding (**radiation cystitis**) can result. Radiation damage to erection chambers within the penis or the erectile nerves could result in severely impaired erections. The **bladder neck,** which contains the muscular trapdoor known as the **internal urinary sphincter,** connects to the top—confusingly called the base—of the gland. At their juncture the two organs are enmeshed like zipper teeth and are virtually indistinguishable. Unless the bladder neck is adequately removed during surgery for prostate cancer, the malignant cells left at the edge could grow back. When we perform a radical prostatectomy to cure cancer, the **external urinary sphincter** takes over the job of holding back urine, so this muscular structure must be carefully preserved to avoid urinary incontinence.

The prostate is so closely intertwined with adjacent structures that the inflammation of prostatitis readily causes rectal and perineal pain, lower abdominal aches, burning at the tip of the penis, and the need to urinate frequently.

HOW WAS THE PROSTATE DISCOVERED?

Considering the prostate's remote location and obscure function, it is not surprising that scholars who worked to map human anatomy centuries ago were late to recognize the gland's very existence. In fact, we are still struggling to divine some of its mysterious secrets and fully understand its strikingly eccentric ways.

Though references to urological diseases—most notably, bladder and kidney stones—date back to an ancient Egyptian papyrus written in 1550 BC, the prostate was first described by an Italian physician, Niccolo Massa, nearly 3,000 years later in renaissance Venice. The gland's given name, "prostate," derives from a Greek term, meaning "to set before," a reference to the prostate's position in relation to the bladder. The word "prostitute" derives from similar Greek roots, meaning "to place before" or "to offer." Given the gland's persistent obscurity, its name is commonly confused with the similar sounding "prostrate," which actually refers to a posture of submission or humility, lying flat with one's face to the ground.

In sixteenth-century Europe, a French military surgeon named Ambroise Paré frequently took embalmed cadavers home to study and practice new medical techniques. Though his family might not have appreciated such unorthodox houseguests, medical science—and urology in particular—owe Paré a considerable debt. He was the first to recognize that the prostate gland is a distinct organ, separate from the bladder. He detailed the gland's intimate relationship to the seminal vesicles and **ejaculatory ducts** and explained how it operates during ejaculation. His work added immeasurably to our understanding of how the prostate functions.

WHAT ARE THE PARTS OF THE PROSTATE?

In a top-down view of a prostate that has been sliced horizontally across the middle and had its top half removed, you would see the urethra at the center. Moving outward, you'd notice many tiny tubelike ducts, akin to a thicket of tree branches, with microscopic glands strewn about the tips like a profusion of leaves.

The portion of the prostate immediately surrounding the urethra is called the **transition zone**. This area of the gland is most infamously known as the site of BPH (benign prostatic enlargement), which often constricts urinary flow as men age.

Continuing out from the transition zone, we come to the **peripheral zone**, which lies beneath the outer covering, or **capsule**, of the gland like an orange rind. In another rich potential source of misunderstanding, the prostate's "capsule" is actually soft and membranous like the skin of a plum, not a hard, impervious barrier as the name might seem to imply. Most prostate cancers arise in the peripheral zone, directly beneath the capsule. If left alone long enough, these tumors tend to spread outward through the capsule into surrounding tissues. Still, about one in four prostate cancers arise in the transition zone. Although the transitional zone and the peripheral zone are anatomically distinct, many men with prostate cancer have malignant disease in both zones.

In addition to these zonal divisions, the prostate can be divided down the middle into left and right lobes, a distinction enhanced by the median sulcus, a groove that runs down the rear surface of the gland and can be felt during a digital rectal exam (DRE). These anatomical landmarks play an important role in describing the location of prostate diseases and in planning for their treatment.

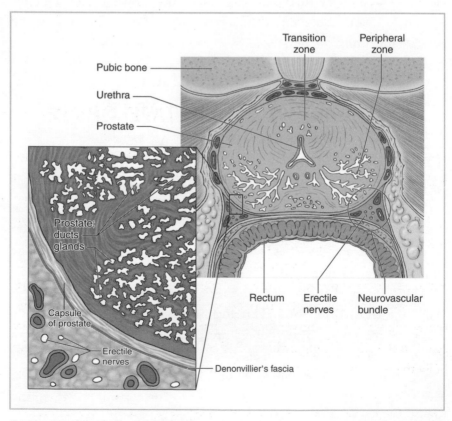

Cross-section through the prostate showing its key parts, the nearby neurovascular bundles (erectile nerves), and the rectum. An enlarged view to the left shows the microscopic ducts and glands.

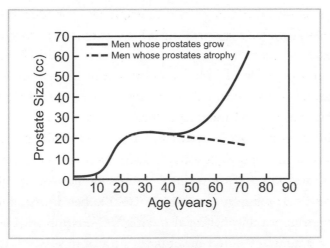

Growth of the prostate with age. After most men reach age 40, the prostate begins to enlarge with BPH, but in some men, the gland remains the same size or shrinks (atrophies).*

HOW DOES THE PROSTATE GROW?

In a young boy, the minuscule prostate weighs a paltry 3 to 6 grams (a nickel weighs 5 grams) and has no known function. At puberty, the gland grows to about 20 grams—the weight of a medium-sized strawberry—and begins to produce part of the seminal fluid. For decades thereafter, the prostate holds steady at this size and goes uneventfully about its business. Except for the problems some have with the inflammation or infection known as prostatitis, most young men remain happily oblivious to the workings of this gland. Then, with appalling frequency, this formerly innocuous bit player on the reproductive stage begins to grow again in the fifth decade or beyond, developing into a strident, intrusive bully that can seriously erode a man's quality—or even quantity—of life.[1]

---

* Source: Modified from Greene, D. R., et al. "Sonographic Measurements of Transition Zone of Prostate in Men with and without Benign Prostatic Hyperplasia." *Urology* 36, no. 4 (1990): 293–9. © 1990. Reprinted with permission from Elsevier.

WHAT PROBLEMS DEVELOP
IN THE PROSTATE?

The prostate could be considered the biblical Job of internal organs, destined to suffer one crushing misfortune after another. From puberty, the gland is highly susceptible to various forms of acute or chronic **prostatitis**, an infection, inflammation, or enigmatic noninflammatory syndrome that lands many men in the doctor's office in search of relief. Experts estimate that fully half of all men suffer from prostatitis at one time or another. Though it almost never poses a threat to survival, the condition can make men miserable. In the most severe cases, patients have likened the pain, urinary symptoms, and general malaise of prostatitis to the chest pain of angina, the abdominal cramps of inflammatory bowel disease, or the aftermath of a heart attack. (See Chapter 4, Prostatitis.)

Benign prostatic hyperplasia (BPH) is another all-too-common source of prostate-induced misery. For reasons we still don't fully understand, the gland, which reaches full size at puberty, frequently undergoes a second growth spurt in middle age that can provoke a litany of urinary woes. Symptoms may include a slow urinary stream with hesitancy in starting, frequent urination with the uncontrollable urge to void immediately, and the need to get up at night to urinate (**nocturia**). In extreme cases, the urinary obstruction becomes so severe that a man cannot urinate at all (**acute urinary retention**) and requires emergency catheterization or surgery for relief. (See Chapter 5, BPH [Prostate Enlargement].)

In addition to benign enlargement, the prostate is also remarkably prone to developing malignant tumors (**cancer**) as men age. It is often said, and not far from the truth, that if you're a man and live long enough, you're bound to develop some cancerous cells in your prostate (though many of these are microscopic and would never cause a serious problem in your lifetime). (See Part Three for a more detailed discussion of prostate cancer.)

WHY DO MEN DEVELOP PROSTATE PROBLEMS?

The prostate's troublemaking potential is unique. No other secondary sex organ develops cancer or enlarges with aging. We don't see benign or malignant overgrowth in the seminal vesicles, vas deferens, or Cowper's glands, though these organs are exposed to many of the same environmental conditions, genetic factors, and hormonal influences as the prostate.

Despite our best research efforts regarding the prostate's function and what can go wrong with it, questions and conundrums abound. We don't know why the prostate is so prone to benign and cancerous growth or why the gland so often gets infected or inflamed. Nevertheless, we have come a very long way from the meager state of knowledge about the gland that greeted me twenty-five years ago when I first became a urologist. Perhaps most critically, we've learned that early detection and appropriate intervention can reduce the chances of dying of prostate cancer and often mitigate the symptoms of BPH and prostatitis. We're making steady inroads toward understanding prostate diseases and learning how to treat them with better outcomes and far fewer negative, lasting effects.

IN SUMMARY

The prostate is a small gland with an outsized capacity to cause problems, notably prostate cancer, prostatitis, and BPH, especially as men age. Because of the gland's location, prostate diseases and their treatments carry a risk of damage to urinary, sexual, and bowel functions. Our understanding of the prostate remains incomplete, but our ability to detect and manage prostate problems has evolved remarkably in the past two decades, and the outlook for men with prostate diseases grows brighter all the time.

2

■

Normal Male Function

READ THIS CHAPTER TO LEARN:

- What are the parts of the male genital and urinary systems?
- What do these organs do?
- How do they develop and grow?
- What's the difference between erection, ejaculation, and orgasm?

As a urologist, I specialize in the functions and diseases of the male reproductive organs and in the prevention and treatment of urinary diseases in both males and females. In other words, as Sam Spade might have put it: the genitourinary system is my beat.

Though the penis is unquestionably the sentimental favorite and garners more attention than all of the other male genitourinary organs combined, like any star player the quality of its performance depends on things going smoothly behind the scenes. Male urinary, sexual, and reproductive functions are in many ways intertwined. These systems share common ground and are often called upon to work in concert. When something goes wrong in one area, the others are often affected as well. Urinary problems and their treatments can impair sexual function and damage fertility. Problems with the genital organs—where the prostate, more often than not, is the culprit—can throw urinary, sexual, and reproductive functions out of whack. To grasp how things go wrong, let's have a look at how genitourinary organs come to be and how they are supposed to work.

HOW DO MALE ORGANS DEVELOP BEFORE BIRTH?

The embryonic kidneys begin to form during the first month after conception. While still in a highly primitive state, they commence their life-long assignment of filtering wastes from the blood and producing urine. By the thirty-seventh day of gestation, when the fetus is about the size of an apple seed, the bladder forms by first expanding out like a bubble from tiny tubes called ureters, which branch off from the kidneys, and then coming together to create an elastic, muscular pouch designed to store urine until it is ready to be released.

All embryos have at least one X chromosome, and everyone is female at the outset. During the second month of fetal life, reproductive (germ) cells generate primitive gonads that eventually grow into ovaries in the female and testes in the male. By six weeks into a pregnancy, the testicles' tiny precursors begin to secrete signaling substances that promote the development of the male organs and inhibit their female counterparts. At seven to eight weeks, under the influence of the Y (male) chromosome, specialized Leydig cells arise in the testicles. Their job is to secrete testosterone, the primary male hormone. At first, this production is controlled by the pregnancy hormone HCG (human chorionic gonadotropin), which is produced by the mother's placenta. Gradually, the fetal brain takes over this management task. From then on, the hypothalamus and pituitary glands in the brain provide the signals that keep the Leydig cells pumping testosterone throughout a male human's life.

Male embryos with a genetic inability to suppress female hormones develop a uterus and a vagina, even though they have the XY chromosomal signature that characterizes every boy and man. Males whose cells are genetically incapable of utilizing testosterone are born with a different condition called testicular feminization. Externally, they appear to be normal females, but they have undescended testes, lack a uterus and fallopian tubes, do not menstruate, and, obviously, cannot bear children. Famous, and famously beautiful and voluptuous actresses, such as Jamie

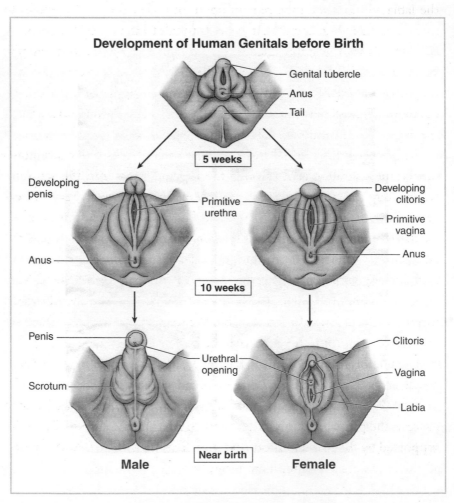

All humans begin life with similar anatomy. Well before birth, a distinctly male or female external appearance develops.

Lee Curtis and the late Kim Novak, are well-known examples of people with this syndrome.

The external genitalia first appear as a tiny nub, called a tubercle, when the embryo is about six weeks old. By ten weeks, the tubercle yields the beginnings of either a penis or a female clitoris (which, like its male counterpart, contains erectile bodies and engorges and enlarges with sexual arousal). Similarly, primitive genital folds develop into either the inner vaginal folds (labia minora) or the male urethra. In the female, the labia and urethral tube remain open. In males, the urethra closes to form an extended channel that passes through to the tip of the penis.

The **seminal vesicles** (glands that produce seminal fluid) develop as an outgrowth of the **vas deferens** (tubes that carry sperm from the epididymis to the prostate), while the pea-sized Cowper's glands, which lie below the prostate and also secrete part of the seminal fluid, arise from a special fold in the embryo, called the urogenital sinus.

At three months, when the fetus is 3 inches long, the testes commence their slow descent through the inguinal canal into the scrotum, where they take up permanent residence. Housing these organs externally allows their temperature to be carefully modulated, a feature essential to the production of healthy sperm. Elastic ligaments adjust the distance that the testes are held from internal body organs, making sure they are kept cool enough to prevent sperm damage. In severe cold, they are drawn closer to the body, where they can be kept sufficiently warm to protect the sperm. In females the counterparts of the scrotal sac are external vaginal folds, the labia majora.

During the twelfth to sixteenth week of gestation, the prostate develops as an offshoot of the urethra. First, many small buds arise from the urinary channel just below the bladder. Gradually they spread and extend to form the prostate's network of ducts and tiny glands (acini). These are supported by the gland's fibrous and muscle tissue (stroma). At this point, all the essential male equipment is in place.

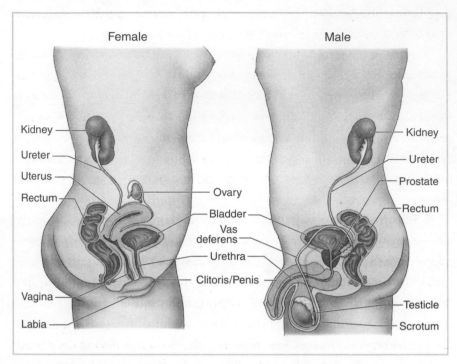

The corresponding parts of the urinary and reproductive systems of males and females.

THE URINARY TRACT

The **urinary tract** functions as a waste management and disposal facility, which helps to maintain the body's critical balance of minerals and fluids. First, the kidneys filter the blood of waste products and excess water, which are excreted as urine—anywhere from ½ to 2½ liters per day in a normally hydrated adult. Average voiding output varies widely, depending on a person's size and activity, the ambient temperature and humidity, the amount of fluids consumed, and a host of other factors.

The **bladder** serves as a holding tank. Urine is stored under very low pressure, though when opportunity and need are at loggerheads, it may seem as if your bladder is positively screaming for attention. As it fills, the urinary reservoir relaxes and offers little resistance. While voiding, pressure in the bladder rises, but at its peak it amounts to a paltry 5 percent of the pressure of beer leaving a properly chilled keg.

The mild-mannered bladder does little to assert itself until it has been stretched very near its limits. Only then does it transmit frantic signals to the brain that emptying and consequent relief are imperative. In a typical adult, a sensation of bladder fullness kicks in when about 200 cubic centimeters (30 cc equals 1 ounce) of urine have accumulated. When 300 to 400 cc have collected, the urge to void grows powerful. Though maximum bladder capacity varies with size and individual urinary habits, the average is about 400 cc.

A full bladder triggers a voiding reflex, which in infants works as automatically as the irresistible jerking response to the tap of a rubber mallet against your knee. The bladder muscle contracts, pulling the inner sphincter open. All resistance gives way as the outer sphincter relaxes, and the urine flows freely through the urinary channel (**urethra**) to the outside. Toilet training derails this automatic feedback loop, modifying the brain's reaction to messages from the bladder. Once urination comes under voluntary control in early childhood, a person wishing to void must consciously let go, releasing the powerful learned inhibitory response that normally keeps us dry.

A newborn urinates two to six times a day for a total output of 30 to 60 cc. By the time a child passes his tenth birthday, four to five daily voiding episodes produce a whopping 800 to 1,400 cc daily urinary yield (about 1 to 1½ quarts). Adult men continue to urinate four to five times per day on average, as long as nothing, such as an enlarged prostate, interferes with normal function. Women void slightly more often, typically five to six times per day, though their stream tends to be stronger and their bladder empties faster than a man's. Men over 40 often notice a gradual slowing of their stream (measured in the doctor's office as the **urinary flow rate**) as the prostate enlarges.

SEX ORGANS

The central responsibility of male genitalia (the penis, scrotum, and testicles) is reproduction. The **testicles**, aka "testes," manufacture sperm, which then pass to the adjacent **epididymis**, a long, slender, tightly convoluted tube that runs along the rear of each testicle. Here, during a ten-day storage period, the sperm mature and learn to swim (become motile). These tiny reproductive road warriors are then deployed through the complex mechanisms of erection, emission, and ejaculation. The testes also churn out male hormones (**androgens**), principally **testosterone**, which is required for normal development. Testosterone also maintains healthy libido, muscle mass, bone density, body and facial hair, and other male characteristics throughout life.

The internal sex organs—including the vas deferens, the seminal vesicles, and the prostate—comprise a critical supporting cast. During sexual climax, these three organs contract vigorously, forcing the sperm and seminal fluid into a staging area within the urethra in a process known as **emission**. To complete ejaculation, the muscles of the urethra and the **perineum** (the area between the scrotum and the rectum) contract rhythmically, propelling the semen out through the penis.

The tasks carried out by the reproductive organs are aided and abetted by a rich blood supply and triggered by carefully choreographed signals from the brain and spinal cord, which in turn rely on the precise action and interplay of many stimulatory and inhibitory nerves. You could liken this to a dazzling theatrical production involving hundreds of dancers, singers, acrobats, and musicians, not to mention props and special effects. The startling fact is not that things occasionally go awry but that they typically proceed without a hitch.

THE BASIC ANATOMY OF ERECTION

The penis contains a pair of large erection chambers (**corpora cavernosa**) on top and one smaller chamber (**corpus spongiosum**) sur-

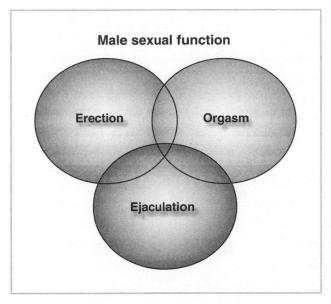

Male sexual function

Erection

Orgasm

Ejaculation

The three parts of male sexual function are interrelated but distinct. For example, orgasm can occur without erection or ejaculation.

rounding the urethra underneath. When sexual arousal is stimulated by a dream, conscious mental imagery, or a sensory stimulus (touch, sight, taste, sound, or smell), arteries leading to the penis relax, allowing a sudden forceful influx of blood. The erection chambers are nonelastic sacs, like tires on a car, so when they're filled to capacity under the pressure of arterial blood, they become rigid. In this state, the penile veins are compressed in a valvelike action, trapping the blood until orgasm occurs or the stimulus that caused the erection ceases.

WHAT IS AN ORGASM?

It may surprise you to learn that an orgasm occurs between the ears, not between your legs. The sensation, which lasts about three to five seconds in a man and five to eight seconds in a woman, takes place strictly in the brain, and the brain is the sole organ required to generate the reflexive flood of pleasure and release. Erection is *not* required for orgasm, and a man incapable of having erections or ejaculating can still experience sexual climax as long as his brain is intact. After **simple prostatectomy** (removal of part of the gland) for an enlarged, obstructing prostate, or **radical prostatectomy** (complete removal) to treat prostate cancer, the ability to reach orgasm should not be impaired despite the loss of ejaculation (**dry orgasm**).

WHAT HAPPENS DURING EJACULATION?

Ejaculation involves the powerful expulsion of fluid through the penis at the startling rate of 28 miles per hour, which, by amusing coincidence, is also the top speed a world-class human runner can achieve during a sprint. In normal males, each ejaculate measures a scant ½ to 1 teaspoon but still contains a whopping 100 million or more sperm—enough to repopulate all of Mexico! Nevertheless, sperm are so unfathomably tiny that this enormous number accounts for a mere 3 percent of the total ejaculatory volume. The seminal vesicles, Cowper's glands, and prostate contribute the other 97 percent in the form of seminal fluids (semen), which help to preserve and protect sperm. Without semen, sperm would never be able to survive the perilous 12-inch journey from the vagina through the uterus and into the fallopian tubes, where, if all goes according to nature's plan, one or more might succeed in fertilizing an egg.

> NOTE: If that 12-inch distance strikes you as no big deal, consider that, given the sperm's minuscule size, the feat is roughly the equivalent of a grueling 70-mile swim for a 6-foot-tall human being.

On their passage through the female reproductive system, sperm, powered by their flickering tail-like flagellum, chug along at about 8 inches per hour, which is actually quite a startling burst of speed for such minute travelers. Since they tend to take a tacking course, rather than making a beeline to the target, the trip toward a rendezvous with an ovum can take several exhausting hours. Then, for any surviving sperm that have managed to go the distance, the daunting work of penetrating the egg and negotiating a successful genetic merger begins. This final phase presents its own considerable challenges. An ovum, though still microscopic, is twenty times as long and forty to fifty times as wide as the male reproductive cell. From a sperm's-eye view, the egg is enormous, significantly larger than the gargantuan 100-foot-long blue whale, the world's largest animal, appears to a typical human adult.

IN SUMMARY

The male genital and urinary systems are complex and intertwined. Normal sexual and urinary development and function hinge on all the component parts running smoothly. Of all the organs involved in male function, the aging prostate is most often the culprit when problems occur.

3

■

Changes with Aging

READ THIS CHAPTER TO LEARN:

- How do sexual and urinary functions typically change as men age, and what can you do to age successfully?
- How do aging hormones affect the prostate?

I n our youth-obsessed society, we are bombarded by the notion that growing older is undesirable and unattractive. If we can't stop the clock, we will do almost anything to stop its effects on our appearance. The resultant costs are staggering. We spend billions annually on "anti-aging" creams and potions, alleged aging "remedies" and reversers, and cosmetics and surgical procedures that promise to preserve or restore youth.

Still, no matter how we attempt to alter or mask our aging exteriors, no matter how doggedly we pursue eternal youth by popping pills or submitting to the scalpel, our internal clocks tick on. Aging is a universal, inescapable fact for all living creatures. It is also a normal process, and *not* a disease to be treated in a desperate attempt at a cure. Despite the deep-seated fear many people have of getting on in years, aging and well-being can, and often do, go hand in hand. While change over time is inevitable, dysfunction and disability are most certainly not.

This is definitely good news for our rapidly graying population. Americans are living longer in ever greater numbers. Thirteen percent of us are now over 65, up from only 4 percent in 1900. People over 75 represent the fastest-growing segment of our population. It was rare indeed to find a centenarian at the turn of the twentieth century. Today, 61,000 of our countrymen have passed the 100-year mark, and that number is expected to swell to over 600,000 by the middle of this century. Though this means that many men will reach their century milestone birthday, 80 percent of centenarians are women. For reasons we have yet to uncover, women continue to outlive men by an average of about seven years.

Americans are not only living longer—they are living longer in good health, thanks to lifestyle improvements, advances in medical science, and an ever-increasing awareness that successful aging is very different from a futile attempt to imitate youth.

Since it began in 1982, the annual National Long Term Care Survey has documented a steady reduction of 1 to 2 percent per year in the number of people who become disabled with age. Increasingly, older citizens remain capable of performing the activities of daily living (e.g., personal grooming, arranging for meals, and paying the bills) that are necessary for independence. The percentage of elderly Americans requiring supervised living arrangements or home care continues to decline. An ever-decreasing proportion now suffers from chronic diseases such as emphysema, arteriosclerosis, arthritis, dementia, stroke, and high blood pressure. Control of these health problems, when they do occur, has improved greatly, allowing older people to enjoy fewer debilitating side effects and better quality of life.

While average life expectancy and long-term well-being continue to increase, the maximum limit of human life remains the subject of considerable speculation and debate. Based on cross-species studies, many scientists set the number at about 108 to 120 years old. In almost all animals, the longest observable life span is about six times the number of years it takes to grow from birth to full maturity.

Biologically this may be related to an enzyme called telomerase, which is responsible for restoring the ends of DNA that are damaged and lost each time a cell is reproduced. Normal cells grown in a culture dish in the laboratory can replicate themselves about fifty times, and then they expire. In every species, the life span ceiling is determined by how many times cells can resurrect themselves before they give out. All animals eventually succumb to death from "natural causes" if they aren't killed or don't die earlier from accidents or diseases.

To age successfully, it's important to understand the normal changes that occur over time and learn what can be done to maintain optimal function and maximal quality of life.

EFFECTS OF AGING ON MALE ORGANS

For many men, an enlarged prostate (BPH) and the changes in voiding habits that can occur as a result are as much a part of aging as is a gradual loss of vision, hearing, and hair. As the prostate enlarges, the flow of urine often weakens, and urination may be difficult to start. The stream may become intermittent, and some men develop a "nervous" bladder— annoying and unpredictable—that demands frequent emptying, even during the night.

When men reach middle age and beyond, gradual changes typically occur in sexual function as well. Older men often notice decreased libido, diminished erections, and reduced staying power during sexual encounters. Orgasm becomes more difficult to achieve. Fertility also slowly declines, and eventually most men lose the ability to father children. (See What Changes Occur in Sexual Function? on page 40 for a more complete discussion.)

These age-related symptoms are common but not inevitable or universal. Some men breeze through life without urinary problems or any perceptible dwindling of sexual powers. Still the vast majority of us will have to deal with some or all of these changes eventually, if we're fortunate enough to live a good long time.

A Word about Balding

While testosterone is the major male hormone circulating in the blood, a higher-octane androgen called **dihydrotestosterone (DHT)** can be found in organs including the prostate and hair follicles. This powerful chemical messenger is produced when a special enzyme, **5 alpha-reductase,** mixes with regular testosterone in the cells. Though testosterone is far better known and gets the banner headlines, it's the relatively obscure DHT that causes the prostate to grow at puberty. DHT also spurs the development of body and facial hair. Over time, 5 alpha-reductase and the DHT it produces are responsible for thickening of the beard, continued growth of the prostate (BPH), and often gradual hair loss that eventually leaves many men with the characteristic horseshoe configuration at the sides and back of the head known as male pattern baldness.

By blocking the activity of 5 alpha-reductase, the drug finasteride (Propecia), at a dose of 1 mg a day, reduces DHT levels, prevents progressive balding, and even causes regrowth of hair in 90 percent of men. In larger doses (5 mg a day in the form of Proscar), the same drug shrinks the prostate and alleviates the symptoms of BPH (see Chapter 5, BPH [Prostate Enlargement]). New evidence suggests that 5 alpha-reductase inhibitors may also be able to prevent prostate cancer.

HOW DOES AGING AFFECT MALE HORMONES?

Testosterone, the predominant male hormone circulating throughout a man's body, is responsible for the development and maintenance of male sex organs and characteristics, including body hair, facial hair, and lean muscle mass. This highly productive hormone also spurs the growth of the prostate gland, penis, and testicles at puberty and, from then on, controls the production of sperm by the testes. Testosterone also plays a role in regulating mood and maintaining **libido**, which we experience as sexual desire.

The testosterone level in a man's blood is regulated by a complex feedback loop. The process boils down to a kind of internal relay race in which hormones are released in turn, triggering a self-regulating chain of events. First, the hypothalamus stimulates the pituitary gland in the brain to secrete a hormone called LH (luteinizing hormone), which behaves

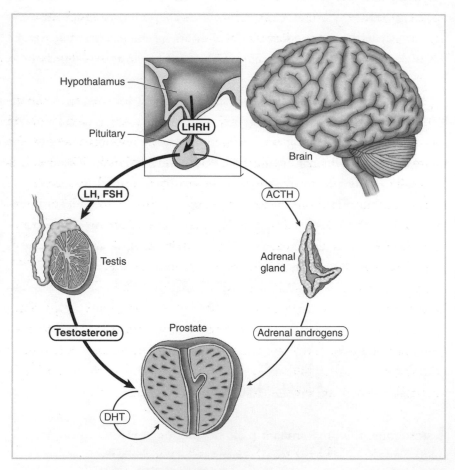

Male hormones (testosterone, DHT, and adrenal androgens), controlled by the brain, regulate the prostate and other sexual functions. LHRH, produced by the hypothalamus region of the brain, stimulates the pituitary to release LH, FSH, and ACTH, causing the testis to release testosterone and the adrenal gland to release other androgens.

like a chemical dispatcher. LH in turn sends out marching orders to the Leydig cells in the testicles, whose job it is to manufacture and release testosterone. This circuit results in an outpouring of testosterone into the bloodstream. Leydig cells discharge testosterone in episodic pulses, so levels of the hormone naturally vary markedly throughout the day.

Generally, testosterone levels follow your circadian rhythms, which are natural fluctuations in such bodily functions as alertness, metabolism, and hormone secretion. In humans, these activities tend to run at higher gear in the mornings than in the evenings, which may explain why some men experience greater sexual arousal on awakening than they do later in the day. Circadian rhythms also vary throughout the year. Testosterone levels are higher in the fall and lower in the spring, exactly contrary to popular notions of when human sap rises and "a young man's fancy lightly turns to thoughts of love."

Starting at about age 40, testosterone levels slowly begin to diminish. This seems to result from a gradual decrease in the secretion of LH from the pituitary, along with a gradual loss in responsiveness of the testosterone-producing Leydig cells to chemical signals. The result is typically a slow but steady reduction in sex drive, arousal, and quality of erections with age. From the beginning of the fifth decade, 10 percent of men report that they no longer have erections adequate for sexual penetration. This percentage increases at the rate of about 1 percent per year, which means 20 percent of men report inadequate erections by age 50, 30 percent by age 60, and 50 percent by age 80 (though it also means that 50 percent of octogenarians are able to function quite well!). Since production of sperm by the testicles also requires testosterone, diminishing male hormone levels also translate into a steady decline over time in the ability to father children. Again, this does *not* mean that infertility is inevitable. There are men who continue to defy the odds.

FSH AND SPERM PRODUCTION

The testicles function like a manufacturing plant with two distinct divisions. On one side of the factory, LH triggers the Leydig cells to pump out testosterone. On the other, FSH (follicle-stimulating hormone) triggers sperm production. In women, the same hormones are responsible for estrogen supply and egg production, respectively.

Historically, some men have been known to father children at unusually advanced ages. Actor Cary Grant, whose only child was born when he was 62, was once considered a remarkable example, though given today's high-tech fertility treatments, the male and female biological reproductive clocks can be drastically reset to run for a far longer time. Still, the level of FSH and the consequent production of viable sperm typically decrease with age. After age 50, the number of sperm-producing cells drops to about half the level found in a 20-year-old. Consequently, fertility, especially in the absence of medical intervention, often steadily declines with advancing age.

IS THERE REALLY
A "MALE MENOPAUSE"?

In women, menopause, which occurs on average at age 51, involves a dramatic shutdown of the production of ovarian stimulatory hormones (LH and FSH) by the brain. Ovulation and menstruation cease, and a host of other physical changes typically follows. Many women suffer hot flashes or other menopausal symptoms for a time. After the body adjusts to the drastic hormonal change, it's common for women to find that they are prone to the bone loss of osteoporosis, rising cholesterol levels, increased risk of stroke and heart attack, and altered sexual function, including thinning of the vaginal walls and vaginal dryness.

Many women and their physicians embraced hormone replacement therapy as a means to "cure" menopausal symptoms. Extravagant claims that hormone replacement therapy could deliver smoother skin, a healthier heart, stronger bones, greater emotional well-being, and improved mental acuity led to the common belief that the hormonal component of female aging could be slowed, arrested, or even reversed by taking a simple pill.

The profit potential of expanding the hormone supplement market by including the male half of the population did not escape corporate notice for long. Male menopause crept into common parlance, as did its more recently introduced equivalent, andropause. Many health care practitioners, drug companies, and supplement manufacturers, with their eyes firmly fixed on the bottom line, would like men to believe that a dramatic male hormone decline analogous to female menopause occurs routinely as we age. Symptoms of andropause, said to include diminished muscle mass, reduced libido and sexual function, fatigue, decreased energy level, and depression, are alleged to be cured by testosterone replacements and other substances designed to boost male hormone levels.

SHOULD YOU CONSIDER HORMONE SUPPLEMENTS?

Administered in small doses, testosterone has been shown to boost flagging libidos, improve erections, and increase men's feelings of well-being, but this only works in those uncommon cases where the problems stem from an abnormally low testosterone level. For men with adequate testosterone, using a simple gel or patch may sound like an irresistibly easy fix for diminished desire or other natural changes that often accompany aging, but there are significant downsides to these drugs.[1]

Over time, testosterone replacements can shut down the normal hormonal feedback loop, silencing the signals that ordinarily cue the testicles to get to work. Sperm production stops, as does the normal production of testosterone. The testicles can shrink, as they often do in athletes who abuse anabolic steroids to boost muscle mass and increase performance on the field. Taken long enough and in large enough doses, testosterone replacements can shut down the testicles permanently, causing irreversible infertility and irrevocably shrunken testes.

While not definitively proven, there are studies that suggest that testosterone supplements may increase the risk of prostate cancer, especially in older men. Since testosterone definitely makes existing cancers grow faster, you should be carefully evaluated to rule out prostate cancer before you consider hormone replacement therapy. A careful digital rectal exam (DRE) and PSA test should certainly be done. I recommend a biopsy of the prostate before beginning testosterone replacement, though not all doctors agree. Testosterone can also raise the risk of heart disease, so it's unwise to take these hormones without first consulting with your internist, family doctor, or cardiologist.

Except in rare cases, a gradual decline in male hormone levels is an expected part of normal aging, not a medical condition that requires treatment. By medicalizing menopause, countless women were actually found to be put at *increased* risk of serious medical conditions, including breast cancer and blood clots, along with the heart attacks and strokes they were purported to prevent. Testosterone replacement therapy should be reserved for men with troublesome symptoms and abnormally low testosterone levels, and then only taken after a thorough medical examination and a careful consideration of the pros and cons.

WHAT CHANGES OCCUR IN SEXUAL FUNCTION?

Mr. Jones complained to his doctor that he was not able to make love the way he used to. Checking the chart, the doctor noted that his patient was 92 years old. "When did you first notice this problem?" he asked. "The first time was last night," said Mr. Jones. "And then it happened again this morning."

While the randy nonagenarian may be the stuff of jokes, aging is not, as is commonly presumed, synonymous with sexual disinterest or incapacity. Many men remain sexually active throughout their lives. For those who do not, sexual dysfunction often results from disease, cultural factors, emotional issues, or the lack of a partner, rather than from aging alone.

This is not to say that sexual performance and experience remain unchanged over time. The primary job of male biological machinery is to facilitate reproduction, not to sustain sexual activity into old age. While there are wide individual variations, most healthy men experience progressive, gradual sexual changes as they get older. The exact mechanism

DHEA

Dehydroepiandrosterone, a steroidal hormone similar to testosterone, is produced naturally by the adrenal glands. Peak production starts to decline in one's early 30s, and sinks to a mere 20 percent of the lifetime maximum by age 75. The function of DHEA in the body remains unclear. All that researchers agree on completely is that the hormone can be converted into either testosterone or estrogen.

A synthetic form of DHEA has been touted as a veritable fountain of youth in handy, over-the-counter pill form. People marketing the drug claim that it improves erectile function, causes weight loss, and increases muscle mass without diet or exercise. Banner ads in the media and on the Internet maintain that this wonder substance cures chronic diseases, including Parkinson's disease, lupus, diabetes, and Alzheimer's. Purveyors also tout DHEA as a cancer preventative, an immune-system booster, and a quick fix for depression and fatigue.

As with anything that sounds too good to be true, there is ample cause for serious skepticism. Synthetic DHEA is sold as a dietary supplement, not a medication, and is therefore not subject to regulation by the Food and Drug Administration. Despite the hype about its potential to halt or even reverse many signs of aging, the safety and effectiveness of DHEA have not been proven. Also, because the supplements are unregulated, the purity and dosage of what you may be getting are not guaranteed. DHEA supplements may also carry significant health risks, including a possible increase in prostate cancer, worsening of BPH, and possible liver damage.

for the common age-related decline in erectile function has yet to be proven, but aging laboratory rats have a reduced ability to produce nitric oxide, the crucial chemical signal that dilates the blood vessels in the penis, allowing the critical inflow of blood that causes rigidity.

In general, older men take longer to achieve erections. Their erections are less rigid than those of young men and do not last as long. Ejaculations tend to become less forceful and lower in volume. The refractory period increases, meaning that it takes more time after orgasm to achieve an erection again. Some researchers have reported decreased tactile sensitivity of the penis with advancing age, and others have noted a reduced incidence of spontaneous nocturnal erections, even in men who continue to have regular intercourse while awake. Young men have an average of four to five erections each night during sleep, each lasting more than thirty minutes. Associated with the REM (rapid eye movement) sleep that accompanies dreams, these nocturnal erections are thought to help maintain healthy erectile tissue by providing a regular supply of highly oxygenated arterial blood to the penis. Erections during sleep continue throughout the life of a healthy man, but their frequency and duration slowly decline as he gets older.

Andro

Like DHEA, androstenedione ("Andro") is produced by the adrenal glands and can be converted into testosterone. Andro supplements have been promoted as a "natural" alternative to anabolic (muscle-building) steroids for increasing athletic performance. Allegedly, Andro accomplishes this by increasing testosterone levels. St. Louis baseball star Mark McGuire made headline news in the late nineties when he touted his regular ingestion of Andro as a key to his on-field prowess.

In fact, studies have failed to support the extravagant claims of Andro promoters, and no significant increase in testosterone levels has been found in users. The hormone does increase estrogen levels, which could result in heart or pancreas problems. Changes in blood cholesterol have also been observed, with a rise in LDL ("bad") cholesterol and a reduction in HDL ("good") cholesterol, both of which are associated with an increased risk of heart attacks and strokes.

Thankfully, in 1999, McGuire backed off from both his use and support of Andro, likely saving legions of impressionable fans from following his dubious lead in taking such an unproven and potentially risky drug. Note: In 2005 Andro was declared a controlled substance.

CAUSES OF AGE-RELATED ERECTILE DYSFUNCTION

THE USUAL SUSPECTS

While the incidence of serious **erectile dysfunction (ED)**, the consistent inability to get or maintain an erection, increases as men age, aging alone is rarely the cause of the problem. Many things, including hormonal imbalances, vascular or neurological problems, diseases and the medications used to treat them, psychological factors, and situational issues such as the loss of a partner, can lead to a loss of effective erections.

PSYCHOLOGICAL FACTORS

The mechanics of erection are extremely complex, and many crucial elements were not recognized or understood until the past decade. Earlier, the majority of erectile dysfunction was thought to be psychological. If no obvious organic cause could be identified, the problem was presumed to reside in the patient's mind. This common misconception arose from studies of nocturnal erections. Many men who complained of erectile problems were put in a lab where their erections were measured during sleep. A strain gauge placed on the penis would register **nocturnal penile tumescence** (penile swelling that occurs during sleep), or—in an odd source of revenue for the postal service—a line of stamps would be placed around the penis. If the stamp "bracelet" broke, it was presumed that an erection had occurred.

Often, using a strain gauge or stamp test, nocturnal tumescence was found to be normal. From this, investigators concluded that there was no physical reason for the reported sexual dysfunction. If a subject had erections while asleep, logic suggested that everything physical was in proper working order.

We now know that the neurological control of nocturnal erection is different from the nerve pathways involved in arousal from physical contact or other sensory stimulation when a man is awake. In addition, the testing of nocturnal erections measures tumescence (swelling), not rigidity. The penis might swell during sleep and still lack sufficient rigidity for sexual penetration. Also, in some men there can be a decrease in arterial blood flow to the penis with active movement, despite the fact that normal blood flow may occur passively during sleep.

Of course, psychological issues can and do affect sexual performance. Depression, relationship problems, anxiety, and stress, all common in the aging male, can lead to loss of erections. Performance anxiety can hamper sexual function at any age, but it can be a greater problem for older men, especially after the loss of a partner (widower's syndrome). The telling difference is that physical problems tend to persist without treatment, while psychological ones are usually temporary and clear up once the underlying issue is resolved.

Vascular Problems

Normal erectile function requires adequate blood flow into and out of the penis. Hardening of the arteries, diabetes, or the negative health effects of smoking, all of which are associated with aging, may impair the necessary influx of blood. A venous leak, which allows the trapped blood in the penis to escape, may make it impossible to maintain an erection. Injury to penile arteries, which can result from an accident or surgery, can also hinder adequate blood flow. In one vascular condition, known as pelvic steal syndrome, blood is diverted from the penis to supply necessary circulation to other organs that are more critical for survival.

Hormone Abnormalities

As discussed above, levels of the hormones that affect libido and sexual performance decline with age, but many older men continue to enjoy healthy erectile function nonetheless. A loss of erections may signal a hormonal abnormality or imbalance, and checking hormone levels is certainly indicated when erectile problems occur. Abnormally low testosterone or a thyroid imbalance can impair erectile function. Increased prolactin (which spurs milk production in females but has no known function in males) may signal the presence of a prolactin-secreting tumor.

Many effective treatments are available for erectile problems. (See Chapter 18, Sexual Side Effects.)

AGING AND THE PROSTATE GLAND

BPH

Beginning at about age 40, the level of male hormones (**androgens**) slowly declines. At the same time, there is a small, gradual increase in female hormones (**estrogens**), which all normal men have in meager amounts. The result is a significant shift in the critical ratio of these two hormones. Current thinking points to this change in hormonal balance as the prime suspect in facilitating benign enlargement of the gland (BPH).

During puberty the prostate grows from its minuscule 3- to 6-gram childhood size to the normal adult range of 20 to 25 grams. Starting in middle age, the gland often begins to grow again, frequently doubling in size. In extreme cases, an older man's prostate can reach ten or even twenty times the size of a gland we'd find in a healthy 20-year-old. The enlarging prostate can narrow the urethra, slow the voiding stream, and may compel men to awaken at night to void or to urinate with increasing frequency and diminished efficiency during the day. Fortunately, if these symptoms become troublesome, they can often be relieved with simple medications. Good surgical interventions can alleviate the problem in more serious or intractable cases. (See Chapter 5, BPH [Prostate Enlargement].)

PROSTATE CANCER

The incidence of prostate cancer also increases dramatically with age, rising at a faster rate than any other cancer. This represents a major, head-scratching paradox. Since prostate cancers require male hormones to develop, why would they arise with much greater frequency as androgen levels decline and estrogen levels rise?

The prostate's lifetime exposure to testosterone appears to be the cause. From puberty on, the gland is constantly besieged by high levels of male hormones. This is in sharp contrast to women, for whom the menstrual cycle, childbearing, breast-feeding, and menopause create periodic hormonal surges and dips in hormone levels. Still, we have much to learn about the role that androgens play in causing prostate cancer and why prostate cells are so devilishly prone to developing malignant changes over time.

Once a prostate cancer has spread beyond the local area, withdrawal of male hormones (**androgen deprivation therapy**) nearly always puts the tumor into remission. Removal of testosterone through medical means or surgical castration has been the mainstay in treatment of advanced prostate cancer for decades. Unfortunately, these cancers eventually learn how to grow in the absence of testosterone, thus becoming **hormone refractory**. How long androgen deprivation succeeds in arresting a cancer is related, to some degree, to a man's testosterone level at the time of diagnosis. Prostate cancers in men with higher male hormone levels take longer to become resistant to androgen withdrawal. We don't yet understand the reason for these oddities, but clearly the relationship among testosterone, aging, and prostate cancer is far more complicated than we once believed.

IN SUMMARY

∎

Aging is a normal process, not a disease. With continued advances in the management of aging-induced changes, such as prostate enlargement, prostate cancer, and erectile dysfunction, we should continue to see an ever-increasing number of men who not only live longer but do so free of urinary miseries, with the ability to enjoy sexual pleasure and satisfaction for the duration of their natural lives.

Part Two

COMMON PROSTATE
PROBLEMS

4

■

Prostatitis

READ THIS CHAPTER TO LEARN:

- What are the different types of prostatitis, and what causes this painful inflammation in the gland?
- How can prostatitis be treated, and what should you do if your symptoms persist?
- How can prostatitis affect your PSA level?

What's in a name? When the name is prostatitis, the answer is neither simple nor clear. While experts estimate that at some point in their lives half of all men will experience the urinary burning or irritation and pelvic or rectal pain that can result from an inflamed or infected prostate,[1] the condition remains strikingly underresearched, inadequately treated, and poorly understood. Tom Stamey, a Stanford University urologist, summed up the sorry situation aptly when he referred to prostatitis as a "wastebasket of clinical ignorance."[2] In many cases, we remain uncertain about what causes prostatitis, how to prevent it, or what to do to ensure that the symptoms will reliably and permanently resolve.

On a more positive note, recent research efforts have begun to yield some promising answers about this strikingly common complaint. Though we lack strong evidence, some cases of prostatitis may be caused by an underlying bacterial infection that eludes detection by conventional means. Reflux of urine into the prostate may trigger the condition in some men. In other cases the inflammation may result from the body's own dogged, though misguided, attempts to heal itself—the immune system gone awry.

A coordinated national effort is under way to define the various forms of prostatitis more precisely so we can better identify what triggers the problem in any individual case.[3] In addition, we'll soon have the results from several large clinical trials that should yield more information about better means of diagnosis and treatment. These studies will increase our understanding of the value of medications and other therapeutic approaches to alleviate symptoms, promote healing, and prevent recurrences.

WHO IS AFFECTED
BY PROSTATITIS?

While benign prostate enlargement (BPH) and prostate cancer are rare before age 50, prostatitis can strike at any time after puberty. In adult men, the problem is an equal opportunity oppressor, distributed fairly evenly across ages, races, and nationalities worldwide. At any given time, about 10 to 14 percent of all men will have one or more of the myriad symptoms physicians look for when diagnosing the condition. In this country alone, prostatitis accounts for upward of 2 million outpatient visits to doctors per year, at an annual cost as high as $1 billion according to experts.[4] Still, the costs could be even more vividly described on the misery scale. The pain and other symptoms of prostatitis can be disabling. The embarrassing nature of the symptoms, the uncertain cause of the illness, and its tendency to recur repeatedly in some men can induce depression and withdrawal that add to the detrimental effects of the disease.

THE FOUR TYPES OF PROSTATITIS

In an effort to promote better understanding of this widespread malady, the National Institute of Diabetes and Digestive and Kidney Diseases (NIDDK) convened a workshop on prostatitis in 1995. There, experts examined the current state of knowledge about the disease and devised the following classification scheme:

CATEGORY I

Acute bacterial prostatitis is a sudden-onset infection in the prostate. Several strains of bacteria can be responsible for this form of the disease, which typically causes flu-like symptoms, including fever, chills, nausea, muscle aches, and general malaise, along with pain in the pelvic region, genitalia, and/or lower back. Symptoms of a urinary tract infection, such as urinary frequency, urgency, and burning, are also common. Plus, the urine may have a foul smell.

In severe cases, a localized collection of pus (an abscess) forms within the prostate. Before the advent of modern antibiotics, such an abscess could rupture, causing serious, even life-threatening, complications. Today, treatment with powerful antibiotics specific to the bacteria causing the infection can kill the germ, relieve the misery, and effect a cure. The

THE FOUR TYPES OF PROSTATITIS

	Category I Acute Bacterial Prostatitis	**Category II** Chronic Bacterial Prostatitis	**Category III** CP/CPPS	**Category IV** Asymptomatic Inflammatory Prostatitis
How common	Rare	Uncommon	Common	Unknown
Risk factors	Old age, compromised immune system, urinary catheter, prostate biopsy	Prior acute prostatitis or urinary infection	STDs*	Unknown
Symptoms	Fever, chills, urinary burning and frequency, sudden pain in the pelvis and genitals	Prolonged pain in the pelvis, genitalia, or anus; urinary burning and frequency	Intermittent pain in the pelvis, genitalia, or rectum; may be debilitating	None
Signs	Infected urine or prostatic fluid; PSA may be markedly elevated	Prostate tenderness, infected urine or fluid; PSA may be elevated	WBC[†] in prostatic fluid (Type IIIA); PSA may be elevated	Inflammatory cells found in prostate biopsy tissue; mildly elevated PSA
Cause	Bacterial infection	Bacterial infection	Generally unknown, rarely STDs* or other infectious agents; muscle spasms, bladder irritability due to BPH, stricture, stone, or tumor	Unknown
Treatment	Antibiotics (6 weeks), pain medicine	Antibiotics (6 to 12 weeks), pain medicine	Antibiotic trial, short-term anti-inflammatory agents (COX-2 or NSAID), alpha blockers, hot tub baths, stress relief	None needed
Time course	Sudden onset, responds to treatment in hours or days	Gradual onset, intermittent over months or years	Similar to Category II	May be permanent
Relapse	Unlikely	Common	Very common	Unknown

*STD: sexually transmitted disease
[†]WBC: white blood cells

error some patients make is discontinuing the medication when symptoms subside. In fact, a full six-week course of antibiotics should be prescribed and faithfully completed to minimize the very real risk of a relapse.[5]

Category I is a rare type of prostatitis, accounting for only 5 percent of cases. It can occur in young men, sometimes related to one of the sexually transmitted diseases, but it occurs more often in older men who have had a **Foley catheter** inserted through their penis to drain the bladder for any reason, or following a prostate biopsy (in 1 percent of cases), or in elderly men with compromised immune systems, who are susceptible to a urinary tract infection.

CATEGORY II

Chronic bacterial prostatitis describes an infection in the prostate that lingers for three months or more. Though their prostates may be teeming with bacteria, men with this form of the disease are usually asymptomatic. The only potential symptom is an acute urinary tract infection that may develop as a result of the disease.

This type of infection, which is localized to the prostate area, generally responds within a few days to antibiotics such as trimethoprim (Trimpex or Proloprim) or fluoroquinolones such as ciprofloxacin (Cipro). Still, a longer course of six weeks on one of these medications is essential to minimize the risk of relapse. Some types of bacteria responsible for this type of prostatitis can develop a protective biofilm that makes them resistant to treatment, causing the symptoms to recur over and over again.

CATEGORY III

The grab-bag term **chronic prostatitis/chronic pelvic pain syndrome**, also known by its acronym, **CP/CPPS**, accounts for 90 percent of all prostatitis cases.[6] Debilitating symptoms and pain persist for three months or more, despite cultures of urine, semen, and prostatic fluid (expressed by massaging the gland during a digital rectal exam) that yield no evidence of bacterial infection. A standardized questionnaire, the NIH Chronic Prostatitis Symptom Index (see page 63), can be used to evaluate the symptoms and gauge their severity. In 7 to 8 percent of men with this form of the disease, we find trace evidence of troublesome sexually transmitted organisms, such as chlamydia, herpes simplex, human papillomavirus, trichomonas vaginalis, or mycoplasmas, but these are thought to be coincidental and unrelated to the chronic prostate woes.[7]

Category III is sometimes further subdivided into inflammatory and noninflammatory types (though some experts question whether the division makes sense). If there is inflammation in the gland in a man with Category III prostatitis, we tend to presume that the symptoms are emanating from the gland (Category IIIA, inflammatory CP/CPPS). On the other hand, if a patient has no evidence of prostatic inflammation, the symptoms are likely caused by something else, such as problems in the bladder or the muscles of the pelvic sidewall (Category IIIB, noninflammatory prostatitis).

In *Category IIIA, inflammatory CP/CPPS,* a significant number of white blood cells (leukocytes) are found in the semen or fluid expressed from the prostate when a doctor massages the gland. Leukocytes are one of the body's major defenses, and their presence signals that a battle against an injury, foreign protein, or bacteria is under way. Oddly, the severity of prostatitis symptoms appears to be unrelated to the number of white cells found in the gland, suggesting that some other mechanism may be the cause.

Though it's far from conclusive, there is some evidence that "nonbacterial" CP/CPPS might be caused by infectious bacteria after all. One study found that about one-third of men with this form of prostatitis had traces of bacterial DNA within the gland, indicating that they once had, and might still have, a bacterial infection that standard cultures simply failed to detect.[8]

If we find white blood cells indicative of an inflammation, further testing is recommended to rule out other conditions that can mimic the symptoms of nonbacterial prostatitis. This includes a number of sexually transmitted diseases (see page 54), which can be diagnosed through a history of exposure and cultures of urethral discharge. A urine specimen can be checked for blood or malignant cells to rule out a kidney stone or bladder cancer, both rare causes of prostatitis-like symptoms. A cystoscopic examination can determine whether a bladder infection, stone, or tumor is causing the pain and urinary problems. Other possible causes for such symptoms are benign enlargement of the prostate (BPH), thickening of the bladder neck, or scar tissue that narrows the urethra (**urethral stricture**).

In *Category IIIB, noninflammatory CP/CPPS,* few or no white blood cells are found in the semen or **expressed prostatic fluid**. The condition, which used to be called **prostadynia** (literally, "pain in the prostate"), involves the same constellation of urinary symptoms and pain as the inflammatory Category IIIA, but the underlying causes and effective treatments can be even harder to divine.

Though we currently lack hard evidence, Categories IIIA and B may develop differently. Category IIIA may stem from an infection, inflammation, or an autoimmune response (a kind of "friendly fire" in which the body's natural defenses go haywire and launch a misguided attack against its own organs). Category IIIB is probably more akin to a headache of the prostate. It's typically either neurological (**neurogenic**), caused by muscle contractions (**myogenic**), or stress-related (**psychogenic**).

What Are the Treatment Options?

Though we find little or no evidence of active bacterial infection in Category III prostatitis, it's reasonable to try a single three- to six-week course of antibiotics.[9] Bacterial cultures are not infallible, and one round of treatment sometimes cures the problem. If it doesn't, further use of these medications is probably unwise. They can trigger common side effects such as nausea and vomiting, a drug allergy, or a yeast infection.

NOTE: Even when the problem resolves with a course of medication, antibiotics may not be the actual hero in the piece. Symptoms of Category III prostatitis tend to fluctuate over time. You may have seen the same results without any intervention at all.

Antibiotic resistance is also a real concern. Exposure to too many germ-killing drugs can set the stage for an invasion by hard-to-control bacterial infections elsewhere in the body.

This is not to say that you should not seek symptomatic relief. For some patients, simple pain relievers or anti-inflammatory drugs are enough do the trick.★ **COX-2 inhibitors** (e.g. celecoxib [Celebrex] and valdecoxib [Bextra]), which were developed for the relief of osteoarthritis, and **NSAIDs** (nonsteroidal anti-inflammatory drugs, e.g., aspirin, ibuprofen, and naproxen), taken for four to six weeks, may reduce inflammation and eliminate the pain.

If symptoms persist or recur after a course of medication, a more intensive evaluation is indicated. This should involve a comprehensive urinalysis, a blood test for PSA, an ultrasound to assess whether an abnormal amount of urine remains in your bladder after voiding (measurement of the post-void residual urine), and **urodynamic testing**, which measures bladder capacity, bladder function, and urinary flow. Your physician should also do tests to eliminate other possible reasons for the symptoms, such as enlargement of the prostate (BPH), bladder outlet obstruction, or carcinoma in situ of the bladder (cancer contained in the cells that line the urinary reservoir). If all these measures fail to expose the root of the problem and a full course of antibiotics has already been completed, a number of second-line therapies may offer some relief.

★While short-term use apears to be safe, recent studies suggest exercising caution before taking these medicines long-term.

Second-line Medications and Other Therapies

Alpha blockers (e.g., doxazosin, terazosin, tamsulosin, alfuzosin) relax smooth muscles of the prostate and the bladder neck, allowing urine to flow more freely. Up to 50 percent of men with chronic prostatitis symptoms—especially those with diminished flow rate, post-void residual urine, or bladder outlet obstruction—experience some relief with these drugs. Alpha blockers are particularly effective for men with a diminished urinary stream or high post-void residual urine that results from bladder outlet obstruction. We're not sure whether the benefits result from a direct effect on prostatitis or from the muscle relaxation these drugs cause.

5 alpha–reductase inhibitors (e.g., finasteride, dutasteride) can shrink the prostate and alleviate urinary symptoms in men with BPH. Some prostatitis patients have also found these medications helpful, though we lack good scientific confirmation of their effectiveness for this use.

Pentosan polysulfate, which is FDA–approved to treat bladder pain and symptoms of the painful bladder condition known as interstitial cystitis, has been tested for effects against CP/CPPS in a few small studies. Though the evidence is meager, some promising preliminary results have been reported.[10]

Because Category III prostatitis causes so much misery and the symptoms can be so difficult to resolve, many men eventually try alternative remedies, including herbs. Quercetin, a bioflavonoid (natural pigments found in vegetables and fruits), and Cernilton, a derivative of pollen, have both shown some benefits in small, limited studies. Flaxseed or soy (isoflavones) may also be helpful, though we don't have solid evidence as yet. The effectiveness of other commonly used substances, such as saw palmetto, *Pygeum africanum* (African prune), and zinc, is largely anecdotal and remains to be proven.[11]

In their long and often frustrating quest for symptomatic relief, typical victims of prostatitis try five or more different approaches. Soaking in a warm bath can relax the prostate and pelvic floor muscles and provide some transient respite. Patients have reported benefits from biofeedback, local applications of heat to the affected area, or acupuncture. In some cases prostatic massage through the rectum has been useful. **Thermal therapy** delivered through the urethra (transurethral microwave thermotherapy, or TUMT) is another potentially helpful therapeutic tactic, as is supportive counseling to relieve the depression and anxiety that can accompany intractable malaise.[12]

There is no evidence that prostatitis, in any of its forms, is caused or relieved by frequent sexual activity or regularity of ejaculation, despite age-old clinical wisdom to the contrary. Scientifically rigorous trials are still needed to determine which, if any, of the many therapeutic approaches available today offer any real and lasting benefits.

CATEGORY IV

Asymptomatic inflammatory prostatitis is a silent form of prostate inflammation, meaning there are no symptoms. The condition is discovered by chance when a microscopic examination of prostatic fluid or prostate tissue taken on biopsy or examined after the prostate is removed shows abnormal numbers of inflammatory white blood cells.[13] Unless a man has an elevated PSA or problems with infertility, no treatment is required, and this condition causes no known adverse effects.

DOES PROSTATITIS AFFECT PSA?

Under normal circumstances, PSA is contained in the prostate, and only minute levels are detectable in blood. The inflammation that accompanies some forms of prostatitis breaks down tissue barriers in the gland, allowing PSA to leak into the circulatory system. This can lead to a much higher number on the screening test for prostate cancer. An acutely inflamed or infected prostate can send the PSA soaring to a stratospheric 50 to 100 nanograms per milliliter (ng/ml), or even higher. With effective treatment, the level should return to normal, though it can take up to six months. Even a minimally inflamed prostate (Category III or IV prostatitis) can cause an increased PSA level in the blood.[14]

For very young men in their teens, twenties, or early thirties, a PSA level that is elevated for a brief time is no great cause for concern, and testing men in this age group is questionable. Prostate cancer is almost never a consideration in this situation, with the possible exception of men in their thirties who have strong family histories of prostate cancer. In men over 40, an elevated PSA is worrisome and calls for medical evaluation. An extreme, rapid rise in PSA almost always comes from infection or inflammation, not prostate cancer. Still, the same man can have both prostatitis and prostate cancer, so abnormally high PSA levels should not be ignored, especially in men over 50. A medical evaluation followed by treatment and retesting can often

NOTE: If the PSA level is elevated in a man with signs or symptoms of prostatitis, he should be treated with a course of antibiotics and have his PSA retested after six to eight weeks. If the PSA falls to its previous level or returns to normal in a man who has never had the PSA test, no further action is necessary and the PSA level can be monitored annually. (See Chapter 8, Detecting Prostate Cancer with PSA and Other Tests, for a detailed discussion of the nuances of PSA testing.)

In a man with an elevated PSA level and no other signs or symptoms of prostatitis, it makes little sense to prescribe powerful antibiotics. I recommend simply waiting four to six weeks and repeating the test. If the PSA level remains elevated, a biopsy to rule out prostate cancer is probably wise.

determine what caused the level to rise. If prostatitis was the culprit, the PSA should return to normal after the infection or inflammation is resolved.

The real dilemma is what to do when the PSA suddenly rises from normal—say, 2—to 6 or 7. Such an increase can cause enormous anxiety, and most men find it hard to wait a month or more before taking action. Still, a prostate biopsy is not a trivial procedure, and it does carry a risk of side effects. It's important to keep in mind that PSA levels can fluctuate from day to day for no apparent reason by as much as 30 percent.[15] An elevated PSA caused by prostate inflammation can be slow to subside, so it's generally prudent to wait four to six weeks and repeat the test before submitting to a biopsy. The exceptions to that rule are cases where there's another reason to suspect cancer. If your PSA spikes and the doctor feels an abnormality on DRE, having a biopsy sooner makes sense.

CURRENT STATUS

We have many miles to go on the road toward understanding the causes and establishing reliable cures for the varied and often enigmatic forms

NOTE: If you have an elevated PSA but no cause can be found, it makes little sense to use medications or herbal remedies to drive the PSA down. Drugs like finasteride or dutasteride will reduce the PSA level and yield more comforting test results, but these medications have no effect on the underlying cause of the elevation. Some men convince themselves, ostrich-style, that a "normal" PSA, even when achieved by artificially masking the actual level, means that they have no cause for concern. Wise medical decisions depend on careful consideration of all the real and relevant facts.

of prostatitis. Studies sponsored by the National Institutes of Health (NIH) have taken critical first steps by developing a questionnaire that can rate symptoms and objectively gauge the effectiveness of various therapies in managing the disease. (See the NIH Chronic Prostatitis Symptom Index on page 63.)

These studies have also established standardized definitions for various forms of the disease, documented the damaging effect of prostatitis on quality of life, and begun to either verify or refute the alleged benefits of many treatments commonly used in an attempt to vanquish the vexing symptoms. Hopefully, we'll learn much more about this common, troubling condition in the near future.

THE FUTURE

Recently, molecular biologists have identified signaling proteins called cytokines that can unleash the scourge of prostate inflammation, along with its highly disagreeable sidekicks: irritation and pain. This discovery may lead to the development of medications capable of inhibiting cytokines and relieving symptoms in cases where prostatitis is caused by inflammation and not a germ.[16]

Meanwhile, bear in mind that while prostatitis may cause discomfort, or even misery, with modern treatment it is *not* a dangerous or deadly medical condition. Though living with persistent or recurrent symptoms may be an inescapable fact of life for some men, the way you deal with these symptoms can make all the difference. A positive attitude and equanimity will go a long way toward minimizing the impact of this disease. If chronic prostatitis is pummeling your quality of life, you might want to consider short-term counseling or even long term psychotherapy to restore your sense of control and keep the condition from looming disproportionately large.

IN SUMMARY

∎

Though half of all men develop prostatitis at some point in their lives, our understanding of the condition remains woefully incomplete. Typically, patients try several treatments in the quest for symptomatic relief, and the process can be difficult and frustrating. Thankfully, given modern medicine, prostatitis is no longer a dangerous or lethal disease.

NIH CHRONIC PROSTATITIS SYMPTOM INDEX (NIH-CPSI)

PAIN OR DISCOMFORT

1. In the last week, have you experienced any pain or discomfort in the following areas?

	YES	NO
a. Area between rectum and testicles (perineum)	$\square_1$	$\square_0$
b. Testicles	$\square_1$	$\square_0$
c. Tip of the penis (not related to urination)	$\square_1$	$\square_0$
d. Below your waist, in your pubic or bladder area	$\square_1$	$\square_0$

2. In the last week, have you experienced:
   a. Pain or burning during urination? $\square_1$ $\square_0$
   b. Pain or discomfort during or after sexual climax (ejaculation)? $\square_1$ $\square_0$

3. How often have you had pain or discomfort in any of these areas over the last week?
   $\square_0$ Never
   $\square_1$ Rarely
   $\square_2$ Sometimes
   $\square_3$ Often
   $\square_4$ Usually
   $\square_5$ Always

4. Which number best describes your AVERAGE pain or discomfort on the days that you had it, over the last week?

$\square$ $\square$ $\square$ $\square$ $\square$ $\square$ $\square$ $\square$ $\square$ $\square$ $\square$
0　1　2　3　4　5　6　7　8　9　10
NO PAIN　　　　　　PAIN AS BAD AS YOU CAN IMAGINE

URINATION

5. How often have you had a sensation of not emptying your bladder completely after you finished urinating, over the last week?
   $\square_0$ Not at all
   $\square_1$ Less than 1 time in 5
   $\square_2$ Less than half the time
   $\square_3$ About half the time
   $\square_4$ More than half the time
   $\square_5$ Almost always

6. How often have you had to urinate again less than two hours after you finished urinating, over the last week?
   $\square_0$ Not at all
   $\square_1$ Less than 1 time in 5
   $\square_2$ Less than half the time
   $\square_3$ About half the time
   $\square_4$ More than half the time
   $\square_5$ Almost always

IMPACT OF SYMPTOMS

7. How much have your symptoms kept you from doing the kinds of things you would usually do, over the last week?
   $\square_0$ None
   $\square_1$ Only a little
   $\square_2$ Some
   $\square_3$ A lot

8. How much did you think about your symptoms, over the last week?
   $\square_0$ None
   $\square_1$ Only a little
   $\square_2$ Some
   $\square_3$ A lot

QUALITY OF LIFE

9. If you were to spend the rest of your life with your symptoms just the way they have been during the last week, how would you feel about that?
   $\square_0$ Delighted
   $\square_1$ Pleased
   $\square_2$ Mostly satisfied
   $\square_3$ Mixed (about equally satisfied and dissatisfied)
   $\square_4$ Mostly dissatisfied
   $\square_5$ Unhappy
   $\square_6$ Terrible

SCORING THE NIH CHRONIC PROSTATITIS SYMPTOM INDEX DOMAINS

Pain: Total of items 1a, 1b, 1c, 1d, 2a, 2b, 3, and 4 = _____

Urinary Symptoms: Total of items 5 and 6 = _____

Quality of Life Impact: Total of items 7, 8, and 9 = _____

The NIH-CPSI is a patient questionnaire developed by the National Institutes of Health (NIH) to measure the severity of symptoms caused by prostatitis or related conditions.

5

■

BPH (Prostate Enlargement)

READ THIS CHAPTER TO LEARN:

- Why does the prostate enlarge as men age, and what problems can an overgrown prostate cause?
- How can we diagnose and treat BPH?
- What effect does benign prostate enlargement have on PSA?

Benjamin Franklin famously opined that nothing is certain but death and taxes. But if you are a normal male and live long enough, you can likely add benign prostatic hyperplasia (BPH) to the list. In fact, Franklin himself is believed to have suffered from bladder stones, urinary obstruction, and other advanced symptoms of the disease, as did his brother. In a classic case of necessity breeding invention, this resourceful founding father devised the flexible urinary catheter to manage the problem.[1]

The first recorded accounts of attempts to relieve men's urinary blockage date from an Egyptian papyrus, written in the fifteenth century BC.

One remedy from that era involved a complex tea brewed from the bark of juniper and cypress trees, and beer.

Despite the best efforts of physicians, little progress in treating the condition was made for the next thousand years. The famous Greek scientist Hippocrates, who became the father of medicine when he founded the discipline in the fifth century BC, expressed extreme pessimism about patients with voiding troubles. He characterized urinary obstruction as a dire condition with a very poor prognosis and held out no hope for permanent relief. Sufferers were forced to rely on the painful insertion of harsh metal catheters of varying composition (depending on a man's financial means), which often caused life-threatening injuries or infections.

Over subsequent millennia, doctors have tried a staggering array of therapies—including heat, irrigation, galvanic cautery, electrical stimulation, injections designed to shrink the prostate, drugs, and acupuncture—in a desperate quest for the elusive cure. Elaborate, expensive, and highly questionable approaches sprang up to solve the frustrating problem. In the early twentieth century, a popular regime prescribed for men with obstructive voiding symptoms involved abundant fresh air, avoidance of sexual excess and constipation, regular holidays in favorable climates, and frequent rounds of golf.[2]

Before the discovery of effective treatments, chronic urinary obstruction could result in permanent bladder and kidney damage and, in extreme cases, death. **Acute urinary retention**, where a man could not urinate at all, was a real and very serious concern. In Victorian times, the condition even spawned a fashion statement. Men with severe urinary symptoms carried the catheters they needed to empty their bladders in the hollow shafts of walking sticks or umbrellas or beneath the band of the popular bowler hat. Cowboys tucked them inside their ten-gallon hats when they set out to ride the range.

In 1891, a doctor aptly named George Goodfellow is said to have performed the first **perineal prostatectomy** for urinary obstruction, removing excess prostate tissue through an incision between the scrotum and rectum. In 1895, Eugene Fuller performed the first procedure to clear the urinary channel using a lower abdominal "suprapubic" approach. Soon afterward, Hugh Hampton Young—who also pioneered **brachytherapy** (seed implants) and **radical prostatectomy surgery** (to remove the gland) in cases of prostate cancer—devised a punch that could remove the overgrowth through the urethra, eliminating the need for open surgery in most cases. One of Young's most famous patients, "Diamond Jim" Brady, was so grateful for the relief he got from this operation that he funded the Brady Urological Institutes at Cornell University and Johns Hopkins University, devoted to the study and cure of urological diseases.[3]

Today, a refined **transurethral resection of the prostate (TURP)** is the most common surgery for prostatic enlargement. Medicines that relax or shrink the gland and minimally invasive surgical approaches have transformed this ubiquitous disease from a potentially grave or even fatal condition into a manageable problem whose impact on quality of life can be minimized and often completely overcome.

WHAT IS BPH?

Benign prostatic hyperplasia (BPH) can be devilishly difficult to understand. Technically, the term refers to microscopic changes in the prostate. "Benign" indicates that the growth is not cancer, which by definition has the ability to escape its organ of origin and spread to other parts of the body. "Hyperplasia" means overgrowth of cells. In BPH, new prostate cells proliferate while the old ones somehow lose their way and fail to die off as they should. Still, no matter how much BPH a man develops, the abnormal overgrowth remains within the gland. Ironically, because it grows in close quarters, pressing inward on the urethra, BPH often causes bothersome urinary symptoms, while prostate cancer, which can spread outward to other organs, usually causes no symptoms at all until it is well beyond a cure.

BPH *does not* become cancer or predict that a man will develop a malignancy. Though some men are diagnosed with both BPH and prostate cancer, the two diseases are distinct and typically arise in different parts

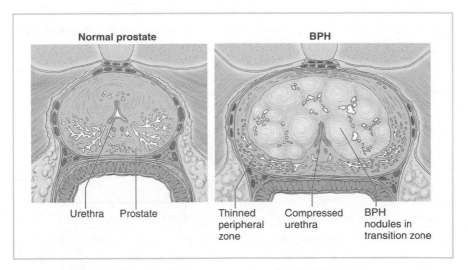

Normal prostate

BPH

Urethra   Prostate

Thinned peripheral zone

Compressed urethra

BPH nodules in transition zone

Compared to the normal prostate (left), a prostate enlarged with BPH (right) compresses the peripheral zone and narrows the urethra, causing urinary symptoms.

of the gland. BPH affects the transition zone, the core of the prostate that surrounds the urethra, while the vast majority of prostate cancers develop in the peripheral zone, which lies under the outer skin (capsule) of the prostate.[4]

Though BPH actually refers to microscopic overgrowth, doctors also commonly use the term to describe a wide range of physical changes and symptoms that may occur as a result. BPH can cause enlargement of the prostate, **lower urinary tract symptoms (LUTS)**, and **bladder outlet obstruction,** though any of these conditions can exist without the others. Some men with the disease have enlarged prostates, and some don't. Voiding problems may be mild, involving a slight increase in frequency or a minor decrease in the force of the urinary stream, while other patients experience severe urinary frequency or incontinence. In the worst cases, a man cannot urinate at all (acute urinary retention) and requires emergency catheterization or surgery to relieve the blockage. Though BPH is a chronic, progressive disease, symptoms can vary over time, sometimes clearing up on their own, for no apparent reason.[5]

The severity of urinary problems hinges as heavily on where the BPH is located as on the extent of the overgrowth or how large the prostate becomes. If the enlargement occurs in the lateral (side) lobes, they may be able to swing away like the flippers on a pinball machine, allowing good urinary flow. On the other hand, an enlarged median (middle) lobe can act like a cork in the neck of a wine bottle, blocking the stream altogether. Eventually, if this benign tumor grows extremely large, it forms strange-looking, knobby protrusions that resemble cauliflower.

WHAT CAUSES BPH?

HORMONES

We still don't fully understand why BPH develops, but hormones are a strong suspect. All males have a tiny supply of the female hormone, estrogen. As men age, testosterone, the male hormone, naturally declines, while the amount of estrogen increases slightly. This change in hormonal balance may trigger benign overgrowth in the prostate, and studies are under way to test this hypothesis.[6] Why only the transition zone of the prostate (and not the peripheral zone or the seminal vesicles or other secondary sex organs) enlarges so much with age remains a medical mystery.

BPH is a disease of aging males, and every normal aging man is at risk. "Normal" is the operative word here. The condition only develops in the presence of circulating male hormones. Men castrated before puberty do not develop BPH. Neither do men with a hereditary enzyme deficiency that affects androgen metabolism.

During the early 1970s, Dr. Julianne Imperato-McGinley, a Cornell epidemiologist, traveled to the Dominican Republic to investigate reports of a tribe in which many female children seemed to develop magically into men at puberty. Called *guevedoces* ("penis at twelve"), these people were genetically male, with an X and a Y chromosome, but they had scant body hair and poorly developed genitalia, with a small penis and only one testicle, which was undescended. Intriguingly, they were also immune from acne and balding. Their prostates never grew to adult size, and they never suffered with benign prostate enlargement later in life.[7]

On examination, these men were found to have a deficiency of the enzyme **5 alpha-reductase**, which is needed to convert testosterone to its more powerful form, **dihydrotestosterone (DHT)**. Without this enzyme, some male sexual features—the prostate, seminal vesicles, and the tendency to baldness—do not develop. This revelation eventually led to the development of finasteride (Proscar), which shrinks the prostate, reduces the need for surgery to alleviate BPH symptoms, and lowers the risk of acute urinary retention.[8]

Many men taking the medication reported an unexpected reduction or even a reversal of balding, and studies ensued to test its safety and effectiveness for this use. At a much lower dose than that prescribed for BPH, finasteride, marketed as Propecia, was approved by the FDA in 1997 as the first oral medication for the treatment of hair loss.[9]

Aging

Aging is another major cause of BPH, and the incidence of the disease increases dramatically as men grow older. While other body parts have the good sense to reach full size at maturity and then remain stable or shrink slowly over time, the prostate undergoes a second growth spurt starting in middle age. Twenty percent of 40-year-olds, 60 percent of 60-year-olds, and 90 percent of men in their 80s have the overgrowth of glandular and muscle cells in the prostate that is characteristic of BPH.[10] (See the graph on page 70.) In about a quarter of all men, the condition causes urinary symptoms that are sufficiently troubling to land them in a doctor's office. The annual bill for treating BPH in the United States alone is estimated to be $9 billion and growing rapidly as the average age of our population continues to rise. By 2020, an estimated 11.2 million American men each year will seek treatment for symptoms of the disease.[11]

Other Risk Factors

Researchers have explored a host of possible causes of BPH, including level of sexual activity, general health, race, diet, exercise, exposure to tox-

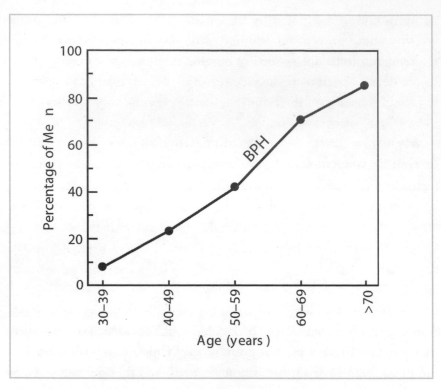

The percentage of men with BPH at each age. Most of these men will have no symptoms.*

ins, and presence of other diseases. None of these has been found to correlate significantly with whether a man is likely to develop urinary symptoms. In a small percentage of cases, the disease appears to run in families, though we have yet to identify the underlying genetic mechanism.[12]

HOW DOES BPH AFFECT URINATION?

The characteristic overgrowth of BPH occurs in the transition zone, the part of the prostate surrounding the urethra, which channels urine from the bladder to the outside. Think of a fist squeezing a drinking straw and

*Source: Modified from Carter, H. B., and D. S. Coffey. "The Prostate—an Increasing Medical Problem." *Prostate* 16, no. 1 (1990): 39–48. © 1990. Reprinted with permission from Wiley-Liss, Inc., a subsidiary of John Wiley & Sons, Inc.

The urethra in males has two distinct sections. The part of the urethra that runs through the penis is a tube. The prostatic urethra is a channel, carved like a tunnel through the gland and covered by protective lining (epithelial) cells. When the prostate is removed to treat cancer, a new connection (anastomosis) is sewn between the bladder and the tube that leads to the outside. A Foley catheter keeps the channel clear while the connection heals and the lining regrows.

you can imagine what happens as the urethra is progressively narrowed. The bladder must work harder and harder to force stored urine past the resistance created by the constricted outlet.

Early on, the bladder compensates by building more muscle so it can contract with sufficient force to void successfully. Over time, this muscular buildup thickens the bladder wall, limiting its ability to expand to store urine. With less and less storage capacity, the bladder must empty more often. As a result, BPH may lead to a constellation of symptoms we call prostatism, with frequent urination during the day and awakening to urinate at night (nocturia). This should be distinguished from awakening for some other reason and deciding to use the bathroom while you're awake. (See page 73.)

Eventually, the overtaxed bladder gets worn out and weak, a situation known as bladder decompensation. Daytime frequency increases, along with more trips to the bathroom during the night. When you get to the bathroom, it may take a while to get the stream started (hesitancy). This is different from the bashful bladder some men have, characterized by difficulty urinating in public restrooms.

Once urination begins, you might notice a decreased urinary flow rate, which is the equivalent of poor water pressure in the sink. The bladder may not be able to contract forcefully enough to empty all at once, and the stream becomes intermittent. The flow stops and starts again unpredictably, sometimes after you've zipped up (dribbling). As the situation worsens, the bladder might become incapable of emptying

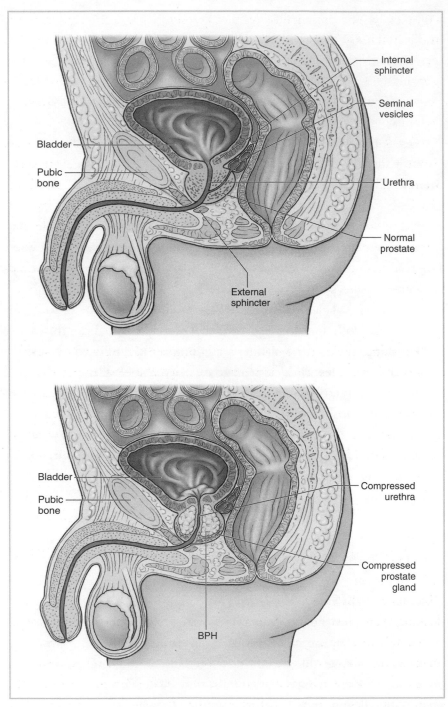

A side view of the normal prostate (top) compared to BPH (bottom), showing the effects on the urethra.

completely. The presence of post-void residual urine (PVR) leaves less room in the holding tank for new fluid to enter, and some men need to urinate with alarming frequency. Standing urine is a bacterial breeding ground, and a bladder that is never fully emptied sets you up for recurrent urinary tract infections. Painful bladder stones are more likely to form under these conditions as well.

As the bladder overfills, it loses the capacity to hold additional urine. Some patients develop **overflow incontinence**. Like **stress incontinence**, this causes leakage when you cough, strain, or stand. The bladder is so full—even though you may not be aware of it—that urine is forced out with any increase in abdominal pressure. Other men develop **urge incontinence**. When they feel the need to go, it has to be *immediately*. They may plan their lives around the availability of a bathroom and still can't always make it on time.

Prostatism refers to the urinary symptoms of BPH, including a weak urinary stream, hesitance, intermittency, frequent urination, and awakening at night to urinate (nocturia). **Prostatitis** is an inflammation or infection in the gland that can cause pain in the **perineum** (the area between the scrotum and rectum), lower abdominal pain, pain in the tip of the penis, as well as urinary symptoms such as frequency, urgency, and pain on urination.

WHEN SHOULD BPH BE TREATED?

Tolerance for BPH symptoms is highly individual. One man might find leaking even a few drops unbearable, while another may consider this an acceptable or even expected fact of life. Getting up during the night to urinate may strike you as a minor annoyance, a major disruption, or a nonissue. Increased frequency could have a very different meaning for a man with a desk job and a bathroom down the hall than for a long-haul truck driver.

You alone can judge what impact your symptoms are having on your quality of life. If you are bothered by urinary changes, it's probably time to see a doctor and explore your treatment options. If you have severe symptoms, such as blood in your urine, recurrent urinary tract infections, bladder stones, or trouble emptying your bladder, toughing it out is *not* a good idea. The longer you ignore the problem, the more likely you are to develop acute retention or incur bladder or kidney damage, which could be irreversible.[13]

Appropriate medical or surgical intervention often resolves bothersome symptoms and may also avert more serious problems later on. Mild or moderate cases can generally be managed by more conservative, less aggressive and invasive measures that carry a lower risk of side effects.

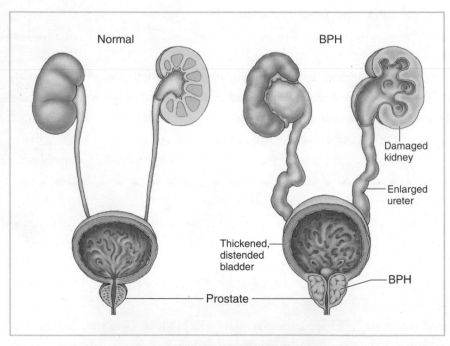

Advanced BPH can cause severe urinary obstruction. The blocked ureters become dilated, and the kidneys are damaged. Given modern treatment, this need not occur.

HOW DO YOU KNOW YOU HAVE BPH?

Troublesome symptoms of BPH call for a careful medical evaluation. Your doctor should take a focused medical and surgical history to rule out conditions like diabetes, Parkinson's disease, and stroke that cause similar symptoms. The physical checkup includes a digital rectal exam to gauge the size of the prostate and check for abnormalities that might signal the presence of prostate cancer or prostatitis. If you've ever had surgery or injury to the area or had a catheter inserted for any reason, a **urethral stricture** (narrowing of the urethra by scar tissue) could be causing your symptoms. To check for this, the doctor can examine the urethra by inserting a thin, flexible **cystoscope** through the penis under local anesthetic. Certain sexually transmitted diseases (STDs), such as gonorrhea, can also cause a stricture, and testing for such conditions should be part of the visit if you are at risk.

The BPH workup includes urinalysis to rule out urinary tract infection, prostatitis, or bladder cancer. We check the PSA for warning signs of prostate cancer and take a blood creatinine level, which can alert us to abnormalities in kidney function.

A number of simple, noninvasive tests can confirm the presence and degree of urinary obstruction. To check **urinary flow rate** (uroflowmetry), a patient urinates into an electromechanical device that measures the voiding pattern at various points in the stream. Ultrasound can determine the presence of post-void residual urine, a sign that the bladder isn't being emptied completely. **Urodynamic testing**, which measures the function of the bladder and other parts of the lower urinary tract, is more invasive and expensive, and we generally reserve it for men with confusing or intractable symptoms.

DOES BPH AFFECT PSA?

A larger prostate is a bigger manufacturing plant, which predictably churns out more PSA (prostate-specific antigen). Prostate diseases can break down

INTERNATIONAL PROSTATE SYMPTOM SCORE (IPSS)

Name: _____ Date: _____

	Not at all	Less than 1 time in 5	Less than half the time	About half the time	More than half the time	Almost always	Your score
Incomplete emptying Over the past month, how often have you had a sensation of not emptying your bladder completely after you finish urinating?	0	1	2	3	4	5	
Frequency Over the past month, how often have you had to urinate again less than two hours after you finished urinating?	0	1	2	3	4	5	
Intermittency Over the past month, how often have you found you stopped and started again several times when you urinated?	0	1	2	3	4	5	
Urgency Over the past month, how difficult have you found it to postpone urination?	0	1	2	3	4	5	
Weak stream Over the past month, how often have you had a weak urinary stream?	0	1	2	3	4	5	
Straining Over the past month, how often have you had to push or strain to begin urination?	0	1	2	3	4	5	

INTERNATIONAL PROSTATE SYMPTOM SCORE (IPSS) *(continued)*

	None	1 time	2 times	3 times	4 times	5 times or more	Your score
Nocturia Over the past month, how many times did you most typically get up to urinate from the time you went to bed until the time you got up in the morning?	0	1	2	3	4	5	
						Total IPSS score _____	

Total score: 0–7 mildly symptomatic; 8–19 moderately symptomatic; 20–35 severely symptomatic

	Delighted	Pleased	Mostly Satisfied	Mixed—about Equally Satisfied and Dissatisfied	Mostly Dissatisfied	Unhappy	Terrible
Quality of life due to urinary symptoms If you were to spend the rest of your life with your urinary condition the way it is now, how would you feel about that?	0	1	2	3	4	5	6

The International Prostate Symptom Score (IPSS) is a questionnaire given to patients to assess the severity of their urinary symptoms and how bothersome the symptoms are.

normal tissue barriers, allowing PSA to leak out of the gland where it belongs and into the bloodstream. This can translate into a high or rising number on the PSA screening test for prostate cancer.[14]

The major issue is what happens next. An elevated level (over 4 ng/ml) or a steadily rising PSA level in the blood should trigger a prostate biopsy to determine whether cancer is the cause. PSA levels between 4 and 10 represent a troubling gray area. Elevations in this range may result from either BPH or malignant disease.

If BPH is the culprit, you could be put through the discomfort and anxiety of a prostate biopsy only to discover that you don't have cancer at all. Still, if cancer is the cause, we'd want to find it while it is still contained and curable.

The tests for **PSA density (PSAD)** and percent of **free PSA (%fPSA)** were devised in an attempt to improve our ability to predict whether an elevated PSA is caused by BPH or prostate cancer. To determine PSA density, we measure the prostate volume in grams by transrectal ultrasound and then divide the PSA by that number. If BPH is causing the elevation, we'd expect the PSA to be directly proportional to the size of the prostate, i.e., bigger gland equals higher number. PSA density greater than 0.07 is suspicious, and a level over 0.15 indicates an increased likelihood that prostate cancer is present. Free PSA (PSA that is unbound to protein) is secreted mainly by BPH cells, not cancer. A high percentage of free PSA (over 25 percent) means you're less likely to have a malignancy. Still, these measures are not perfect, and relying on

NOTE: Some people mistakenly assume that having surgery for BPH means that you can no longer get prostate cancer. In fact, after a simple prostatectomy for BPH, the peripheral zone, where prostate cancer most often arises, is left in place, and prostate cancer remains a very real possibility. No matter what treatment you have for symptoms of an enlarged prostate, you should continue to have digital rectal exams, have your PSA tested regularly, and take appropriate action if the numbers are steadily rising or abnormally high.

them too heavily to rule out a cancer is unwise. Any time the PSA level is elevated, it's important to have a careful evaluation by a urologist. (For more on how PSA testing is used to screen for cancer, see Chapter 8, Detecting Prostate Cancer with PSA and Other Tests.)

After successful treatment for BPH with surgery, your PSA level should fall markedly within six to twelve weeks.[15] If the level remains elevated, your doctor should be alert to the possibility that something else, including prostate cancer, may be responsible. Some BPH treatments—such as finasteride, which shrinks the prostate, as well as certain herbal and holistic therapies—can lower PSA levels artificially. Finasteride typically drops PSA production to less than half the previous level and does not seem to affect the total free PSA ratio (% f PSA). This could mask the presence of a cancer and lead to a potentially harmful delay in diagnosis and treatment. Men taking these agents should notify their doctors and be extra vigilant.

WHAT ARE THE TREATMENT OPTIONS FOR BPH?

WATCHFUL WAITING

Whether, when, and how we treat BPH depend on the severity of the symptoms it causes and the impact those symptoms have on a patient's quality of life. Men with mild symptoms (a score of less than 12 on the **International Prostate Symptom Score (IPSS)**, see pages 76–77) are good candidates for **watchful waiting**. Simple lifestyle changes, such as restricting liquids a couple of hours before bedtime and taking care to empty the bladder before a movie or long car ride, may be enough to alleviate the situation. With moderate or severe symptoms, active treatment is the wiser course, both to reduce urinary problems and to prevent progressive urinary obstruction.[16]

MEDICAL TREATMENTS

Urinary symptoms may respond to medication, and doctors typically recommend trying these more conservative therapies before resorting to more aggressive treatment, such as surgery.

Alpha blockers, such as doxazosin (Cardura) or terazosin (Hytrin), were originally developed to treat high blood pressure by relaxing smooth muscles in blood vessel walls. By the same action, these drugs can lower muscle tension in the prostate, bladder neck, and urethra, allowing urine to flow more freely. Newer agents, like tamsulosin (Flomax) or alfuzosin (Uroxatral), have a more specific effect on relaxing only the prostate and may have fewer side effects. Also, unlike earlier alpha blockers, they do not need to be built up gradually to find the appropriate dose. All of the alpha blockers appear to be equally effective.[17]

About two-thirds of men with symptomatic BPH experience a mild to moderate reduction in voiding problems with the use of alpha blockers, though since they are relatively new, the long-term effects of these drugs on symptom management and whether they prevent the progression of the disease are not yet known.

Alpha blockers take effect quickly, providing relief in a matter of days or weeks. They work best in patients with small prostates whose BPH nodules largely arise from the smooth muscle tissue of the gland. Five to 10 percent of men on these drugs experience unpleasant side effects, including fatigue, headache, nasal stuffiness, and postural hypotension, where a change in position causes a sudden drop in blood pressure with resultant dizziness. **Retrograde ejaculation**, where the sperm is harmlessly discharged up into the bladder on orgasm, rather than out through the penis, and decreased ejaculatory volume may also occur in men taking these drugs.

Finasteride (Proscar) was approved for the treatment of BPH by the FDA in 1996. This medication and its chemical cousin dutasteride (Avodart) gradually shrink the prostate by blocking production of the enzyme 5 alpha-reductase that converts testosterone into its more powerful form, dihydrotestosterone (DHT). For men whose symptoms are caused by an enlarged gland, these drugs have been proven highly effective in reducing symptoms and preventing the need for more invasive, aggressive treatments down the road.

Though early studies suggested that alpha blockers were more effective than these drugs in relieving symptoms, more recent investigations, including the landmark Proscar Long-term Efficacy and Safety Study (PLESS) trial—a four-year study involving over 3,000 men—confirmed that finasteride was equally effective for symptom relief and better at preventing acute urinary retention and the need for surgery to relieve symptoms.[18] Finasteride takes longer to work than alpha blockers, so a lengthy trial of at least six months on the drug may be necessary to gauge its effects.

> There are two forms of the enzyme 5 alpha-reductase that is required for prostate growth. Drugs that block this enzyme can shrink the gland and alleviate urinary symptoms in men with BPH. Finasteride blocks Type II of the enzyme. A new drug, dutasteride, blocks both forms of 5 alpha-reductase: Types I and II. Theoretically, you might expect that blocking both forms would be more effective, but so far, studies have demonstrated no significant difference between these drugs.

The Medical Therapy of Prostatic Symptoms (MTOPS) study, a large trial reported in 2002, compared the effectiveness of finasteride taken alone, the alpha blocker doxazosin taken alone, and both of these drugs used in combination. Using both of these medications proved superior in halting progression of the disease and relieving symptoms, but of the two, finasteride was more effective in reducing the risk of acute urinary retention or the need for surgery over a five-year period.[19]

Finasteride is approved for the treatment of BPH, but we have long speculated that it might prevent prostate cancer.[20] Indeed, the Prostate Cancer Prevention Trial (PCPT), published in 2003, demonstrated that finasteride can reduce the incidence of tumors in the gland, but at the cost, it seemed, of allowing more high grade, potentially aggressive cancers to flourish (see Chapter 7, Risk Factors and Prevention). Until this issue is completely resolved, I would not recommend finasteride for cancer prevention alone. Still, this drug is so effective for BPH, and it so markedly reduces the risk that men with BPH will need surgery, that I strongly recommend that men with BPH continue to take it. Of course, anyone on finasteride should inform his doctor that he's taking the drug and continue regular screening for prostate cancer.

While taking finasteride, 4 percent of patients experience a loss of libido, and 3 percent develop erectile dysfunction or reduced ejaculatory volume. Some men on this medication report breast swelling or tenderness, and some have allergic reactions. In most cases, the symptoms resolve promptly when the drug is stopped.

Medications for BPH can cost up to $5 per day, and their effectiveness depends on careful compliance in taking the recommended dose.

NOTE: While 5 alpha-reductase inhibitors reduce the risk that a man with BPH will need surgery over time, the reduction among all men treated was small, from about 10 percent to 5 percent over four years.[21] We need better ways to determine which high-risk patients would benefit most by taking medication permanently, so the other men can avoid the side effects and expense of the drugs. A collaborative project between Dr. Kevin Slawin of Baylor College of Medicine and our doctors at Memorial Sloan-Kettering is developing mathematical models called **nomograms** (see Chapter 12, Deciding How to Treat Localized Prostate Cancer) that can predict which men are likely to see their BPH progress and cause serious problems, so we can identify who needs these drugs and should take them early.

Phytotherapy

These supplements, derived from plant extracts, have not been proven effective in managing the urinary symptoms of BPH. Despite extravagant claims, some of these substances may, in fact, do nothing more than shrink the size of your wallet. Still, some patients do report symptomatic relief when taking such herbal remedies as saw palmetto. Though we don't yet have scientific support for their effectiveness, they appear to be pretty benign and may prove to have some meaningful benefits.[22]

Keep in mind that these agents are unregulated and not subject to manufacturing oversight. Purity and quality can vary widely, and there is no guarantee of safety. If you try any of them, be sure to let your doctor know. Certain supplements can artificially lower your PSA, altering the results on the screening tests for cancer. Also, there is always a possibility of drug interactions, even with nonprescription "natural" or herbal substances.[23]

SURGICAL TREATMENTS

If your symptoms persist or worsen on medications, if they severely affect your normal activities, or if you develop recurrent urinary tract infections, repeated bleeding in the urine, bladder stones, or acute urinary retention, you should strongly consider surgical treatment for your BPH.

> NOTE: All the surgical approaches to BPH involve some trade-off. Not surprisingly, the more effective and durable the treatment, the greater the risk of side effects.[24]

SURGERY DESIGNED TO REMOVE BPH TISSUE

Transurethral Resection of the Prostate (TURP)

Long considered the surgical gold standard, TURP (sometimes colloquially known as "Roto-Rooter" surgery) accounts for 95 percent of the surgical procedures done to relieve the symptoms of BPH. Though the development of medicines to treat the disease has reduced the number of TURPs by 60 percent in the past decade, it remains one of the most commonly performed operations in the United States.

TURP is dramatically effective and can restore your urinary tract to

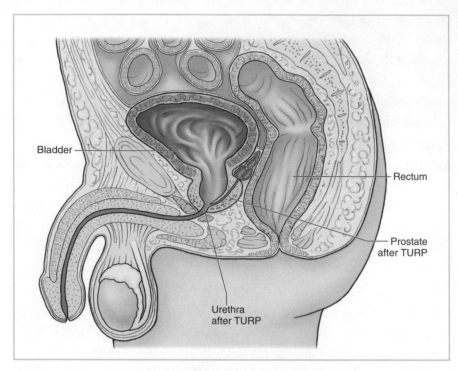

Bladder

Rectum

Prostate
after TURP

Urethra
after TURP

With TURP, laser prostatectomy, or traditional open surgery, the goal is to remove all the BPH tissue obstructing the urinary tract. The normal prostate gland (peripheral zone) is not removed.

the way it functioned when you were 18 years old.[25] Under general, epidural, or spinal anesthesia, a small electric loop is introduced into the urethra through the penis. Excess tissue blocking the urinary channel is chipped away, and then electrical current is applied to cauterize the wound. TURP requires a hospital stay of one to three days.

SIDE EFFECTS AND COMPLICATIONS. Immediate complications include bleeding that may require transfusion in about 4 percent of cases, acute urinary retention (in 6 to 7 percent of cases), and infections in 2 percent. TURP syndrome, a very rare and serious, though highly treatable complication, can cause mental confusion, visual and digestive disturbances, and cardiac symptoms. Men with prostates larger than 60 grams, who require a longer time on the operating table and more fluids introduced to flush out the excised tissue, are at greater risk for TURP syndrome. Experienced surgeons know how to avoid the problem.

> NOTE: It's *always* wise to put yourself in the best possible hands.

Although reported in about 13 percent of cases, a properly performed TURP should not cause erectile dysfunction. About 5 percent of patients develop a urinary stricture, and about 1 percent report some incontinence. Over half of men treated with TURP develop retrograde ejaculation, where semen is harmlessly expelled into the bladder rather than out through the penis during orgasm. As a result, most men are infertile after the procedure. If this is of concern, plan to bank sperm before the operation.

Though TURP often proves to be a permanent fix, about 1 percent of patients per year experience a recurrence of symptoms, requiring further treatment.

Open (Traditional) Prostatectomy

In men with very large prostates or those for whom hip or other medical problems preclude the physical positioning required—legs spread and elevated—during the TURP surgery, excess prostate tissue can be removed through an incision in the abdomen. Although it is as effective as TURP in relieving symptoms, open prostatectomy results in a longer hospital stay and increases the risk of bleeding that requires a transfusion.

SIDE EFFECTS AND COMPLICATIONS.   Retrograde ejaculation (see TURP complications above) occurs in 80 to 90 percent of patients after an open procedure, and 2 to 3 percent develop erectile dysfunction or a narrowing of the bladder neck. Open prostatectomy also carries a small risk of more serious surgical complications, such as pulmonary embolism, deep vein thrombosis, heart attack, or stroke.

Transurethral Electrovaporization of the Prostate (TUVP)

A specially designed roller-ball electrode rapidly heats excess prostate tissue and turns it to steam. Because the tissue is vaporized and rapidly cauterized using electrical energy, TUVP avoids the irritative urinary symptoms we see with other procedures, where tissue dies and is sloughed away.

Though we don't yet have the data to gauge long-term effects, TUVP has shown early promise as a means to eliminate prostate overgrowth with minimal side effects, low blood loss, and a short, overnight hospital stay.[26]

SIDE EFFECTS AND COMPLICATIONS. Retrograde ejaculation is as common as it is with TURP, and incontinence is equally rare (less than 1 percent), but about 12 percent of patients experience blood in the urine and irritation when urinating for up to three weeks after surgery.

Laser Prostatectomy

During the past decade, several laser delivery systems have been developed to vaporize and cauterize prostate tissue. The new KTP high-energy laser shows particular promise as a means to relieve urinary symptoms with a low risk of serious complications and side effects.[27]

Laser prostatectomy involves a shorter hospital stay, generally overnight, and more rapid removal of the catheter than TURP. The procedure carries a low risk of serious complications, such as incontinence or the need for transfusion. This is especially important for patients with congestive heart failure or medical conditions requiring blood thinners or anticoagulants, who may be more vulnerable to the risks of the traditional TURP.

Symptom improvement in the short term appears to be comparable to TURP. Because laser treatment is so new, we don't yet have long-term results.

SIDE EFFECTS AND COMPLICATIONS. Though the side effects vary depending on the type of laser used and the means by which the energy is delivered, some patients have irritative voiding symptoms for a month or two as tissue destroyed by the procedure is sloughed off. About 11 percent experience painful urination (dysuria) for a time. Retrograde ejaculation seems less common than with TURP, perhaps because more of the bladder neck tissue can be spared. A loss of erections is equally rare.

The Bottom Line

These procedures remove all the overgrowth. To the extent each is done successfully, relief of urinary obstruction is comparable, as are side effects. None of these treatments, properly performed, should cause a loss of erections. The erectile nerves lie outside the peripheral zone of the gland, which is not removed to treat BPH. None should cause incontinence, either, since the external urinary sphincter is left intact. In all cases, there's a risk of retrograde ejaculation, but the more thorough the removal of BPH, especially from the bladder neck, the greater that risk becomes. Blood loss and the need for transfusions seem less with the laser and TUVP procedures, and recovery appears to be a bit quicker.[28]

If you need surgical relief of BPH, my advice is to seek a highly experienced, trustworthy surgeon and have the procedure with which he or she is most comfortable.

SURGICAL PROCEDURES DESIGNED TO IMPROVE SYMPTOMS WITHOUT REMOVING ALL THE BPH[29]

Transurethral Incision of the Prostate (TUIP)

For men with prostates smaller than 30 grams, TUIP may be a good, less invasive alternative. Under general or spinal anesthetic, the surgeon passes a special scope through the urethra and uses electrical current or laser energy to make small incisions in the prostate near the bladder neck that allow urine to flow more freely.

Typically, TUIP requires a shorter hospital stay than TURP, and it can sometimes be done on an outpatient basis. A catheter remains in place for one to three days until the area heals. About 80 percent of men report an improvement in urinary symptoms. On the downside, TUIP offers less improvement in urinary flow rate and other BPH symptoms than does TURP, and it carries a greater risk of symptom recurrence with the need for additional procedures.[30]

SIDE EFFECTS AND COMPLICATIONS. Blood loss is low, and only 1 percent of patients require transfusion. Retrograde ejaculation is low as well, affecting only 10 percent. About 1 percent of patients report a loss of erections, and about 1 percent of men develop urinary incontinence.

Transurethral Microwave Thermotherapy (TUMT)

The prostate is heated by microwave energy, which is delivered via an antenna inserted through a catheter in the penis. Cooling fluid protects the urethra during this simple procedure, which can be done on an out-patient basis and takes thirty minutes to an hour. Excess prostate tissue is effectively cooked. Full effects are seen after the dead tissue sloughs off, generally in about three to six months.[31]

At that point, more than 50 percent of men experience symptomatic improvement that lasts for up to three years. Longer-term effects are questionable. The procedure works best for men with prostates smaller than 30 grams.

Because tissue is simply heated and not destroyed, TUMT does not cause retrograde ejaculation. Bleeding is kept to a minimum, as are surgical complications and side effects. The trade-off is a greater risk that symptoms will recur and further surgery will be required.

SIDE EFFECTS AND COMPLICATIONS.   Complications include a high incidence of acute urinary retention (70 to 80 percent) for up to two weeks after the procedure, requiring the use of a catheter. As the dead tissue is sloughed away, it can get lodged in the urethra, creating the equivalent of a plugged drain. Some patients have blood in the urine or urinary tract infections, and some men have sexual dysfunction after TUMT. In rare cases, if this approach is improperly performed, severe damage to the penis or urethra can result.

Transurethral Needle Ablation (TUNA)

The prostate is heated by microwave needles that are placed into the BPH nodules through a cystoscope. The operation can be done under local anesthetic or sedation in the doctor's office or in the hospital. The precise placement of the needles requires a transrectal ultrasound for treatment planning. The heated tissue sloughs off slowly over days or weeks. Maximum symptom improvement is generally seen after one to two months. Because the technique is fairly new, we don't have good evidence that it offers a durable, long-term effect.[32]

Side Effects and Complications. Because urinary retention is common right after the operation, patients go home with a Foley catheter that remains in place for three to seven days, depending on the size of the gland. Other immediate complications may include painful urination, which is often worse for men with chronic prostatitis. Some men have mild urinary bleeding for twenty-four to thirty-six hours, and some develop acute urinary retention or a urinary tract infection.

One-third of men develop retrograde ejaculation. A small percentage has erectile dysfunction, and less than 1 percent of men develop some degree of urinary incontinence.

High-Intensity Focused Ultrasound (HIFU)

HIFU quickly cooks prostate tissue. An ultrasound transducer placed in the rectum heats the prostate overgrowth to 80 to 90°C for about a second. The procedure must be done under heavy sedation or general anesthetic.[33]

Fifty percent of men experience some symptomatic improvement, but results are modest and not very durable. Ten percent of patients per year require re-treatment. HIFU equipment is expensive, and the procedure requires considerable training. Good comparative studies to other treatments are not yet available.

Other Procedures Designed to Offer Mechanical Relief

Prostatic Stents

For elderly patients or men with serious medical conditions, who are not good candidates for other surgical interventions, inserting a stent can relieve urinary obstruction and improve voiding. Basically, this is a mechanical metal mesh device, which is inserted into the portion of the urethra that runs through the prostate and keeps the channel clear.

On the downside, stents have to be replaced periodically and can become encrusted with stones, so this fix is only temporary.

THE FUTURE

Now that we know that drugs like finasteride and dutasteride lower the risk of urinary blockage and the need for surgery in men with symptomatic BPH, new studies are needed to see which men with BPH are most likely to benefit from taking these drugs. We are working on new nomograms to predict the long-term risks for patients with BPH so we can identify those who most need the drugs. New blood tests such as bPSA (PSA produced by BPH)[34] may help find patients at high risk as well as help distinguish between BPH and cancer. Better imaging techniques will also help us visualize the prostate and determine whether a cancer is present or not.

If patients stop taking these drugs, the prostate regrows and symptoms reappear. Could there be a permanent way to block the production of the DHT hormone that induces growth of prostate? Will minimally invasive procedures be refined so that all men with budding BPH could have their transition zone ablated at an early age without causing retrograde ejaculation or other unpleasant side effects?

IN SUMMARY

Benign enlargement of the prostate is remarkably common as men age. Effective treatment with drugs or, if need be, surgery can alleviate urinary symptoms caused by BPH and prevent permanent bladder or kidney damage. Often, early medical treatment can avert the need for surgical intervention later.

Part Three

PROSTATE CANCER

6

■

Prostate Cancer Facts

READ THIS CHAPTER TO LEARN:

- How common is prostate cancer, and who is most likely to
  get this disease?
- What is cancer?
- How does prostate cancer develop, progress, and spread?

HOW COMMON IS PROSTATE CANCER?

Prostate cancer strikes with remarkable frequency, and the incidence continues to rise. In 2004, 230,110 new cases were diagnosed in the United States, and 29,900 men died of the disease, making it the second most common cancer in American men (after skin cancer) and the second leading cause of male cancer deaths (after lung cancer). This pattern holds true throughout the Western world, except in Scandinavia, where prostate malignancies (another word for cancer) have surpassed lung cancer, both in sheer number of cases and in fatalities.

Prostate tumors account for one-third of all internal cancers diagnosed in men, and the risk of the disease is greater than that of breast cancer in women. One man in six will be diagnosed with prostate cancer in his lifetime, while a woman's risk of developing a malignancy in the breast is one in eight. Though fatality rates for these diseases are virtually the same, government research funding for breast cancer has historically been far higher than for prostate cancer.[1]

Through the Herculean efforts of Michael Milken and his dedicated colleagues at the Prostate Cancer Foundation, private research funding has made great strides toward equalizing the situation. This remarkable organization, with Milken at the helm, has also worked tirelessly and effectively to promote public awareness of this disease.

WHO GETS PROSTATE CANCER AND WHY?

Nobody knows precisely why prostate cancer develops. Several factors may work individually or in concert to cause normal cells in the gland to undergo malignant changes. One man's prostate cancer may have a strong genetic component, while another case might stem primarily from high levels of dietary fat or exposure to toxins or both. Still, though we can't point the finger at any single universal cause, age, diet, race and ethnicity, and certain environmental factors all appear to play a significant role.

THE AGING CONNECTION

Prostate cancer and aging go hand in hand. Though I see an increasing number of patients with malignant prostate tumors in their 30s and 40s, the disease is relatively rare before age 50. After that, the numbers begin to spike dramatically, and in men over 70, the incidence increases faster than that of any other cancer. Since the average age of men in industrialized countries is rising steadily, prostate cancer is a burgeoning problem throughout the developed world.

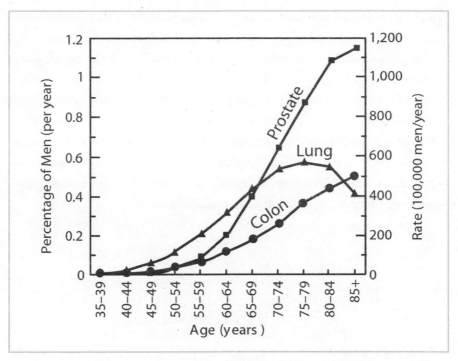

The incidence of prostate cancer increases with age faster than that of any other cancer.*

Despite steady inroads in early detection and treatment that have led to a 20 percent decrease in mortality in the United States since 1992, the swelling volume of prostate cancer patients is expected to result in an ever-increasing number of fatalities. Experts estimate that by 2025, unless we find a way to prevent this disease, 380,000 new cases will be detected annually in this country alone, and patient deaths will more than double to 60,000, unless we find better ways to treat it.[2]

THE ROLE OF DIET

Though all the relevant factors have yet to be proven, a lack of adequate exercise coupled with excessive fat and caloric intake and the resultant

*Source: Modified from Carter, H. B., and D. S. Coffey. "The Prostate—an Increasing Medical Problem." *Prostate* 16, no. 1 (1990): 39–48. © 1990. Reprinted with permission from Wiley-Liss, Inc., a subsidiary of John Wiley & Sons, Inc.

epidemic of overweight and obesity are all prime suspects in the mounting frequency of the disease.

The evidence for a nutritional link is compelling. Prostate cancer is ten times more common in the United States than it is in Japan. When Japanese men move to the States and trade their traditional low-fat, soy-rich diet for fatty American favorites such as pizza, burgers, and fries, their risk of developing the disease soon escalates. By the next generation, the incidence shoots up markedly, and the adult grandchildren of Japanese-Americans develop prostate cancer only slightly less often than the average American man of European descent.

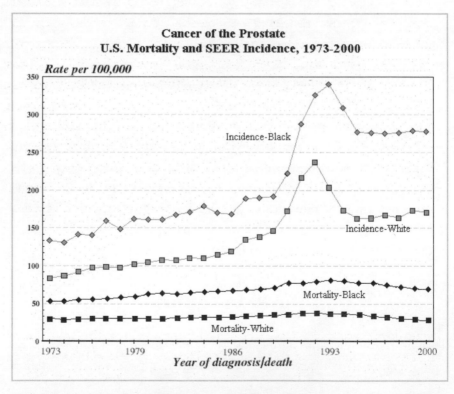

The incidence of prostate cancer, by year, corrected for age. Note that the incidence (number of cases per 100,000 men per year) increased markedly in the late 1980s with the introduction of PSA testing, and then declined as many existing cases were discovered, but has been rising again since 1995. African-Americans are more than twice as likely to die of prostate cancer at any given age.

RACE AND DEMOGRAPHICS

Race and ethnicity appear to play a role as well. A 50-year-old European-American has a 16 percent chance of developing prostate cancer in his remaining lifetime and a 3.6 percent chance of dying of the disease. African-Americans have the highest prostate cancer incidence in the world. Their risk of developing and dying from the disease is more than twice as high as it is in European-Americans.[3] Though the causes remain unproven, genetic factors, coupled with less aggressive screening and treatment, are likely to blame. It is noteworthy that prostate cancer is less prevalent in black Africans than in African-Americans, pointing to a possible dietary or other lifestyle link rather than race alone. Asians run the lowest risk of developing the disease, and among Asian countries, Koreans have the lowest occurrence of all. The risk is lower for Hispanics than non-Hispanic whites. These differences can be dramatic. The average African-American has a seven times greater risk of having a positive prostate biopsy than does a recent Korean immigrant to the United States.

Geographic differences are evident as well. Men in Sweden have nearly double the prostate cancer incidence of German men, who, in turn, have a far higher risk than Israelis of developing the disease. A host of variables may be responsible, including diet, soil content, and sun exposure. (See Chapter 7, Risk Factors and Prevention, for a further discussion of the factors that affect prostate cancer risk.)

What Do Fred and Fido Have in Common?

The only species known to develop prostate cancer are men and domestic dogs. Anecdotal evidence suggests that the culprit is diet. Domestic dogs often dine on human table scraps. They are also the only mammals aside from men who have the genes for PSA and its close relative, hK2, both members of a family of enzymes called kallikreins and both strongly suspected of playing a role in the development of prostate cancer.

WHAT IS CANCER?

The disease we call cancer has two distinctive features: uncontrolled growth and the capacity to escape the area in which it arose and invade other parts of the body.

For organs to maintain health, old cells must step aside to create the space new ones require to grow and thrive. Normal cells have a limited life span and then undergo a process of programmed cell death called **apoptosis.** This phenomenon is dramatically evident in nature when autumn leaves explode with vivid color and then fade and wither. What we see as a glorious show of foliage is in fact an example of the cyclical death of old leaves required to make eventual room for new ones. In the life of cells, this process happens without such fanfare, but it is crucial nonetheless. Cancer cells, profoundly resistant to apoptosis, are virtually immortal.

Having lost the critical balance of cell birth and death, cancer grows exponentially. One cell becomes two; two yield four; four spawn eight, etc. If one cell doubles ten times, 1,024 cells result. Double that number ten more times, and the total is over a million. We refer to the rate of this geometric proliferation as a cancer's **doubling time.** The faster a malignant tumor doubles in size, the more dangerous and difficult it is to control. Some highly virulent brain tumors double in size in as little as twelve days. Early prostate cancers have an average doubling time of two to four years, though some grow far more slowly, and others, which we refer to as **high grade** or **poorly differentiated**, typically run a far swifter and more perilous course (see Chapter 9, Biopsy). Keep in mind that doubling times may not remain constant. As a tumor progresses, its growth rate often accelerates.

The faster a cancer grows, the sooner it's likely to spread. By the time some very rapidly doubling cancers trigger positive test results or cause symptoms, many have already spread to distant organs (metastasized) and are beyond our ability to cure with surgery or radiation. Systemic treatment with hormones, chemotherapy, immune therapy, or experimental approaches would be our only hope of controlling or delaying the progress of the disease at that point.

> NOTE: Like normal cells, cancer cells depend on blood to deliver the oxygen and nourishment they need. Without an adequate blood supply, a tumor cannot grow beyond the size of a BB (about ⅛ inch). To survive at all, cancer cells must be in extremely close proximity to blood vessels, no farther away than the width of a grain of sand. Cancers recruit the blood vessels they need through a complex process called angiogenesis.[4] Researchers have been trying to develop drugs and other therapies that might arrest this process and cut off a cancer's essential blood supply.

In addition to unregulated growth, cancers eventually develop the ability to penetrate normal barriers in the body and spread. Normal cells are like peaceable neighbors who respect property lines and keep to their side of the fence. **Benign** tumors can grow, but no matter how large they become, they are not capable of escaping the organ in which they arise. A benign kidney tumor remains in the kidney. A **malignant** kidney tumor, if left untreated long enough, eventually escapes.

Cancer cells act like greedy, land-grabbing marauders. Their pattern of invasion can be straightforward or unpredictable. As a malignant tumor grows, it may break through biological fences such as the capsule of the prostate and spread into the adjacent seminal vesicles or erectile nerves. Alternatively, some of the cancer cells may enter the blood or lymphatic systems, which circulate throughout the body. If they survive in the circulation, these malignant cells eventually attach themselves to lymph nodes, bones, or other distant organs, where they thrive as metastases. No matter where they are in the body, these cells retain their identity as prostate cancer cells. They don't become bone cancer, even though they attach themselves to bone.

NOTE: The way a cancer spreads has a crucial bearing on whether any given therapy will succeed or fail. Invasion of cancer through the capsule of the prostate means that the cancer is no longer confined to the gland, but this *does not* necessarily mean that the cancer has spread beyond the local region or become incurable. As long as the area removed surgically or treated with radiation is large enough to include the area of **extracapsular extension (ECE)**, the cancer can still be cured. On the other hand, a cancer that shows no extracapsular extension and appears to be confined within the gland may in fact have sent microscopic clusters of cancer cells into the bloodstream, which then become established in distant sites such as the bones of the hips or spine. In this case, radiation or removal of the prostate alone will not arrest the disease, but removal of the primary tumor in the prostate may stop the seeding of more metastatic cells.

Observing cancer cells under a microscope yields valuable clues about how a tumor is likely to behave. Compared to their normal counterparts, malignant cells look odd, irregular, or even bizarre. Cancers arise from mutations that alter the cell's genetic blueprint, also known as **DNA**. Imagine a builder working from an abstract sketch by Picasso, and you get the sense of what strange structures might result. Cancer cells have striking abnormalities, including enlarged, irregular nuclei and a generally disorganized appearance. As the disease progresses, the cells become ever wilder. The architecture of the tissue is increasingly disrupted, like a building that has been sacked and abandoned for many years. The more abnormal (poorly differentiated) the cancer looks, the more abnormally and aggressively it's likely to behave. So-called "high grade" cancers, which bear little or no resemblance to normal cells, tend to grow rapidly and metastasize.

ARE ALL PROSTATE CANCERS SERIOUS?

Conventional wisdom holds that any man who lives long enough will develop prostate cancer eventually. This statement is based on the ubiquitous presence of minuscule clusters of malignant cancer cells that are not picked up by prostate cancer screening with the PSA test or digital rectal exam, often go undetected, and would rarely pose any serious threat if left alone. Autopsy studies have demonstrated that these tiny clusters would be found in one third of men over 50 if their prostates were removed and examined under the microscope.[5] The presence of these microscopic cancers rises dramatically among men in their 80s and 90s, when as many as 80 percent have what we call autopsy or **incidental** cancers, names designed to indicate that these tiny malignant tumors are found only by chance when prostate tissue is examined after it is removed on autopsy or during surgery to treat urinary obstruction. Incidental also means that because these cancers are so minuscule, they have no effect on one's health.[6] Another term we use to describe these tiny tumors that pose no current or immediate risk is **indolent** (sometimes referred to as clinically unimportant).[7]

The nearly universal presence of malignant cells in the prostates of older men leads some people to view the disease as inevitable and to adopt an attitude of potentially dangerous apathy: *Everyone gets this,* they think, *so I may as well simply ignore it and hope for the best.* The oft-repeated statement that more men die *with* prostate cancer than *of* it can reinforce the risky notion that a laissez-faire approach to the disease is as good as any.

In fact, there are enormous differences between these common incidental cancers and the clinical cancers diagnosed when a pathologist examines tissue removed from the prostate during a biopsy. While prostate biopsies occasionally turn up tiny, insignificant (incidental) clusters of cancer cells, the typical cancer found on biopsy is ten to one hundred times larger.[8]

It takes a long time for a tiny acorn to yield a giant oak tree, and the same holds true for prostate cancers. Because this disease is typically so slow-growing, most incidental cancers never grow large enough to pose a threat to health or life.

Still, finding tiny cancer clusters in the prostate does raise the risk that a man will eventually develop a serious cancer in the gland. Eight to 9 percent of incidental cancers do eventually grow, develop the capacity to spread beyond the prostate, and turn lethal. While active treatment for these tiny cancers is typically unnecessary at the time they are discovered, ignoring them is not a good idea. Regular PSA tests, digital rectal exams, and other testing where indicated should provide ample time to success-fully treat a growing tumor. (See Chapter 13, Watchful Waiting.)

LIFETIME RISK OF DEVELOPING OR DYING OF PROSTATE CANCER FOR A 50-YEAR-OLD MAN IN THE UNITED STATES

LIFETIME RISK OF	RISK (%)	RISK RATIO	PROPORTIONAL RISK
Developing incidental cancer	42	11.7	100
Developing clinical cancer	16.7	4.4	38
Dying of prostate cancer	3.6	1	8.6

For every 100 men who develop cancer cells in their prostate during their lifetime, only 38 of them will ever be diagnosed with prostate cancer by biopsy, and only 8.6 are at risk of dying of prostate cancer.*

The picture is considerably worse for men whose biopsy results lead to a diagnosis of clinical cancers. Despite the best modern medical inter-vention, 20 percent will eventually die of the disease. You don't want to be on the losing end of that statistic. Prostate cancer can be a fearsome

---

*Source: Modified from Scardino, P. T., R. Weaver, and M. A. Hudson, "Early Detection of Prostate Cancer," *Human Pathology* 23, no. 3 (1992): 214, table 3, © 1992, reprinted with permission from Elsevier; Scardino, P. T., "Early Detection of Prostate Cancer," *Urol Clin North Am* 16 (1989): 646, table 11, © 1989, reprinted with permission from Elsevier; Greenlee, R. T., T. Murray, S. Bolden, and P. A. Wingo, "Cancer Statistics, 2000," *CA Cancer J Clin* 50, no. 1 (2000): 13, tables 1 and 2, reprinted with permission from Lippincott Williams & Wilkins; and Seidman, H., M. H. Mushinski, S. K. Gelb, and E. Silverberg, "Probabilities of Eventually Developing or Dying of Cancer—United States, 1985," *CA Cancer J Clin* 35, no. 1 (1985): 51–52, tables 4 and 5, reprinted with permission from Lippincott Williams & Wilkins.

adversary whose lethal potential should not be underestimated. Your best defense is to have regular screening with PSA and DRE so we can catch the disease early in its course and treat it while it can still be cured.

CANCER IN OTHER MALE ORGANS

One question that continues to confound scientists is why the prostate is so prone to developing cancers, while other similar organs are virtually immune to tumor development. Cancers almost never arise in the seminal vesicles or Cowper's glands, though, like the prostate, both secrete seminal fluid and both come in regular contact with testosterone. Cancers do develop in reproductive cells in the testicles, but not because of male hormones. Testicular cancers are markedly different from prostate cancers. They do not respond to hormone withdrawal as prostate cancers do, but are exquisitely sensitive to chemotherapy, which has not been a traditional part of the prostate cancer treatment arsenal (though this is changing). Penile cancers, which occur rarely in this country, have no hormonal basis, either. Infections with the human papilloma virus and poor hygiene in uncircumcised men are seen as probable causes.

Something about the prostate gland makes it uniquely vulnerable to the effects of male hormones, and once we determine what that is, we may finally be able to unravel the mystery of why this disease develops with such staggering frequency and learn how to stop it before it starts.

WHERE DOES CANCER DEVELOP IN THE PROSTATE, AND HOW DOES IT SPREAD?

Seventy-five percent of all prostate cancers and 90 percent of serious ones develop in the **peripheral zone**, which lies just beneath the outer rim or capsule of the gland like an orange rind.[9] As they grow, these

tumors spread out toward the capsule as well as inward toward the urethra. Because they are located within millimeters of the rectal wall, peripheral zone tumors—if they are large enough—can be felt during a
digital rectal exam.

Eighty-five percent of prostate cancers are multifocal, meaning they
arise in several parts of the gland at once. In about 85 percent of cases,
adenocarcinomas (the type of cancer most common in the prostate)
are found on both sides (**lobes**) of the prostate. This explains why many
men have positive biopsies on both sides of the gland. It also explains
why radiation therapy must adequately treat the entire prostate to be successful, and why surgeons must remove the entire gland and the seminal
vesicles cleanly, leaving no cancer cells behind.

About 25 percent of prostate cancers start in the **transition zone**,
which encircles the urethra and is the part of the gland that develops
BPH. These tumors tend to be less aggressive and less likely to metastasize than peripheral zone cancers, but they are also trickier to diagnose.[10]
Transition zone cancers often arise in the part of the prostate that is far-

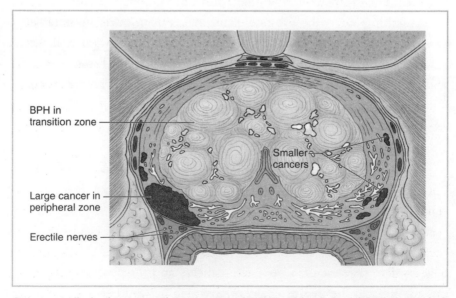

BPH in
transition zone

Smaller
cancers

Large cancer in
peripheral zone

Erectile nerves

Cancer typically develops at several sites at once within the peripheral zone of the prostate, which
lies just inside the capsule. Large, peripheral zone cancers can usually be felt during a DRE.

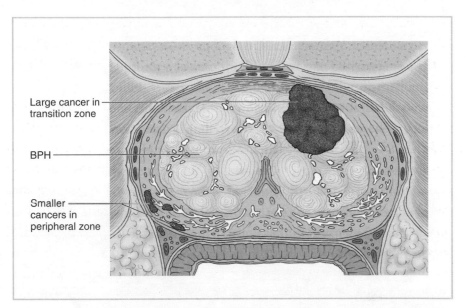

About one in four prostate cancers arise in the transition (BPH) zone. Because they are at the front of the prostate, they usually cannot be felt during a DRE or seen on ultrasound or MRI. Transition zone cancers are often accompanied by smaller but more aggressive cancers in the peripheral zone.

thest away from the rectum, toward the front of the body (anterior), so they are often missed on digital rectal exam and biopsy. On ultrasound or MRI, such cancers can be hidden by or confused with BPH. Still, as standard practice shifts toward sampling an increased number of biopsy cores, more and more transition zone cancers are being discovered (see Chapter 9, Biopsy). I am particularly suspicious that a man has an anterior transition zone cancer if his PSA is high for the size of his prostate, and one or two previous biopsies have found no tumor or a cancer that is too small to account for the PSA elevation.

In addition to being difficult to detect, transition zone cancers are challenging to treat, no matter what method is chosen. A surgeon must take extra care to excise the cancer completely and avoid cutting into the cancer, resulting in a **positive surgical margin**, which means that cancer cells are present at the edge of what is removed. To avoid damaging the urethra, seed implants tend to focus on the outer peripheral portion of the prostate, and the radiation dose they deliver may be inadequate to destroy a transition zone cancer. With anterior cancers becoming

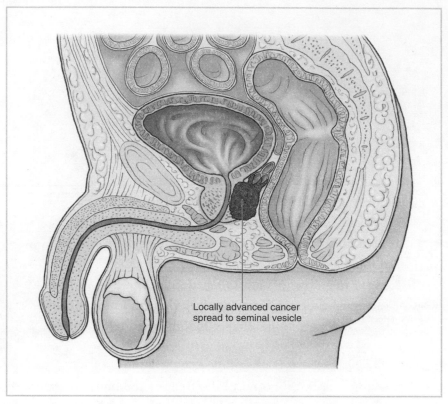

Locally advanced cancer
spread to seminal vesicle

A large, locally advanced prostate cancer may spread through the capsule and into the seminal
vesicles.

increasingly common, treatment must focus on the whole gland, not just
the rear or peripheral zones.

If prostate cancer grows unchecked, it may spread to the seminal vesicles, which are soft, fluid-filled sacs above the prostate. **Seminal vesicle
invasion (SVI)** is an ominous sign, signaling a locally advanced cancer
(see Chapter 10, Understanding Your Cancer). While malignant cells
can migrate to the seminal vesicles from anywhere in the prostate, most
cancers invade these sacs by direct extension from the base (top) of the
prostate. Because SVI can be difficult to detect, the seminal vesicles
should be included in the radiation field or surgically removed whenever
a prostate cancer is treated.

Eventually, untreated prostate cancers invade lymphatic and blood
channels, sending cells off to colonize in lymph nodes, bones, or other sites.

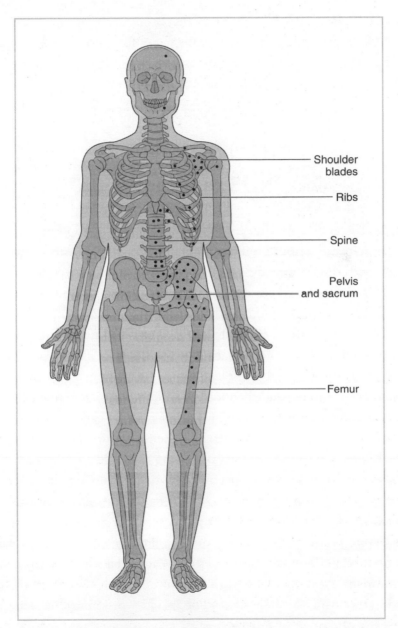

Shoulder
blades

Ribs

Spine

Pelvis
and sacrum

Femur

Bones, especially the spine, hips, and ribs, are the most common sites of spread
when prostate cancer metastasizes.

By growing directly into blood vessels, a tumor may travel through the circulation to bones in the hips or spine without ever involving the lymph nodes, so a negative pelvic lymph node biopsy is no guarantee that the cancer has not spread. Bones are a prime target for prostate cancer metastases. Like enriched soil, bone marrow appears to provide a particularly hospitable environment in which these malignant cells can settle and thrive.

THE SYMPTOMS OF PROSTATE CANCER

Prostate cancer is typically slow-growing and can take years, or even decades, to cause serious problems. More like the fabled tortoise than the hare, it tends to run a steady, persistent course. The disease is highly curable while still localized but difficult to interrupt once spreading cells become firmly established beyond the gland.

Early prostate cancer is silent, meaning it offers no warning in the form of symptoms. As the tumor grows, however, it can trigger a variety of problems. Once the disease is advanced enough to cause symptoms, it has spread beyond the local area and is no longer curable.

Urinary symptoms of locally advanced prostate cancer may include diminished size or force of the stream, a sense of incomplete emptying of the bladder, or the need to get up during the night to urinate. If cancer is the culprit, these symptoms tend to develop rapidly, over six months or less, compared to the slowly worsening urinary problems that are more characteristic of BPH. As prostate cancer progresses, some patients develop acute urinary retention, requiring emergency catheterization or surgery. The disease sometimes causes bleeding in the urine (**hematuria**), typically at the beginning or end of the stream. If there is blood in the urine throughout voiding, bladder or kidney problems are more likely the cause.

Blood in the sperm (**hematospermia**) is rarely a sign of prostate cancer, though if it occurs, you should consult with a doctor to rule out a different malignancy or other serious condition. Usually, the problem is a ruptured varicose vein within the prostate or an infection or trauma to the area.

As a tumor grows within the prostate, it may extend upward and block the ureters, the small tubes that carry urine from the kidneys to the bladder. Ureteral obstruction can cause flank or abdominal pain, or fever and chills if the blockage leads to infection or signs of reduced kidney function such as an increased blood creatinine level. The problem puts a patient at risk for kidney damage or even kidney failure. Treatment may involve the insertion of a stent or tube to open up the channel and restore the flow.

If prostate cancer spreads to the lymph nodes, obstruction of the lymphatic drainage system may result. This can lead to intractable swelling of the scrotum, penis, feet, and legs. In the pelvis, a spreading cancer can surround nerves and cause sciaticlike pain.

Bone pain is the most common symptom of advanced prostate cancer. In addition to causing discomfort, metastases in the hips and vertebrae can lead to spontaneous fractures (see page 107). Some patients experience sudden weakness or radiating pain to the legs that can signal spinal cord compression. *Immediate* medical intervention is essential to avoid permanent paralysis.

> NOTE: Prostate cancer spreads to central skeletal bones in the hips and spine, not to peripheral bones like those of the hands and feet.

Advanced prostate cancer can also metastasize to other sites, including lymph nodes in the abdomen or chest, the liver, and the lungs. Anemia caused by invasion of cancer into the bone marrow may also accompany advanced disease, as can appetite changes, fatigue, and increased susceptibility to infections. When men die of prostate cancer, it's usually due to a constellation of system failures.

HOW FAST DOES PROSTATE CANCER GROW AND SPREAD?

Early prostate cancers grow very slowly, typically taking two to four years to double in size. Over time, as the tumor grows and the cells become wilder and more aggressive, the growth rate accelerates. Think of a small, peaceful assembly of protesters that attracts a steadily spreading groundswell of support and eventually spawns a huge, uncontrollable mob.

If we don't treat prostate cancer while it is still curable, the disease will take an average of ten to twelve years to metastasize and fifteen to seventeen years to cause death.[11] If the tumor is large and locally advanced, invading the seminal vesicles or surrounding organs, life expectancy drops to the eight- to twelve-year range. If the lymph nodes are grossly involved, meaning they are recognizably enlarged on a CT scan or MRI, or seen as enlarged by the surgeon in the operating room, the cancer generally takes six to eight years to cause death. Once there are bone metastases, the average patient lives about five to six years.

NOTE: All these figures are averages. Actual outcomes vary widely for individuals, depending on the features of their particular cancer—including stage, grade, PSA level, etc.—so you should not view statistical averages as literally predictive of what may in fact happen to you. (See Chapter 10, Understanding Your Cancer.)

THE FUTURE

With widespread screening and earlier diagnosis, the prostate cancer timeline is getting longer. If only a few metastatic spots are found in the lymph nodes at the time of radical prostatectomy, average life expectancy is more than fifteen years. The goal of a treatment program is to cure the disease when possible, but if it is not curable, to control it for as long as possible, with luck for the remainder of a man's natural life.

With this objective in mind, our philosophy at Memorial Sloan-Kettering is to treat a cancer in the prostate even if the disease has spread to other areas. If lymph nodes are found to contain cancer during surgery, we still recommend removing the gland. Doing so will stop further metastatic spread from the primary tumor and avoid debilitating symptoms that can come from a cancer growing deep in the pelvis.

Modern radical prostatectomy and radiation therapy have far fewer side effects than they did fifteen to twenty years ago. Further refinements in surgical technique (see Chapter 14, Surgery) and radiation delivery (see Chapter 15, Radiation Therapy) are constantly being introduced.

Because prostate cancer has a tendency to spread to bones, one important research focus is on bone-protective agents. Another is chemotherapy. While chemotherapeutic drugs have commonly been used to treat many cancers, they have not traditionally been part of the treatment protocol for prostate cancer. That is changing as emerging studies show that certain drugs, such as docetaxol, are in fact effective against this disease. Researchers are also looking at novel treatments such as vaccines, gene therapies, monoclonal antibodies, and variations in the way we administer hormone therapy that may slow or even arrest the progression of advanced prostate cancer, while maintaining the best possible quality of life.

IN SUMMARY

Prostate cancer is the most common internal cancer in men and the second leading cause of male cancer deaths. One man in six will eventually develop the disease, though not all cases need to be treated. Fortunately, this malignancy is typically very slow-growing and highly curable while it is still locally contained. Awareness and vigilance can ensure that we will catch the disease before it takes a lethal turn.

7

■

Risk Factors and Prevention

READ THIS CHAPTER TO LEARN:

• What are the risk factors for prostate cancer?
• Can anything be done to prevent this remarkably common disease?

f you have prostate cancer, you may be asking: *Why me?* If you are worried about developing the disease someday or living with the anxiety of an elevated PSA of uncertain origin, you may be wondering: *What, if anything, can I do to prevent it?*

Being concerned about prostate cancer is completely understandable. If you are an American man, your lifetime risk of being diagnosed with the disease is 1 in 6, and the chance that you'll subsequently die of it is 1 in 28. In stark contrast, only 1 person in 4,000 is killed in an automobile accident, 1 in 30,000 succumbs to drowning, 1 in 100,000 dies in an airplane disaster, and lightning claims a mere 1 in 2,000,000 (though fear of flying and anxiety about being struck during a lightning storm far exceed those rare-as-hen's-teeth odds).[1]

Of course, the risks are not equal for everyone. A stunt pilot is far more likely to die in a plane crash than someone who flies frequently on large commercial airliners. The regular business flyer in turn is obviously at greater risk than a traveler who always drives. Naturally, road warriors on wheels trade the slim possibility of an airline crash for an increased probability of a fender bender.

Certain risk factors, such as an inherited predisposition to develop an illness, might be difficult, if not impossible, to circumvent. Someday, gene therapy may allow us to simply reprogram or disarm our genetic time bombs, but that remains a distant dream. Other risks can be reduced, and perhaps eliminated, by simple lifestyle changes. Standing under a tree in a thunderstorm is asking for trouble. If you want to avoid a lightning strike, you can simply seek appropriate shelter until the danger passes. If the storm you're trying to escape is death from prostate cancer, crucial first steps include understanding your risk of developing the disease and learning the facts about prevention, early detection, and treatment alternatives.

WHAT PUTS A MAN AT RISK FOR PROSTATE CANCER?

GENDER AND HORMONES

Every normal man is at risk for developing prostate cancer. The disease does not develop in the absence of male hormones, so men castrated before puberty and those born with severe androgen deficiencies are not susceptible. Without the most common male hormone, testosterone, or 5 alpha-reductase, the enzyme required to convert testosterone into its more potent form, DHT, the prostate will never grow to normal size, enlarge with aging, or become malignant.

Androgens are manufactured by the testicles. They circulate in the bloodstream and then attach to special receptors in organs that rely on

NOTE: This is not to suggest that a testosterone drought is desirable. Male hormones play a crucial role in lean muscle development, bone growth and health, virility, libido, and mood.

these hormones, including the penis, prostate, skeletal muscles, and hair follicles. The degree of hormone exposure depends on how much testosterone is floating in the circulation and on how efficient a man's cells are at taking it up.

RACE AND NATIONALITY

African-American men have the highest prostate cancer incidence in the world. They are seven times more likely to be diagnosed with the disease than Asian men, who run the lowest risk. African-Americans have positive prostate biopsies 70 percent more often than do white Americans. On average, their cancers are detected at younger ages. They are more likely to present with advanced disease, and their mortality rate is more than twice as high as whites'.[2] Several factors may account for these racial differences. Young African-American men tend to have higher levels of prostate cancer–promoting testosterone than whites, whose levels are higher, in turn, than Asians. In addition, many blacks have a quirk in their androgen receptor genes, called a short CAG repeat, which renders them more vulnerable to testosterone's effects, including the promotion of prostate cancer. Other prime suspects in the more ominous picture for African-American males include high levels of dietary fat, low vitamin D synthesis (see page 126), and less access to medical care.

North American and northwest European countries have the highest rates of prostate cancer, while far fewer men develop the disease in South and Central America, Africa, and Asia. Though geographic variations may be partially due to genetics, environmental factors such as diet, sunshine, and soil selenium content (see page 124) may be responsible for some of the differences as well.

AGE

The incidence and death rate from prostate cancer rise faster with age than any other malignancy.[3] Though I have treated a 32-year-old with prostate cancer, and men in their 40s are now a regular part of my practice, the overall percentage of new cases rises sharply after age 50 and skyrockets in men over 70. The median age at diagnosis is 69, as opposed to age 63 for breast cancer. The median age for prostate cancer death is 77. With breast cancer, fatalities rise dramatically in the 50s, 60s, and early 70s, and then steadily decline.

Age and prostate cancer appear to be bound together in some fundamental biological way that we don't yet understand. Either through a cancer-promoting factor or a reduction in the body's normal ability to inhibit cancer development, nearly all men eventually develop some microscopic cancers in their prostates if they live long enough. Many of these are never detected, and most will never grow large enough to present a real risk or cause problems in a man's lifetime, but some pose a highly significant danger, and we must make every effort to detect and treat them before they get out of hand.

DIET

Prostate cancer is far less common in countries like Japan, where the diet is low in fat and rich in soy. When Japanese men immigrate to America and adopt a typical meat-and-potatoes Western diet, their risk of prostate malignancy soon increases. Their sons have an even higher incidence, and their grandsons develop the disease at a rate much closer to that seen in Americans of European descent.[4]

> NOTE: "Median" means that half the men are over and half are under this age.

Such epidemiological evidence suggests that greater fat consumption is strongly associated with a higher risk of prostate cancer. Still, we can't leap from this observation to the conclusion that eating fat is ill-advised or that reducing fat intake will solve the prostate-cancer problem. In heart disease, the issue is not simply the overall amount of fat in the diet, but the particular type of fats consumed. Saturated and trans fats—found in foods like margarine—have been implicated in elevating the risk of atherosclerosis and heart attacks, while certain unsaturated fats, such as olive oil and omega-3 fatty acids, are thought to be protective. Fat intake itself may increase the risk of prostate cancer, or the crucial link may be the total number of calories consumed or the higher ratio of weight to height—also known as body mass index (BMI)—that often results from a diet laden with high-calorie fatty foods, especially in the absence of an exercise program to burn them off.

Being overweight strongly affects how well men fare once they get the disease. A recent large, long-term study found that the mortality rate for prostate cancer increased in direct proportion to body mass. The heaviest subjects were nearly 30 percent more likely to die of their cancers than were patients whose weight/height ratio fell within normal limits.[5] Hormones may play a role in this as well. High body fat is related to increased testosterone levels, and testosterone is a powerful driving force for prostate-cancer growth.[6]

Genetic factors render certain men more susceptible than others to the effects of dietary fat and obesity. The cholesterol in animal fats is converted to testosterone through the action of an enzyme, which some men produce in greater-than-average quantity.[7]

There is some evidence that a diet low in protective antioxidants such as Vitamin E and selenium may increase prostate cancer risk, while a regime rich in fruits and vegetables might help ward off the disease (see Prevention, starting on page 121).

FAMILY HISTORY

Having close family members with prostate cancer considerably increases your risk of developing the disease. If a first-degree relative (your father or brother) has had the disease, you are two and a half times as likely to be diagnosed. With two first-degree relatives, your risk soars to five to ten times higher than that of a man with no family history. Three first-degree relatives elevate your risk by a multiple of eleven. Closer relatives increase your odds of getting the disease more than distant ones do, but, nevertheless, a strong familial strand, even among uncles and cousins, may be significant.[8]

> NOTE: Prostate cancer is inherited just as often via the maternal side, so if your mother's father, uncles, or brothers were diagnosed with a malignancy in the gland, extra vigilance is in order. Many studies have sought a link between breast and prostate cancer inheritance, but as yet there is no evidence that the two go hand in hand.

About one of every eleven men with prostate cancer reports that a family member also has had the disease. These patients have what we consider to be familial prostate cancer. By studying identical twins that have been reared apart, researchers have determined that about 40 percent of familial cases of prostate cancer are caused by mutated genes.[9] Based on this, only one in twenty-eight men with prostate cancer—less than 4 percent—have an inherited form of the disease, which is somewhat less than the percentage of women with the inherited form of breast cancer.

To date, human genome studies have identified nine separate genes that appear to have some correlation with prostate cancer, though none has proven as important as the mutated BRCA1 and -2 genes, which are strongly predictive of breast cancer and can be identified through a sim-

NOTE: Families tend to be exposed to similar environmental, lifestyle, and dietary influences. Many cases of familial prostate cancer appear to result from exposure to these shared factors, rather than genes. For example, familial prostate cancers might be caused by all men in the family eating the same high-fat diet or living in a northern climate where they are rarely exposed to the sunshine required to produce vitamin D. The inherited form of the disease, resulting from mutated genes, affects far fewer men. As a consequence, even identical twins reared apart, with totally different environments and lifestyles, tend to get prostate cancer if they share the genetic predispositions.

ple blood test. None of the prostate cancer genes accounts for more than about 1 percent of cases, and to date we have no reliable means to screen for them.[10] Prostate cancer, whether inherited, familial, or sporadic, as we call all other cases, seems to develop through multiple pathways. Just as it might take a combination of bad economic news, skittish consumers, foreign turmoil, epidemic disease, and adverse climatic conditions to trigger a recession, prostate cancer requires a confluence of adverse events within a man's cells.

NOTE: Men with a strong family history tend to develop prostate cancer at younger and younger ages in succeeding generations. In patients diagnosed with the disease below the age of 55, half are thought to have the familial form. One of my patients, diagnosed at 62, has three sons in their 30s with prostate cancer. If your family tree hangs heavy with prostate cancer, you and your brothers and sons might do well to begin screening far earlier than standard guidelines typically suggest (see Chapter 8, Detecting Prostate Cancer with PSA and Other Tests).

OTHER RISK FACTORS

SEXUAL FUNCTION

Studies attempting to demonstrate a link between prostate cancer and various sexual issues have universally struck out. We've found no association between the incidence of the disease and the age at which a man reached puberty. The same is true of sexual behavior, including frequency of sexual encounters, frequency of masturbation or orgasm, number of partners, types of sexual activities, sexual orientation, or marital status.[11] The risk is no different for heterosexual and homosexual men. Celibate priests get the disease just as often as men who have frequent sex with multiple partners.

For a time, it appeared that having a vasectomy might somehow increase a man's risk of getting prostate cancer. After further, more carefully designed studies, researchers concluded that the link was strictly coincidental. Men who had vasectomies were simply being checked by urologists more often, and that extra scrutiny led to the detection of more cancers.

NOTE: Sexually transmitted diseases (STDs) such as gonorrhea may increase the risk of inflammation or prostatitis, but there is no evidence that they raise the odds of developing prostate cancer.

LIFESTYLE

Rodeo cowboys, motorcycle riders, long-distance cyclists, and long-haul truck drivers all put extra stress on their prostates, but while that can result in the perineal or pelvic pain typical of prostatitis, none of these activities has been found to contribute to the development of BPH or prostate cancer.[12]

NOTE: Researchers have found some evidence that inflammation at the molecular level may contribute to malignant changes in prostate cells, but whether these findings will translate into a causative link between inflammation and prostate cancer remains to be seen.[13]

A sedentary lifestyle contributes to increased body mass—a prime suspect both in promoting prostate cancer and in increasing the risk of dying from the disease. Regular exercise makes sense for many reasons, and reducing your risk of prostate cancer may well be one of them.

EXPOSURE TO TOXINS

A few early studies suggested that workers exposed to the heavy metal cadmium in mining or in nickel cadmium battery manufacturing plants ran an increased prostate-cancer risk. Cadmium is a known carcinogen that is weakly associated with the risk of developing lung cancer, but more recent, more extensive investigations have failed to confirm any causative link to prostate cancer.[14]

Dioxin is a toxic by-product of Agent Orange, which was widely used as an herbicide during the Vietnam War. Though the issue of whether or not dioxin causes prostate cancer has not been resolved, the government provides benefits for veterans who were exposed to Agent Orange and subsequently develop the disease.[15]

Studies have failed to confirm anecdotal observations that smoking and/or heavy alcohol consumption might increase prostate-cancer risk, though avoiding both is wise for many other health reasons.

Anabolic steroids were developed in the 1930s to treat testosterone deficiencies. Today, they are frequently abused by athletes attempting to boost their performance or beef up their appearance. Some of these drugs, including DHEA, are legally and readily available without a prescription, though they may cause heart disease, testicular shrinkage, breast enlargement, mania, depression, violent behavior, severe acne, and cancers of the kidney, liver, and prostate. In recognition of its dangers, androstenedione was declared a controlled substance by the FDA in 2005. While the precise level of risk posed by anabolic steroids has not been fully documented, androgens are such a powerful stimulus for prostate cancer, and this disease is such a significant risk for all men, that I strongly recommend against using these bodybuilding substances.[16]

THE FIRST LINE OF DEFENSE: PREVENTION

In the public health field, prevention describes a three-pronged assault on a targeted disease. As with a security system, the primary goal is to keep trouble at bay, i.e. maintain health. If that frontline defense fails to work, the aim is to minimize negative effects by catching the problem quickly through early detection and intervention and to resolve it before it can wreak major havoc. If that fails, we seek the most effective, least disruptive means to minimize deaths from the disease and reduce side effects, medically known as **morbidities**. If fireproofing fails, the sprinkler system douses the blaze before it can destroy the building. Once the fire is out, we repair any smoke, heat, or water damage with minimal disruption at the lowest possible cost.

WHAT IS DISEASE PREVENTION?

Primary prevention refers to strategies aimed at keeping people from contracting or developing an illness in the first place. Anti-smoking campaigns that discourage teenagers from taking up the virulent habit are geared toward preventing lung cancer, heart disease, and emphysema down the road. Pesticides are sprayed to kill off the ticks that cause Lyme disease or the mosquitoes that carry West Nile virus. Clean needle exchanges, public education efforts, and condom giveaways endeavor to stem the pandemic spread of HIV.

While many studies in the test tube or on experimental mice suggest a variety of effective preventive strategies, proving that they work in humans is a major challenge. Gaining approval of a drug or treatment by the FDA requires studies lasting seven to fifteen years, at a cost of tens of millions of dollars or more. It's no wonder that to date we have no certain means to prevent prostate cancer. Still, a number of promising strategies are currently being investigated.

Diet

A heart-healthy diet may be prostate healthy as well. The dietary guidelines set forth by the American Heart Association will reduce your risk of heart disease—the leading cause of death for adult men. Even though we lack hard scientific evidence that such a regime reduces your chance of developing prostate cancer, it's a good idea to minimize your intake of salt, excess calories, saturated fats, trans fats (e.g., margarine), and cholesterol. At the same time, be sure to consume plenty of fresh fruits, vegetables, unsaturated oils, low-fat proteins, and grains. Finally, if you consume alcohol, do so in moderation.

Some small studies suggest that vegetable consumption may protect against prostate cancer. Cruciferous greens, such as broccoli and cabbage, are thought to provide the best defense, though eating a wide variety of vegetables has been well-established as making sound nutritional sense.[17]

5 Alpha-reductase Inhibitors

Finasteride inhibits production of the enzyme 5 alpha-reductase, which converts testosterone to its more potent form: DHT. Men born with a genetic lack of this enzyme never develop BPH or prostate cancer. The Prostate Cancer Prevention Trial (PCPT) sponsored by the National Cancer Institute enrolled over 18,000 healthy men over the age of 55 and followed them for nearly seven years. This study found that long-term use of finasteride reduced the overall incidence of prostate cancer by an astounding 25 percent when compared to a placebo.[18]

This would have been groundbreaking news, not to mention cause for celebration, but the trial results had several striking peculiarities. In the control group, 24.4 percent of men were diagnosed with cancer, while only 6 percent were anticipated. Never before have 24 percent of randomly selected men been found to have prostate cancer, except in autopsy studies, which detect tiny, insignificant clusters of malignant cells. More curiously, these were men who should have been at low risk for the disease. Initially, they all had a normal DRE and a PSA level of less than 3! True, finasteride reduced the risk of cancer in those taking it to 18 percent, for an overall reduction of 25 percent. But why did such a high proportion of men in this study develop prostate cancer?[19]

More worrisome, the men in this study who took finasteride developed a higher number and disturbing percentage of intermediate and high grade cancers (see Chapter 9, Biopsy), the kind that pose a serious risk to life and health. But recent analyses of the study data indicate that this troubling effect may simply be an artifact of the way the study results were originally evaluated.[20] Indeed, finasteride may prove to be the first drug capable of preventing prostate cancer. This prescription drug has side effects, so men should not begin taking finasteride solely to prevent prostate cancer without carefully considering the pros and cons with their doctor. Men who have a legitimate reason for taking this drug—to reduce the symptoms of BPH or even to prevent or reverse baldness—should certainly continue, but they should have regular checkups for prostate cancer and exercise a bit more vigilance.

NOTE: Dutasteride, a more recently approved 5 alpha-reductase inhibitor, blocks the action of both forms of the enzyme and is now being studied to see if it is also effective in preventing prostate cancer. (See page 81 for more on dutasteride.)

Vitamins and Other Supplements [21]

SELENIUM AND VITAMIN E.   Antioxidants counteract the damaging effects of oxygen in tissues. Selenium and vitamin E are antioxidants that may work in combination to prevent the development of prostate cancer and impede the growth of the tumors that do arise. The SELECT trial, the largest prostate-cancer prevention study to date, involving more than 32,000 men, seeks to discover whether these two nutrients can reduce the incidence of or mortality from the disease.

> NOTE: You may want to consider enrolling in a prostate-cancer prevention trial. For more information in the United States and Puerto Rico, call the National Cancer Institute's Cancer Information Service at 1-800-4-CANCER (1-800-422-6237) or TTY (for the deaf): 1-800-332-8615, for information in English or Spanish. In Canada, call the Canadian Cancer Society's Cancer Information Service at 1-888-939-3333, for information in English or French. You can also find information about prevention trials online at http://swog.org or http://cancer.gov/select.

Selenium is a trace mineral, meaning that the body requires only minuscule amounts to maintain health. Still, researchers have observed that low selenium levels in the soil, which translate into less of the mineral in the food supply, are associated with an increase in cancers and many other diseases. Heavy rainfall tends to wash selenium out of the soil, so people in areas prone to rainy weather should take note.

In studies aimed at documenting the beneficial effects of selenium supplements on other cancers, notably melanoma, an unexpected finding was a substantial reduction in prostate-cancer deaths. The benefit of supplements seems to be limited to men with selenium deficiencies.

Vitamin E (tocopherol) has been shown to inhibit the growth of prostate-cancer cells in the laboratory. Place this vitamin in a dish occupied by tumor cells, and the cells beat a dramatic retreat. A large study of Finnish male smokers found that men who took small, 50 IU daily supplements of vitamin E were less likely to develop prostate cancer and less likely to die of the cancers that arose. Whether this was pure coincidence or a bona fide effect of vitamin E is unclear, but preliminary findings are encouraging. Because dietary sources of vitamin E are often fatty foods, supplements may be a better bet.

NOTE: All vitamin supplements, as well as so-called "natural" and herbal medicines carry a risk of damaging side effects and many can prove toxic, especially in large amounts. Widely embraced substances such as ephedra, commonly known as herbal ecstasy, which was touted as an appetite suppressant, have turned out to carry significant health risks. You would be wise to discuss the pros and cons, as well as the recommended dosage and administration of *any* supplements, with your doctor before taking them. Also, be sure to advise your doctor of everything you take, no matter how innocuous it may seem. Some supplements or over-the-counter remedies can cause hazardous drug and anesthesia interactions.[22]

PHYTOESTROGENS (ISOFLAVONES, ISOFLAVONOIDS).   A modern cancer-prevention buzzword, phytoestrogens are naturally occurring female hormone–like substances found in plant products such as flaxseed and soy. In countries like Japan, where the diet is rich in soy, the incidence of breast and prostate cancers is strikingly low (though the Japanese have an alarmingly high incidence of stomach cancer, possibly linked to a different dietary factor, yet to be identified). Preliminary laboratory studies suggest that phytoestrogens may reduce the level and tumor-promoting effects of male hormones or even destroy the blood supply that existing prostate tumors need to grow. While not yet sufficiently proven, a diet high in soy or other phytoestrogens, found in such foods and spices as alfalfa, red clover, wild yam, and fennel seeds, appears to be safe and may help reduce prostate-cancer risk.

Soy has also been shown to diminish the incidence of hot flashes in menopausal women. A current study is investigating whether men taking hormone ablation therapy for prostate cancer, which can cause debilitating hot flashes, might enjoy the same symptomatic relief.

LYCOPENE.   A diet rich in this powerful antioxidant, found in tomatoes and certain other fruits, is under study as a possible means of prostate-cancer prevention. The form of ingestion seems to be important, since oil promotes lycopene absorption. Consequently, tomato sauce and pizza would theoretically be more effective than tomato juice. Nevertheless, no studies to date have proven that if men ingest tomatoes, much less lycopene supplements, they can reduce their prostate-cancer risk.

VITAMIN D.   It's possible that a deficiency in this antioxidant might increase prostate cancer risk, while some believe high levels may be preventive. In the lab, vitamin D markedly reduces the growth rate of prostate-cancer cells. The same phenomenon has been observed in animal studies, though a similar effect in humans has yet to be demonstrated.

Dark-skinned African-American men, who have the world's highest incidence of prostate cancer, absorb less sunlight and therefore have lower levels of vitamin D than do people with fair skin. People of all skin tones living in the north, where sun exposure and vitamin D synthesis are generally low, have higher rates of prostate cancer than those living in sunny southern climes. With age, the body's ability to manufacture vitamin D diminishes, while the incidence of prostate cancer increases. Studies are being conducted to test whether these correlations mean that vitamin D offers some protection against the disease and, if so, whether the vitamin is most effectively ingested in foods, given as a supplement, or boosted by some minimal amount of controlled sun exposure that would not increase the health risks associated with sun damage.

Preliminary evidence also suggests that vitamin D slows the growth of advanced prostate cancers. Ironically, because it causes cancer cells to act more like normal prostate cells, therapy with vitamin D can actually cause PSA levels to rise. Advanced cancer cells grow so wild that they to lose their ability to produce PSA, and the level drops. The ironic increase in PSA caused by vitamin D therapy makes it far more difficult to judge treatment effects and the progress of the disease, not to mention fanning the flames of anxiety.

VITAMIN A. Beta-carotene is the best known of a large group of yellow and red pigments called carotenoids, which are stored in the liver, where they are converted into vitamin A. Foods rich in beta-carotene, such as carrots, and those rich in vitamin A, including dried apricots and spinach, may have a direct protective effect against some cancers, or the benefit may simply derive from eating more fruits and vegetables and less animal fat. Supplements of vitamin A and beta-carotene have never been shown to reduce the risk of prostate cancer. In fact, in the study of male smokers in Finland, beta-carotene supplements actually appeared to increase both the risk of developing prostate cancer and the likelihood of dying from it.

GARLIC. One recent study found some correlation between regular garlic ingestion and a lower risk of prostate cancer, but the evidence is weak. While garlic is a popular recipe ingredient, garlic supplements can cause flatulence and gastric distress. If you're going to use garlic in the hopes of lowering your prostate-cancer risk, you should probably do so with the natural form.

PC-SPES. Given as a capsule containing eight Chinese herbs, PC-SPES has powerful estrogenlike effects. This herbal compound and its chemical cousins (PC-CALM, PC-CARE, etc.) are manufactured without regulatory oversight. PC-SPES was recently pulled from the market when investigators found that some batches were contaminated with warfarin (Coumadin), a blood thinner that can cause serious bleeding, and alprazolam (Xanax), a drug used to treat anxiety and panic disorders.

PC-SPES and related herbal preparations contain powerful agents and have the potential to cause serious, life-threatening cardiovascular side effects, including thrombophlebitis (inflammation in a vein caused by a blood clot), heart attacks, and strokes.

> NOTE: While touted as anticancer agents and demonstrably effective and useful in some men with advanced, hormone-refractory prostate cancer, *these herbal concoctions are far too potent and dangerous to be used for cancer prevention.*

TEA.   In Asian countries, where the consumption of tea is high, the incidence of prostate cancer is low. Early laboratory studies suggest that substances in tea, especially green tea, may cause cancer cells to commit suicide and that adding a cup or two of green tea to your daily diet might be a good idea.

SAW PALMETTO.   This herb may have some benefit for BPH and has been widely promoted for the prevention of prostate cancer, though as yet, we have no proof that it works.[23]

THE SECOND LINE OF DEFENSE: CURE

Our second line of defense is early detection and effective treatment to catch a cancer before it spreads or causes needless adverse effects. PAP smears have dramatically reduced deaths from cervical cancer. In prostate cancer, PSA screening, along with modern, ultrasound-guided biopsy, represent a home run in secondary prevention. Today, we discover these cancers far earlier in their natural history, while the vast majority are localized to the prostate and can be cured with surgery or radiation. Further advances in PSA interpretation and the development of other, better markers of this disease should enable us to distinguish the prostate cancers that pose a significant risk from those that are unlikely to do harm or require treatment, at least in the short term. (See Chapter 8, Detecting Prostate Cancer with PSA and Other Tests, and Chapter 10, Understanding Your Cancer.)

THE THIRD LINE OF DEFENSE: MINIMIZING SIDE EFFECTS AND COMPLICATIONS

On the prostate-cancer front, great strides have been made in reducing death from the disease and the risk and severity of treatment side effects. Modern radiation and surgery have lowered the incidence of bowel, urinary, and sexual damage dramatically, and excellent treatments are available for many of the problems that do occur. Improvements in hormone therapy and advances in chemotherapy have doubled the life expectancy for men with advanced disease, and the percentage of patients who die of prostate cancer—which was reduced by 25 percent in the 1990s—continues to decline.

THE FUTURE

Based on the Prostate Cancer Prevention Trial (PCPT), finasteride now appears to have a significant effect in preventing prostate cancer. As we learn more, using finasteride or its chemical cousin dutasteride for this purpose may make sense, especially for young men who are at high risk because of a strong familial history of the disease.

The SELECT trial may prove that vitamin E and/or selenium are effective preventive agents. And vitamin D appears promising as well. Still, the best bet for men wishing to optimize their general health is probably a heart-healthy diet, a regular exercise program, and appropriate medical checkups.

IN SUMMARY

■

While all normal men are at risk for developing prostate cancer, a variety of factors may increase or lower your odds. Men at high risk because of race or family history should be more vigilant and begin screening earlier than standard guidelines suggest.

Recent studies suggest that finding ways to keep men from developing prostate cancer may well be within our grasp.

8

■

Detecting Prostate Cancer with PSA and Other Tests

READ THIS CHAPTER TO LEARN:

- How do we screen men for prostate cancer?
- Why is screening controversial, and should you be screened?
- How do we interpret screening results?

PROSTATE CANCER SCREENING: PROS AND CONS

Though we've had the PSA screening test that can signal the possible presence of cancer in the gland for nearly two decades, public health policy experts and medical professionals continue to debate whether diagnosing these cancers early yields more benefits or risks.

Screening proponents point out that early detection has led to a dramatic 25 percent reduction in prostate-cancer death rates. Since PSA testing came into widespread use in the late 1980s, there has also been a major change in the prostate-cancer patient population. In the pre-PSA era, men typically were not diagnosed until their tumors had advanced to the point of causing urinary symptoms or bone pain from metastases. At that stage, cancer cure was no longer possible, and treatment focused on easing symptoms and attempting to prolong life. Given widespread PSA screening, we now see patients far earlier in the course of this disease, while their cancers are still localized and—in the vast majority of cases—curable with surgery to remove the gland or radiation to kill the tumor. Also thanks to PSA testing, we now discover prostate cancers far more often in young, healthy men, who can be treated successfully with modern therapies that carry a much lower risk of serious or lasting side effects.[1]

Screening opponents counter that early detection is a decidedly double-edged sword. Though the PSA test can help ferret out clinically significant prostate cancers while they are still curable, it can also trigger unnecessary biopsies and lead to the overdetection of tiny clusters of cancer cells that often lurk in the prostates of older men and would likely never cause any problems if left alone. Discovering these minuscule cancers can expose patients to unnecessary invasive tests and treatments and the risk—however small, transient, or reversible—of negative effects on sexual, urinary, and bowel function.[2]

Despite major advances, our knowledge of prostate cancer remains incomplete. To date, we lack unequivocal scientific proof that catching the disease early confers a survival advantage, though we do have compelling statistics to bolster that conclusion (the aforementioned 25 percent reduction in prostate-cancer deaths since PSA screening began in the late '80s). Still, just as screening advocates can cite impressive reductions in prostate-cancer deaths, those opposed to early detection can name studies that failed to find a significant survival difference between men who were diagnosed and treated early and those who were not. Scientific trials often yield such frustrating inconsistencies. Many factors can affect results (see Chapter 21, Treating Metastatic Prostate Cancer, for a discussion of clinical trials).

Nevertheless, certain facts are indisputable. We *do know* that every year nearly 30,000 men die of prostate cancer in the United States alone, and that number is expected to increase steadily as the average age of citizens in all developed countries continues to rise. We know that once established, this disease is a formidable foe that causes debilitating symptoms and, eventually, death. We know that cancers have the capacity to change over time, and that it can be difficult, if not impossible, to tell which small, seemingly harmless tumors might eventually prove to be aggressive and dangerous. We also know that once prostate cancer spreads to organs beyond the prostate, it becomes far more difficult to control and is often lethal. Screening allows us to find these cancers far earlier in their natural course, when they are still curable. Modern treatment for prostate cancer is generally safe, with a very low risk of mortality. Though the side effects of surgery and radiation can be unpleasant and affect quality of life for some men, the problems are often transient and, if not, are generally treatable and remediable.

So should you be screened for prostate cancer? That depends.[3]

Prostate cancer is a highly heterogeneous disease, and the men who develop these tumors have widely varying personal needs and medical profiles. For older patients in poor health whose life expectancy is less than ten years, screening is most often unnecessary and probably inadvisable. It's unlikely that this cancer, which is typically slow-growing, would cause any problems in that remaining lifetime. Learning that they have the disease would only cause needless anxiety.

Healthy younger men need to assess whether the risks inherent in treating some cancers unnecessarily are outweighed by the benefits of catching potentially aggressive, life-threatening tumors before they can spread and do harm. Men at high risk for developing prostate cancer, including African-Americans and those with a family history of the disease, have additional issues to factor into the equation. Because of their increased risk, they are typically advised to start screening earlier than the general population.

Given the persistent controversy about prostate-cancer screening, it's unsurprising that the guidelines from major health organizations are at odds. The American College of Preventive Medicine (ACPM) suggests that doctors inform men age 50 or older, with a life expectancy of ten years or longer, about the potential positives and downsides of screening and help patients make their own informed decisions about whether to undergo PSA and DRE exams. Testing is not routinely recommended.[4]

The American Urological Association (AUA) and the American Cancer Society (ACS) are more positive about the benefits of screening. They advise physicians to offer men annual DRE and PSA testing starting at age 50 (45 for those at high risk) as long as the patient's life expectancy is at least ten years. These groups recommend that doctors present comprehensive information about screening so that men can provide informed consent.[5]

The American College of Physicians (ACP) suggests that doctors provide information about prostate-cancer screening and encourage men to make their own decisions. The U.S. Preventive Services Task Force (USPSTF) currently opposes routine prostate-cancer screening, though this recommendation is under review.[6]

Such generalizations are expected and unavoidable from health policy makers, but they don't necessarily speak to what's right for you. The best way to make that highly personal determination is through a careful, reasoned discussion with a physician who fully understands your particular situation and has knowledge of the ins and outs of this complex disease. Together, you can gauge the risk/benefit ratio of screening in your case and, if it seems appropriate, when to start and how often you should have testing done.

I'd urge you to make sure you're fully informed before deciding to forgo screening for prostate cancer. Blinders are a poor defense against a potentially lethal disease. Certainly, you don't want to undergo unnecessary, invasive treatment, but neither would you wish to die an unnecessary death from a disease that is highly curable if detected in time.

HOW PSA AND DRE HELP TO DETECT PROSTATE CANCER

In the early 1970s, scientists discovered a previously unknown component of human seminal fluid and traced its origins to the prostate gland. One early investigator speculated that this new marker might prove to be a sort of semen signature, unique in each man, that could prove useful in identifying rape suspects (though this theory did not hold up in later studies).

In the early 1980s, researchers found a way to detect minute quantities of this substance in blood, as little as 0.1 nanograms/milliliter. (To get an idea of how astonishingly tiny this is, a mosquito weighs in at a relatively corpulent 2,000 to 2,500 nanograms.)

Scientists observed that while men normally had nearly undetectable levels of what had come to be called PSA, 68 percent of patients with benign enlargement of the gland, up to 79 percent of men with localized prostate cancer, and as many as 86 percent of men with advanced cancer showed elevated concentrations. Finally we had a marker to alert us to the presence of possible prostate cancer while it was still in an early, curable stage!

PSA, which stands for **prostate-specific antigen**, is produced by the prostate and released as part of the ejaculate. Under normal circumstances, the only two places we expect to find significant amounts of PSA are in the prostate gland and in the seminal fluid. Detecting elevated levels in the bloodstream is a clear indication that something is amiss. When things are functioning according to plan, the concentration of PSA in semen is a startling millionfold higher than the minuscule trace there would be in a blood sample.[7]

The term prostate-specific highlights the fact that the prostate gland is the sole organ that manufactures a significant amount of PSA (though, in fact, a tiny bit is produced by the salivary glands). An antigen is a substance capable of provoking a response by the body's immune defenses, as PSA can do when damage or disease in the gland allows it to leak into the bloodstream. Because it causes a chemical reaction, PSA also qualifies as an enzyme. And by chemical composition, it can be classified as a glycoprotein, meaning that it is a sugar and a protein combined.

Though we still have much to discover about PSA, Dr. Hans Lilja discovered in 1985 that it plays an important role in human reproduction. Soon after ejaculation, semen coagulates. PSA returns seminal fluid to liquid form in a process called proteolysis, freeing the sperm it contains to go about their business.

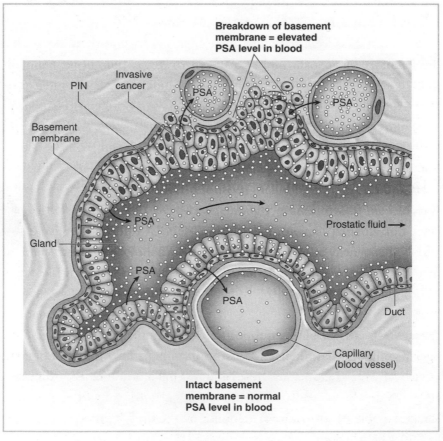

As cancer invades through the barrier (basement membrane) around the glands within the prostate, PSA can leak freely into the blood vessels, causing an elevated level on the PSA test.

We expect to find PSA in the ejaculate. But under ordinary circumstances, this hefty molecule is far too large to penetrate tissue barriers in the prostate and find its way into the bloodstream. Discovering a measurable amount of PSA in a blood sample indicates that something has gone awry in the gland, causing those natural defenses to break down.

Anything below 4 ng/ml (referred to as a PSA of 4) used to be considered insignificant, but it is now clear that levels as low as 2 are associated with an increased risk of cancer.[8] (See the table below.) It's reasonable to adjust for age when evaluating PSA (see page 141 for a discussion of BPH-related PSA-level increase). My suspicions might be raised if a 45-year-old man with a strong family history of prostate cancer had a PSA over 1, while a level of 5.5 in a 75-year-old with an enlarged prostate may not sound a serious alarm.[9]

NORMAL RANGE OF PSA LEVELS FOR MEN IN EACH AGE GROUP*	
AGE RANGE (YR)	PSA NORMAL RANGE (MG/ML)
40–49	0–2.5
50–59	2.6–3.5
60–69	3.6–4.5
70–79	4.6–6.5

THE DIGITAL RECTAL EXAMINATION (DRE)

During a **digital rectal exam (DRE),** the doctor inserts a gloved finger into the rectum to examine the rear of the prostate for abnormalities. Many men, and some physicians, find the test off-putting and would

*Source: Modified from DeAntoni, E. P., Crawford, E. D., Oesterling, J. E., Ross, C. A., Berger, E. R., McLeod, D. G., Staggers, F., Stone, N. N., "Age- and Race-specific Reference Ranges for Prostate-specific Antigen from a Large Community-based Study." *Urology* 48, no. 2 (1996): 234–239. © 1996. Reprinted with permission from Elsevier.

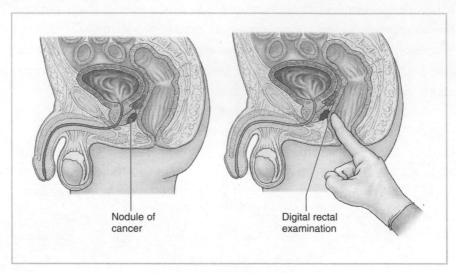

Nodule of cancer

Digital rectal examination

The digital rectal examination (DRE).

just as soon avoid it. The DRE is also highly subjective. A physician examines you and draws an impression about the probability that you have prostate cancer. The level of suspicion and the way a given doctor responds to that suspicion can vary enormously. What one doctor considers an alarming nodule, another might judge to be a harmless, meaningless irregularity in the gland. The DRE is a difficult test to master, and doing so requires a great deal of practice. If a urologist sees fifty or sixty men a day, three or four days a week in the office, it might take six months or more before he really understands all the nuances of this exam. Given all that, you might wonder why we persist in recommending the test at all, especially given the existence of PSA.

PSA is far from perfect. While the test can help to detect prostate cancer, studies that compared screening methods found that one of every five cancers were detected because of an abnormal DRE in patients who had a normal PSA.[10] Part of the reason lies in the uncertain definition of "normal." We've known for years that cancer can be found in some men with a PSA well below the traditional cutoff of 4. In many cases, the cancer is too small to make enough PSA to push the level that high. Sometimes the cancer is large enough, but there is so little PSA made by the rest of the prostate that the threshold of normal is not passed. In rare cases, a high grade cancer functions so abnormally that the cells ironically make very little PSA.

> NOTE: While PSA produced by a cancer and PSA made by normal prostate cells are identical, we can distinguish between these two diseases that raise PSA levels using PSA density, PSA velocity, and the free-PSA test. Newer tests for molecular forms of PSA and related antigens are likely to improve the detection of cancer in the future.[11]

Recent European studies have focused on relying entirely on PSA for prostate-cancer screening. If the test result falls below a predetermined level of 1.5 to 2.5 (depending on the trial), no further testing is done. If the PSA is above the threshold, follow-up with a DRE and a prostate biopsy is recommended. Advocates of this approach argue that cancers found by DRE in men with a very low PSA are rarely dangerous. Theoretically, if they are missed during this screening process, any cancers will be picked up the next go-round in ample time to treat the tumor successfully.

In this country, we still advocate PSA plus a digital rectal exam as the most effective way to detect prostate cancer early.[12]

DRE results can play an important role in treatment planning. If the doctor felt an abnormality, how extensive was it? Did it distort

> NOTE: If you have both tests regularly, it's almost guaranteed that any prostate cancer you develop will be detected while it is still localized and curable.

PROBABILITY OF FINDING CANCER ON BIOPSY ACCORDING TO A MAN'S DRE RESULT AND PSA LEVEL

DRE Result	PSA (NG/ML)		
	2–4	4–10	>10
Normal	15%	25%	50%
Abnormal*	20%	45%	>75%

*"Abnormal" means nodular or suspicious for cancer.

the normal border of the gland? Did it appear to protrude through the capsule? The answers to all these questions will have implications for whether or not you should have a biopsy and, if you do, how it should be done.

If a biopsy confirms that you have prostate cancer, the DRE you had before the biopsy is critically important in determining the stage of your tumor and how it might best be treated. Following a biopsy, the prostate area may be tender and uncomfortable, and the doctor may be reluctant to do a full exam that could provoke bleeding. Also, due to swelling from the biopsy needles, the prostate might not feel normal.

NOTE: While a small percentage of general physicians are excellent DRE interpreters, urologists, in general, have more experience and expertise. If you're at high risk for prostate cancer, if your doctor found an abnormality in your prostate, or if your PSA is creeping up, having a prostate exam by an experienced urologist is probably a good idea.

OTHER THAN CANCER, WHAT CAN CAUSE YOUR PSA TO RISE?

With benign prostatic hyperplasia (BPH), the gland enlarges, and a larger prostate produces more PSA. Though BPH is not cancer, it can cause the same breakdown of tissue barriers in the gland that we see with malignant disease (see the figure on page 136). PSA leaks into the bloodstream and registers as a higher number on the prostate-cancer screening test.

The inflammation or infection of prostatitis can cause a dramatic increase in PSA. By compromising prostate tissues, prostatitis also allows PSA to escape the gland and slip into circulation.

In addition, transient, meaningless increases in PSA can result from inflammation caused by a prostate biopsy or a **cystoscopic** examination of the urethra or bladder through a tube inserted in the penis. Testing for PSA should be postponed for at least three to four weeks after such procedures, to allow the inflammation to resolve.

Some medications, most notably finasteride (see Chapter 5, BPH [Prostate Enlargement]) can lower the PSA artificially.[13] Surgical or medical castration for prostate cancer will also result in an artificially depressed PSA. Herbal remedies, including saw palmetto (a limited effect) and PC–SPES (a profound effect), may affect PSA as well. If you're planning to use such compounds, you should have a careful medical evaluation first and be sure to mention anything you're taking, or planning to take, to your doctor.

Studies have failed to support the common belief that ejaculation or manipulation of the prostate during DRE causes the PSA to rise.[14] Though some doctors caution men to avoid ejaculation for several days before PSA screening and to delay the test for some time after a DRE, I've seen no evidence that either of these practices is necessary.

HOW RELIABLE IS THE PSA TEST?

Though it helps us to catch prostate cancers while they are in an early, curable stage, PSA testing is far from an exact science. In 70 to 80 percent of cases, an elevated PSA that triggers a biopsy uncovers no evidence of cancer. For every man who is found to have a malignant tumor in the gland, four men are subjected to a biopsy needlessly. Perhaps more distressing, 20 percent of existing prostate cancers would be missed if doctors relied on PSA results alone.[15]

To make matters worse, PSA can fluctuate by as much as 36 percent from day to day, for no identifiable reason. If your PSA rises in the absence of other red flags, such as an abnormal digital rectal exam, it's probably wise to repeat the test in a few weeks before submitting to a prostate biopsy.[16]

This is not to suggest that we should abandon PSA screening. Despite some recent warnings to the contrary,[17] the PSA test, properly used, remains the best indicator of a cancer's presence. The test's ability to detect prostate cancer is comparable to or better than mammography at warning us of the possible presence of breast cancer.[18] Unfortunately, measuring PSA is not very specific, meaning it does a good job of alerting us to the fact that there's a problem, but it's far less adept at telling us what kind. Where there's smoke, there may be fire, but it's also possible that an overcooked dinner, a roomful of cigar enthusiasts, woodchips in a roaring barbecue, or even a special-effects machine might be responsible instead.

If an elevated PSA can be compared to a smoke detector, a PSA that rises rapidly over time is more akin to a fire detector. By observing how fast the PSA level increases, we get a better picture of whether cancer is responsible for the rise. (See page 144.) The rate of rise (**PSA velocity**) is much faster in men with cancer than those with BPH or a normal prostate.[19] The problem is the inherent variability in PSA test results. Values vary so much from week to week that detecting a genuine rise can be tricky. Measuring PSA velocity requires at least three PSA tests over a year and a half, and more results allow more accurate calculation of the rate of rise. If the PSA level increases more than 0.75 ng/ml per year, there's an increased risk of finding cancer on a prostate biopsy. A recent study suggested that men whose PSA rose by more than 2 ng/ml per year in the year before radical prostatectomy had a 28 percent chance of dying of prostate cancer within seven years. This alarmed many men who seemed to have a rapidly rising PSA before surgery.[20] Our group tried to duplicate the result but could find no such alarming results associated with a steep PSA rise. In fact, men with a rise greater than 2 over a year did no worse than men with a rise less than 2, and in both groups the chances of dying of prostate cancer within seven years was only 3 percent, not 28 percent. A rapidly rising PSA may be ominous, but more often it is caused by normal variation in PSA levels.[21]

FREE PSA

PSA comes in several varieties. Complex PSA circulates with a companion protein. **Free PSA** is a sort of bachelor antigen that travels on its own. This unbound form of PSA comes from BPH, not prostate cancer.

The widely available test for free PSA (**%fPSA**) indicates what percentage of your total PSA comes from benign enlargement of the gland. From this, we can predict the likelihood that a man with an elevated PSA would be found to have prostate cancer if we performed a biopsy. The test is especially useful for men whose PSA falls between 4 and 10, a gray area where either BPH or prostate cancer might be responsible for the increase. Testing for free PSA improves our ability to predict whether cancer is the cause of an elevated PSA by 20 to 40 percent yet reduces by only about 5 percent the cancers we would otherwise fail to detect. The measure can also be useful in characterizing a cancer after it has been diagnosed.

Readings over 25 percent suggest that the elevated PSA is largely caused by BPH. Any cancer present is more likely to be small and confined to the gland. On the other hand, having a free PSA under 10 percent suggests that your total PSA is mostly elevated by a cancer, which is likely to be large and require active, aggressive treatment.[22] Levels between 10 and 25 percent are harder to evaluate in terms of your outlook for a permanent cure. But, in general, the lower the free PSA, the greater the cause for concern (see the following table).

PROBABILITY OF FINDING CANCER ON BIOPSY ACCORDING TO A MAN'S "FREE PSA" LEVEL, FOR MEN WITH A PSA IN THE "GRAY ZONE" BETWEEN 4 AND 10 NG/ML*†

% FREE PSA	PROBABILITY OF CANCER
0–10%	56%
10–15%	28%
15–20%	20%
20–25%	16%
>25%	8%

*Results are for PSA level of 4–10 ng/ml (25% probability of cancer). Also, note that free PSA is reported as the percentage of total PSA that is "floating free," or not bound to a large protein in the blood. Probability of finding cancer on biopsy according to a man's free PSA level, for men with a PSA in the "gray zone" between 4 and 10 ng/ml, where the elevation may be from BPH or cancer.

†Source: Modified from Catalona, W. J., A. W. Partin, K. M. Slawin, M. K. Brawer, R. C. Flanigan, A. Patel, J. P. Richie, J. B. deKernion, P. C. Walsh, P. T. Scardino, P. H. Lange, E. N. Subong, R. E. Parson, G. H. Gasior, K. G. Loveland, and P. C. Southwick. "Use of the Percentage of Free Prostate-Specific Antigen to Enhance Differentiation of Prostate Cancer from Benign Prostatic Disease: A Prospective Multicenter Clinical Trial." *JAMA* 279, no. 19 (1998): 1542–7. © 1998, American Medical Association.

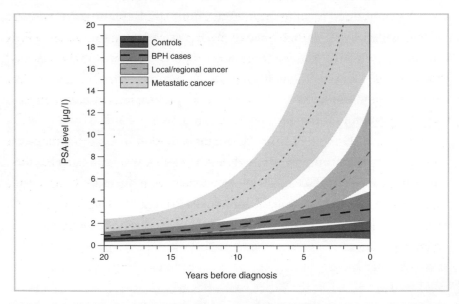

PSA levels in the blood test begin to rise many years before local/regional or metastatic prostate cancer can otherwise be detected. The rate of rise (called **PSA velocity** or **PSA doubling time**) is much faster in men with cancer than in those with BPH or a normal prostate.*

*Source: Modified from Carter, H. B., et al., "Longitudinal Evaluation of Prostate-Specific Antigen Levels in Men with and without Prostate Disease," *JAMA* 267, no. 16 (1992): 2218, fig. 3. © 1992, American Medical Association.

PSA DENSITY AND VELOCITY

PSA density (PSAD) looks at the ratio of PSA to prostate size. The larger the gland, the higher we expect PSA to be. To calculate PSA density (PSAD), simply divide your PSA by the size of your prostate, as measured by ultrasound. The digital rectal exam is *not* the best way to judge how large your gland may be. In fact, it is notoriously inaccurate. Doctors can only feel the side of the prostate that rests against the rectum. Ultrasound, which is also used to guide the needles for your biopsy, measures prostate shape and volume far more accurately, in three dimensions. If you've had a biopsy, you should be able to get a report of your ultrasound results, which would include the size of your prostate.

If your PSA is 6 and your prostate weighs 30 grams, you would divide 30 into 6 and find that your PSA density is 0.2. A PSA of 4 in a 60-gram prostate would translate into 4 divided by 60, or a density of 0.067.

Higher density, meaning more PSA per cubic centimeter of prostate tissue, suggests a higher likelihood that cancer is the cause. We view PSA density under 0.07 as a safe level that strongly suggests that the elevated PSA is coming from BPH; between 0.07 and 0.15 is uncertain. If your density is greater than 0.15, I would be highly suspicious that a cancer is present.[23]

By observing how fast the PSA level increases, we may get a better picture of whether cancer is responsible for the rise. Measuring PSA velocity requires three PSA tests over a two-year period. Studies have shown that if the PSA level increases more than 0.75 ng/ml per year, there's an increased risk that a prostate biopsy would be positive for malignant disease.

THE FUTURE

Scientists are seeking more reliable markers to help us predict the presence and extent of prostate cancers. While PSA remains the cornerstone of prostate-cancer detection, the free PSA test has proven valuable, especially in men with enlarged prostates or those who have had one or two biopsies that have found no cancer. The complex PSA test measures the PSA that is bound to large serum proteins and not free. Advocates argue that this single test gives all the information that we can get from the PSA and free PSA tests combined.

Another promising test measures human kallikrein (hK2), a protein that is closely related to PSA and present in minute quantities in blood. HK2 begins to rise years before cancer would be detected by DRE, and it may eventually be used to supplement PSA as a screening measure for prostate cancer. In one recent study, hK2 showed promise in distinguishing between cancers that were confined to the gland and those that had spread and would not be cured with radiation or surgery to remove the prostate. By combining a number of tumor markers like PSA and hK2, or tracking their levels over time, our ability to detect prostate cancer early and to distinguish potentially dangerous cancers from those likely to remain harmless should be far better in the future.

There are more than fifteen genes in the kallikrein family. Other recently identified members that are produced by the human prostate include hK4, also known as prostase, and hK15, nicknamed prostin. Researchers are exploring the potential value of these markers in screening and early detection of prostate cancer.[24]

IN SUMMARY

■

Screening for prostate cancer has enabled us to catch the disease early and cut the prostate-cancer death rate. Though screening remains controversial and is not appropriate for every man, having these tests regularly can virtually ensure that we'll detect prostate cancers before they become lethal. Hopefully, new and better markers will eventually allow us to predict which prostate cancers are serious and which can be safely monitored.

9

■

Biopsy

READ THIS CHAPTER TO LEARN:

- Why are prostate biopsies done, and when might you need one?
- How can you interpret biopsy results?
- What is the Gleason grade, and how is it significant?

WHEN MIGHT YOU NEED
A PROSTATE BIOPSY?

An elevated PSA level is a warning sign that something might be wrong. The same holds true for an abnormality on a digital rectal exam. Like a storm watch, these tests alert us to potential problems. Still, just as a predicted storm might fail to materialize, troubling results of prostate cancer screening tests often turn out to be simple false alarms.

PSA results are highly variable, with meaningless fluctuations of up to 36 percent from day to day.[1] A PSA of 3 on Monday could rise for no notable reason to 4.1 or sink to 1.9 by Tuesday. An infection or inflammation in the gland can cause a rapid spike in your level that has nothing to do with cancer. A bigger prostate puts out more PSA, so benign enlargement of the gland alone, which happens in most men as they age, can cause your number to rise.[2]

The results of a digital rectal exam (DRE) are highly subjective. The same thing one doctor finds suspicious might be entirely overlooked or deemed insignificant by a different examiner. Tiny lumps or bulges may represent meaningless calcifications or benign enlargement of the gland. Only one in five abnormal DREs turns out to be cancer.[3]

Recommending surgery or radiation on the basis of these uncertain tests would be irresponsible and overreaching. On the other hand, we don't want to miss the chance to identify and evaluate an early curable cancer or stop an aggressive tumor in its tracks. If your PSA or DRE raises a red flag that cancer may be present, a **biopsy** can determine whether or not you have the disease.

NOTE: A biopsy is only appropriate if you would take action as a result of a cancer diagnosis. I would rarely recommend the test for a man whose remaining life expectancy is less than five years, unless he has symptoms of advanced disease, such as voiding problems or bone pain, and some treatment might be useful to alleviate them.

MODERN BIOPSY TECHNIQUES AND HOW THEY DEVELOPED

Before the PSA test was developed, prostate cancers were typically suspected because of an abnormal DRE or symptoms of advanced disease, such as bone pain. As recently as 1985, the biopsies we did were targeted to suspicious thickenings or nodules we felt on the gland during a digital rectal exam. Guided by finger touch, we would insert a needle equipped with a pair of narrow cutting blades into the palpable lesion and remove one to three tissue cores, each about 1 inch long by ¼₄ inch wide. Because the needles were large, the procedure was done under general anesthesia.

The Development of
Ultrasound-Guided Biopsies

During World War I, very high frequency sound echoes in water (sonar) were used to detect enemy submarines and the sort of treacherous submerged iceberg that sank the *Titanic*. After the war, scientists began to investigate how this technology might be used in medical diagnostics. The first medical ultrasound device was developed by an Austrian physicist to visualize brain tumors. During the 1950s and '60s, similar instruments were devised to detect breast, intestinal, and abdominal lesions and to monitor fetal development throughout pregnancy.

In the 1970s, Hiroke Watanabe, a Japanese urologist, designed a highly peculiar device to image the prostate. Patients sat on a chair fitted with a fingerlike ultrasound probe that was cranked into the rectum, allowing the examiner to visualize the gland.[4]

Danish scientists modified the Japanese probe in the 1980s, using a handheld wand that could be inserted into the rectum and manipulated to show the prostate from several angles. This **transrectal ultrasound (TRUS)** produced a clear, detailed picture of the prostate and surrounding tissues (see page 154).

Ultrasound probes had been used to guide needles into other organs, so once we had this flexible transrectal probe, a natural next step was the development of a long, thin, flexible needle that could be guided by ultrasound into the prostate. A further major breakthrough came in the early 1990s, with the production of the spring-loaded, handheld biopsy "gun." This device fires a hollow inner needle into the prostate, then instantly sends a sheath forward to slice off and retrieve a core of prostate tissue.[5]

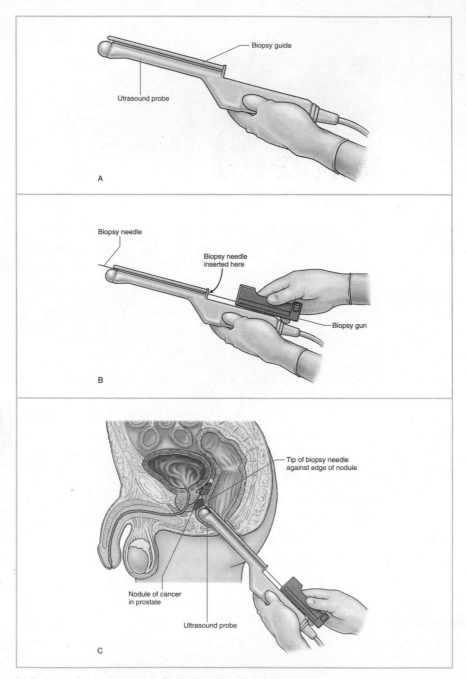

(a) Probe used to guide a biopsy by transrectal ultrasound.

(b) The needle is placed in a spring-loaded gun and inserted through the biopsy guide.

(c) The probe is placed in the rectum.

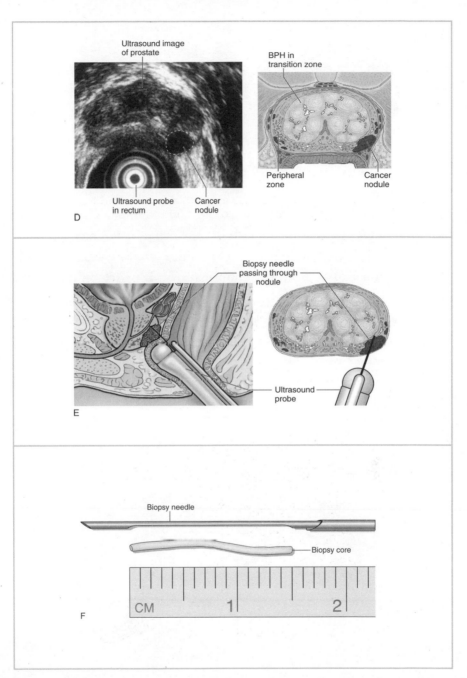

(d) An image of the prostate is produced by ultrasound. The tip of the needle is placed at the edge of the prostate or nodule.

(e) The needle is fired through the nodule.

(f) A core of tissues about 15 mm long is removed.

Virtually all biopsies today are guided by ultrasound, which allows us to see precisely where a biopsy needle is placed into the prostate. Once we've identified the target, the biopsy gun deploys an 18-gauge (18 would fit in an inch) or smaller "true cut" needle—which is sharp, disposable, and minimizes bleeding and pain—to obtain a core of tissue that measures 0.4 mm wide and 12 to 15 mm long.

Most prostate cancers are now discovered early, while they are too small to feel or to see on TRUS. Given the absence of palpable or visible nodules to target, our biopsy approach has shifted to sampling specified areas of the gland. Several studies have confirmed that these systematic segment biopsies are at least as effective at finding cancers as those targeted to suspicious areas. To maximize results, I also take an additional sample or two from any abnormal area that I see on ultrasound or feel on DRE.

It became standard in the field to divide the prostate into sextants and take six samples (cores) from the left and right side of the apex, the middle, and the base of the outer peripheral zone, which is where most cancers arise (see Chapter 1, The Prostate). Needles are inserted at a 30-

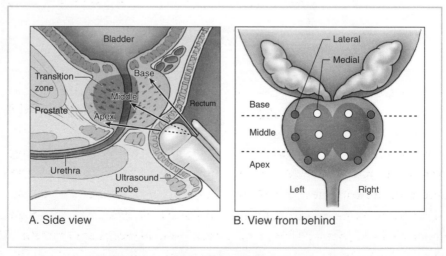

A. Side view   B. View from behind

The location of each biopsy core in systematic segment biopsy. A typical biopsy would sample twelve cores from the peripheral zone and perhaps two from the transition zone.

to 45-degree angle, running from the middle to the side of the prostate as they pass from the back toward the front.

Recent studies have found that the typical six-core biopsy may be inadequate. The more samples we get, the more likely we are to detect existing cancers.[6] Many doctors now advocate eight to fourteen, and some take as many twenty-four cores. Unfortunately, more needles involve greater discomfort and increased side effects. Ten to twelve cores appears to be an optimal number, ensuring a thorough biopsy that most men tolerate well.

> NOTE: If I found no cancer on the first set of biopsies, I might do a second series, adding two cores from the transition zone, where BPH grows and prostate cancers develop less commonly, in addition to directly sampling any abnormal areas I felt on DRE (which is called a finger-guided biopsy).

WHAT DOES A BIOPSY ENTAIL?

PREPARATION

I don't recommend any special diet or bowel preparation such as an enema before the test.[7] If you're taking a blood thinner like warfarin (Coumadin), you'll have to stop it five days before the procedure and have your prothrombin time or INR (which is the ratio of your clotting time compared to a healthy norm) and clotting factors checked to be sure they are back near the normal range to prevent excess bleeding. Short-acting blood thinners, like heparin or its relatives, can be stopped about six hours before a biopsy. I've seen no evidence that eliminating aspirin, NSAIDs, or vitamin E is necessary, though some doctors routinely recommend doing so.[8] If stopping these drugs would cause you troubling symptoms of arthritis or other problems, you may want to question whether it's really necessary in your case.

Since prostate biopsy involves passing needles through the rectum, infection is a serious concern. Most doctors prescribe a broad-spectrum antibiotic, such as ciprofloxacin (Cipro) or levofloxacin (Levaquin). By starting antibiotics the night before the test, you'll build good protective levels in your bloodstream.

Special caution is in order if your immune system is compromised for any reason. This applies if you're taking immunosuppressive drugs because of a transplant or if you have an autoimmune disease or a low white blood count. Steroids, including hydrocortisone or prednisone, and chemotherapeutic drugs can also depress the immune system.

Be sure to discuss any of these situations thoroughly with your doctor before biopsy. The need for the test should be weighed against your increased risk of infection. For example, if an HIV-positive or AIDS patient has a mildly elevated PSA level, it might be preferable to follow the PSA over time and get a sense of the dynamics of change before exposing him to the risks of a biopsy.

Otherwise healthy patients who have artificial heart valves, heart murmurs, or a history of rheumatic fever may be at risk for subacute bacterial endocarditis (SBE), an infection caused by bacteria that enter the bloodstream and settle in the heart valves or heart lining after invasive procedures. To prevent this, the American College of Cardiology recommends a powerful antibiotic regimen, including a high-dose oral ampicillin or amoxicillin along with intramuscular or intravenous antibiotics such as gentamicin or tobramycin. If you have to take antibiotics before dental work or any kind of surgery, or if you have had a joint replacement within the last two years, you should follow the special antibiotic regimen before a prostate biopsy.[9]

The Procedure

Typically, going through a biopsy takes only a bit longer than a standard checkup. You should allow time to visit with the doctor and nurse beforehand. The test itself involves about ten to fifteen minutes for the ultrasound, plus five to ten minutes to harvest the sample cores. If you're going to have a local anesthetic, plan on another ten minutes for the lidocaine to take effect. Prostate biopsy does not require general anesthetic, and there is usually no need for anxiety medications, muscle relaxants, or pain medications. Discomfort from the needles is fleeting, like an injection. You should feel little or no lasting pain.

SIDE EFFECTS AND COMPLICATIONS

The degree of discomfort from a prostate biopsy tends to be directly related to the number of sample cores we take. Recently, there has been a move toward using local anesthetics such as 1 percent lidocaine to numb the gland before the test, especially when we plan to take more than six samples.[10]

After the test, you may feel some soreness in your rectum or penis, but this should resolve within a matter of hours, and most men are able to return to work and resume most normal activities the same day.

About 50 percent of men notice blood in the urine and may pass small clots after a prostate biopsy. In most cases this clears up in about three days, though occasionally it continues for weeks. Rest and increased fluid intake to flush the system usually take care of the problem.

Bleeding from the rectum is common for the first day or two but rare after that. Occasionally, a biopsy needle hits a small artery in the rectal wall, causing more severe bleeding. About 1 in 1,000 patients needs to be admitted to the hospital for a blood transfusion or requires cauterization, fulgeration (a radiofrequency that causes coagulation), or sutures to resolve rectal bleeding.

I advise patients to avoid vigorous exercise for a few days after the test until any rectal or urinary bleeding stops. For five to seven days, it's wise to be cautious about activities that might exert pressure on the prostate, such as riding a bicycle, a motorcycle, or a horse.

What you should or should not do depends on the specifics of the situation. For example, riding a very narrow bicycle seat on bumpy roads for several hours may be ill-advised, but sitting on a very well-padded seat on an exercise bicycle and peddling might not be a problem at all. The goal is to avoid trauma to the prostate until it heals.

It's a good idea to wait until rectal and urinary bleeding has stopped for at least twenty-four hours before you have a sexual climax after a biopsy. Orgasm causes the gland to contract, which can promote bleeding. Blood in the ejaculate is common for a month or more and should not be a cause for alarm.

If your bleeding has stopped but starts again after sex, it will almost always clear up uneventfully. Rest and increased fluid intake should help. Serious bleeding from sexual activity after a biopsy is very rare. Some men report a temporary problem with erections following a prostate biopsy. This should resolve on its own within a few months.

Be aware of rare but significant complications that can develop during the first week or two after the test. About 3 percent of men who take antibiotics—and 6 to 10 percent of those who don't—come down with a urinary tract infection or develop bacterial prostatitis, a serious infection of the gland.[11] During this time period, if you experience symptoms such as a fever of 101°F or higher, chills, muscle aches, or urinary problems (frequency, urgency, or burning), you should go to your doctor or emergency room *immediately* for a round of cultures. Be sure to tell the examining physician that you had a transrectal biopsy of the prostate and might need intravenous antibiotics. With appropriate treatment, the infection will be arrested promptly, and you can go home within a day or two. A wait-and-see approach is definitely unwise. If you allow an infection to build for even six to twelve hours, you can become overwhelmingly septic, which could result in a long hospitalization and serious health risks. Fortunately, this occurs in less than 1 of every 200 cases.

People who have an enlarged prostate or difficulty urinating before a biopsy are at risk of developing a sudden inability to urinate, medically known as acute urinary retention, because of swelling from the needles. As a preventive measure, your doctor may prescribe alpha-blocking drugs (see Chapter 5, BPH [Prostate Enlargement]). Still, if urinary symptoms worsen after the test or you are unable to urinate, let your doctor know.

Given the risk of infection or bleeding, I advise patients not to take any plane flight that lasts more than four to five hours until a week to ten days after the test. If you do travel, avoid remote or underdeveloped areas. You'll definitely want to have access to top-notch medical care if complications occur.

BIOPSY RESULTS: "POSITIVE" MEANS CANCER

While heart disease can be established by clinical means through an electrocardiogram (ECG), and we have chemical tests for diseases like diabetes, biopsy is the *only* currently available tool for diagnosing cancer. To make the call, a pathologist must examine tissue taken from the suspect organ under a microscope and decide whether cancer is present or not. There is no magical passing number, no blazing indicator light, no unequivocal reading on an electronic monitor.

A positive biopsy means the pathologist has found cancer. In one of the many ironies of medical terminology, "positive" in this case turns out to be what you don't want to hear, while a "negative" result is desirable. Still, knowing that you have a malignancy is far from the whole picture. Prostate cancers vary widely, and you have to understand the specifics of your particular disease to make a sound decision about whether, when, and how to treat it.

CAN BIOPSIES MISS A CANCER?

Because biopsies test a tiny fraction of prostate tissue, any given biopsy will detect about 75 percent of existing cancers. If the result is negative, with no cancer found, a second biopsy session would pick up many of the remaining malignancies, bringing the total to 91 percent. With a third series, 97 percent of cases will be detected, and at four biopsies, we'll find 99 percent of prostate cancers.[12] Biopsies can be scheduled six

NOTE: You may wonder why your doctor might recommend another biopsy if the first one (or the second) finds no cancer. Studies have shown that the more biopsy samples we take, the greater the chance we'll find an existing cancer. If an elevated PSA and/or an abnormal DRE suggests that you might have a malignancy in your prostate, we don't want to miss the chance to find, evaluate, and treat it appropriately. A first biopsy detects 75 percent of existing cancers. That means one out of four will go undetected. By the third set of biopsies, we'll pick up 97 percent of prostate cancers. For that reason, I recommend doing three good, thorough sets of biopsies to rule out cancer if our level of suspicion remains the same. Some doctors do saturation biopsies, which take forty to fifty cores. Given that these require general anesthesia, I see them as riskier and don't recommend them. Also, saturation biopsies may be overkill, picking up tiny, insignificant cancers that don't require treatment.

weeks to three months apart, allowing time for swelling and bleeding from the previous test to resolve, so the prostate can be examined anew.

Occasionally, it can take five or six or even more attempts to find a prostate cancer. There was one patient at Memorial Sloan-Kettering whose cancer was not detected until the twelfth biopsy. Still, in the overwhelming majority of cases, three good sets of biopsies using modern techniques are sufficient. On the second set, I'd add two transition zone biopsies and a targeted biopsy to any suspicious areas I felt on DRE. For the third biopsy, I would consider imaging the prostate with an **endorectal MRI with spectroscopy**[13] or color duplex Doppler ultrasound,[14] with or without contrast. These highly sophisticated studies may yield better information about where a cancer might be. I'd be especially inclined to use these tests if a patient has a high PSA level given the size of his prostate (PSA density over 0.15), or a low free PSA level (less than 10 percent) in combination with an elevated PSA, both of which point to a higher likelihood that a cancer exists (see Chapter 8, Detecting Prostate Cancer with PSA and Other Tests).

After three properly performed biopsies, I recommend testing the PSA and free PSA every six months and doing a periodic digital rectal exam. I would only suggest another biopsy if any of the test results raised my level of suspicion.

NOTE: Though some people worry that a biopsy might spread cancer, there is no evidence that this is true with modern biopsy techniques.[15] With the old technique using large needles, cancer was sometimes spread along the needle track.

THE PATHOLOGY REPORT AND GLEASON GRADING

The standard report will include your diagnosis, a description of what was found on gross and microscopic inspection, and a summary comment about the findings.

Adenocarcinoma

Ninety-eight percent of prostate cancers are **adenocarcinomas**, from the Greek root *adeno,* meaning gland, and *carcinoma,* which describes a cancer that arises in epithelial cells, the biological equivalent of wrapping paper that covers or lines internal organs, including the skin. Prostate cancers develop in the lining cells of the ducts and glands that secrete seminal fluid. When these malignant cells are contained within the individual ducts and glands, they are called **high grade PIN (prostatic intraepithelial neoplasia)**.[16] Once they invade through the surrounding basement membranes, internal fences that separate the ducts and glands, they are considered to be invasive adenocarcinomas, commonly known as prostate cancers.

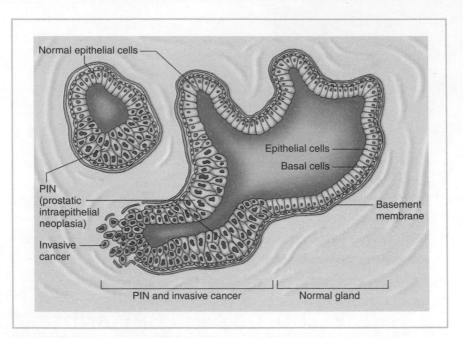

Microscopic view of a prostate gland showing normal cells and premalignant changes seen in high grade PIN, and cancer cells invading through the basement membrane.

Grade

The term **grade** refers to the degree to which cancer cells resemble the normal cells from which they arose. Low grade cancers are well-differentiated. Under the microscope, they look very much like their normal counterparts with many features of the normal cell still recognizable. Moderately differentiated, intermediate grade cancers still have some identifiable features, but they are more disrupted and disorganized than low grade cells. High grade, poorly differentiated cancers are wild and bear little, if any, semblance of their original form.[17] Compared to a box of berries, low grade cells would be pretty regular with some minor variations in shape and size; intermediate grade cells would have some fairly normal-looking elements and some that were crushed or distorted; and high grade cancer would be very irregular with some unusually large cells, some abnormally small, and many distorted by lumps or otherwise misshapen.

The concept of grade arose from looking at cancers under a microscope and recognizing that the more normal a cancer cell looks, the

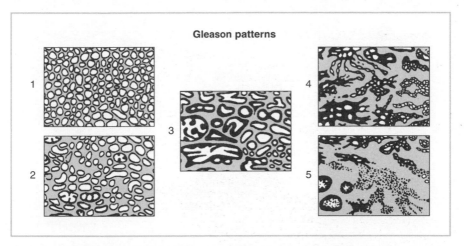

Gleason patterns

The microscopic appearance of prostate cancer typical of each Gleason pattern. Patterns 1 and 2 are well differentiated and closest to normal; pattern 3 (the most common) is moderately differentiated; and patterns 4 (the next most common) and 5 are poorly differentiated.*

slower it grows and the better it's likely to behave. Cancer cells with close to normal architecture pose less of a risk and are less likely to spread beyond the original organ than are higher grade cells. Wilder, stranger-looking cells are more likely to escape their local confines, set up camp in distant sites (metastasize), and prove lethal.

Gleason Grading

In prostate cancer we use the Gleason grading system as a simple means to characterize the seriousness of the cancer. The system is named after its inventor, a pathologist named Donald Gleason. After studying countless prostate cancers under a microscope, he devised a scale of patterns ranked from 1 to 5, where 1 is closest to normal glandular architecture and 5 is the wildest, most poorly differentiated, and highest grade.[18]

Gleason observed that the same man frequently had more than one malignant pattern within his biopsy sample. To reflect this, his grading system reports on the primary pattern plus a secondary pattern if it represents at least 5 percent of the cancer. The grades of the dominant and

---

*Source: Modified from Tannenbaum, Myron. *Urologic Pathology: The Prostate.* Philadelphia: Lea & Febiger, 1977. © 1977. Reprinted with permission from Lippincott Williams & Wilkins.

NOTE: Many experts today believe that patterns 1 and 2 may not be cancer at all, so it's rare to have a Gleason sum of less than $3 + 3 = 6$. If your biopsy report indicates that you have a Gleason 5 or lower, I'd be very wary. A review of your slides by a highly skilled pathologist may find that you don't have cancer at all, and you don't want to have treatment unnecessarily. Another possibility is that the first pathologist underestimated your Gleason sum, and a review will find that you have a higher-grade, more serious cancer.

secondary patterns are added together to yield the **Gleason sum**, **score**, or **grade**, which can range from 2 to 10. If there is no secondary pattern, the primary pattern is added to itself (e.g., $3 + 3 = 6$).

Gleason grouped his grades into 2 to 4 (well differentiated and highly favorable), 5 and 6 (moderately differentiated and highly curable), 7

NOTE: Analyzing biopsy slides is highly subjective. What appears to one pathologist to be a Gleason pattern 3 may strike another as a pattern 2 or 4. What one doctor considers normal tissue may be deemed cancer by a different pathologist. Sometimes a biopsy finding of cancer is reversed by a reviewing expert. Often, the doctor who first reviews the slides is not a prostate specialist at all.

For all these reasons, *I strongly urge you to have a second pathologist review your biopsy slides!* I advise against having this done by a different practitioner in the same office or department, because there may be pressure—no matter how subtle or subconscious—for colleagues to agree. To get the most valid second opinion, ask your diagnosing physician to send the slides to a recognized expert in the field. So-called "referee centers," such as the Armed Forces Institute of Pathology, Memorial Sloan-Kettering, or Johns Hopkins, have pathologists whose sole job is analyzing prostate tissue.[19] Make sure that all of your slides are sent and that you get a complete report of all findings.

(moderately to poorly differentiated), and 8 to 10 (poorly differentiated and likely to have spread beyond the gland). It is best to note the primary and secondary Gleason patterns separately, since the presence and amount of poorly differentiated pattern 4 or 5 cells tends to drive the behavior of the cancer. A Gleason 2 + 4 would cause more concern than a 3 + 3, even though both patients would have a Gleason score of 6. And a 4 + 2, where the predominant finding is poorly differentiated cancer, would be far more worrisome than a 2 + 4, with a smaller amount of high-risk cancer.

TIPS ON INTERPRETING YOUR BIOPSY RESULTS

After you've had your slides reviewed, be sure to ask whether there was any poorly differentiated component to your cancer. Generally, that would mean you have been assigned a Gleason score of 7, 8, 9, or 10, but sometimes less than 5 percent of what the pathologist sees is poorly differentiated, and that would not be included in your Gleason score.

If your cancer shows any pattern 4 or 5 cells, ask what percentage of the cancer this represented. Your doctor may report your grade as Gleason 3 + 4 for a sum of 7, indicating that more than 50 percent of your tumor was a pattern 3, but that does not tell you whether the pattern 4 cells constituted 49 percent or 6 percent of the remaining cancerous tissue. At the very least, if your grade is a Gleason 7, you'll want to know whether your biopsy findings were 4 + 3, which means that the dominant pattern was poorly differentiated, or 3 + 4, with a majority of more moderately differentiated cells.[20]

If all this seems unreasonably confusing, try to focus on the two critical issues in grading: *Was there any poorly differentiated cancer in your biopsy, and if so, how much?* A poorly differentiated cancer should be treated with all deliberate speed, not watched. While you should wait for the prostate to heal following a biopsy, aim to begin treatment within six to eight weeks after diagnosis.

At the time of your biopsy, the doctor probably took at least four, more commonly six, and quite possibly as many as twelve or fourteen sample cores from your prostate. The pathologist who read the slides reported on every core, whether it contained cancer, and if so, the nature and percentage of the primary and secondary Gleason patterns. You'll want to know these specific results. Cancers tend to behave according to their worst components. The presence of poorly differentiated cells suggests that a cancer is growing quickly. The more high grade cancer there is, the faster the tumor is likely to grow.[21]

HOW RELIABLE IS THE PATHOLOGY REPORT?

Most often, the Gleason grade of the cancer found in the biopsy cores accurately reflects the grade of all the cancer in the prostate. Nevertheless, in 30 percent of cases, the tumor will turn out to be higher grade than it appeared to be in the biopsy, and 5 percent of the time, the grade will be lower.[22] A biopsy session, even one where twelve or more cores are taken, randomly samples only a tiny fraction of prostate tissue, so complete accuracy can't be guaranteed. Sometimes we repeat a biopsy to

NOTE: Gleason grade is not the only important information you can get from a biopsy report. You should also ask whether there was any evidence of **perineural invasion (PNI)** (cancer in the prostatic nerves), which means that the cancer is more likely to penetrate through the capsule, escape the gland, and invade surrounding tissues.[23] Did the pathologist see cancer cells outside the prostate gland? Were cancer cells detected in the fatty tissue surrounding the gland (periprostatic fat)? If a biopsy was done of the seminal vesicles, was any cancer found there? If there is evidence that the cancer has spread beyond the prostate, standard local treatments may not be enough to arrest the disease.

learn more about the nature of the tumor. In about a third of cases, we find no cancer the second time, not because the cancer has disappeared but because the needle cores missed a small malignancy that was hit the first time.[24] Think of a biopsy as a good approximation, but not an exact replica of what is actually in the prostate gland.

RARE TYPES OF PROSTATE CANCER

NEUROENDOCRINE (SMALL-CELL) CARCINOMA

These extremely rare tumors are very aggressive. They grow rapidly and metastasize early. Small areas of neuroendocrine carcinoma can be found in many prostate cancers, especially large, poorly differentiated tumors with a high Gleason sum (8 or more), but these tiny findings do not have any special significance. However, when the predominant element is neuroendocrine, the prognosis is poor, and chemotherapy to shrink the tumor is generally the treatment of first choice.[25]

TRANSITIONAL CELL CARCINOMA

The prostatic ducts and the urethra running through the prostate are lined by the same cells as the bladder. A cancer arising in these lining cells can spread into the prostate. If you have this rare carcinoma, you'll need a thorough evaluation to determine where the cancer arose and whether it should be treated as a prostate cancer or a bladder cancer.

DUCTAL CARCINOMA

Adenocarcinomas that arise in or invade the ducts of the prostate have a characteristic appearance, are usually high grade, and have a worse prognosis, but are otherwise typical prostate cancers.[26]

Endometrial Carcinoma

Most of these unusual prostate cancers are moderately to poorly differentiated. Their treatment and prognosis are similar to other tumors of similar grade.

Other Rare Cancers of the Prostate

In a tiny fraction of cases, a biopsy of the prostate finds sarcomas, melanomas, or cancers that have spread from the kidney, bowel, stomach, or lung. Each case must be evaluated thoroughly to determine the appropriate treatment.

ASIDE FROM CANCER, WHAT OTHER IMPORTANT FINDINGS MIGHT THE PATHOLOGY REPORT CONTAIN?

Prostatitis

If the pathologist sees many white blood cells within the prostate tissue, he or she may report prostatitis. **Chronic prostatitis** indicates that the type of white blood cells found are typical of lasting inflammation, while **acute prostatitis** means the white cells are more likely due to recent infection. Such a finding does not necessarily mean that you have an infection, in fact. There seems to be little relationship between these microscopic observations and the troublesome symptoms of clinical prostatitis or chronic pelvic pain syndrome that lead men to seek medical treatment (see Chapter 4, Prostatitis). Some men simply have higher levels of white blood cells in their prostates, which tends to mean higher PSA levels, and thus these men are more likely to be referred for biopsy.

NOTE: Though prostatitis may cause an alarming increase in PSA, men with an active infection in the gland *should not* undergo a biopsy. Wait until you complete the course of antibiotics and your prostate has time to heal.

PROSTATIC INTRAEPITHELIAL NEOPLASIA (PIN)

Low grade PIN, also called mild dysplasia, indicates some small, insignificant changes in the cells. This has no clinical importance and does not lead to prostate cancer. Many pathologists have dropped the designation altogether.

With high grade PIN, on the other hand, the cells resemble cancers, except that the basement membrane, which functions like the skin around a grape, remains intact. (See page 162.)[27] There is no invasion of the abnormal cells into surrounding tissues, so we refer to this condition as carcinoma in situ (cancer cells that remain in their site of origin). High grade PIN is comparable to carcinoma in situ (intraepithelial neoplasia, or IEN) of the cervix or the breast. In those organs, fairly aggressive treatment of carcinoma in situ is common, but current thinking in the prostate field is that treatment would be overkill. Having high grade PIN *does not mean* you'll inevitably develop prostate cancer. We view it as an early forewarning, similar to an elevated PSA. Fifty percent of men with high grade PIN will be found to have prostate cancer on a subsequent biopsy over the next five years, and 85 percent of patients diagnosed with prostate cancer also have areas of high grade PIN. The overwhelming evidence is that most malignant lesions in the prostate start out as high grade PIN.

High grade PIN is a cancer precursor and calls for vigilant monitoring, but it is not a disease or pressing emergency. The condition *will not* suddenly develop into an aggressive cancer or metastasize. If your pathology report shows areas of high grade PIN but no cancer, your doctor may recommend a repeat systematic biopsy within a few months, depending on your particular situation. Your chances of eventually being diagnosed with cancer depend on your age, your family history of prostate cancer, your PSA level, and many other factors.[28]

ATYPICAL SMALL ACINAR PROLIFERATION (ASAP, ATYPIA)

The pathologist sees a cluster of cells with malignant features, but the suspect sample is too tiny or uncertain to warrant a cancer diagnosis. A finding of ASAP means you are at increased risk of having a cancer. A second pathologist's opinion is particularly important in these cases, and a repeat biopsy is in order if both doctors agree that the cells are atypical and suspicious. You should wait six weeks to three months until the effects of the previous biopsy have resolved. The repeat biopsy should pay special attention to the region of the prostate where the abnormal glands were found.[29]

ADENOSIS (ATYPICAL ADENOMATOUS HYPERPLASIA, AAH)

This is not cancer and does not suggest an increased cancer risk. An inexperienced pathologist might mistake this overgrowth of benign abnormal cells for a low Gleason score cancer of 3 + 3 or less.

THE FUTURE

A needle biopsy of the prostate is nobody's idea of fun, and the procedure can seem even more onerous for men who need to go through it several times. You may be wondering why we can't find a kinder, gentler way to diagnose prostate cancer without having to pierce the gland with needles. In fact, researchers are exploring possible alternatives to traditional biopsy that would enable us to do just that.

Semen contains thousands of prostate cells as well as a number of distinctive proteins that are secreted by the gland. One promising approach would be to examine the ejaculate or fluid expressed by prostate massage for the presence of malignant cells or specific proteins that might prove as useful in diagnosing cancer as a biopsy specimen. Some studies have focused on the levels of an enzyme called telomerase in prostatic fluid or semen. Telomerase—which is absent from normal adult cells—increases markedly in the presence of a cancer. If we can find ways to accurately test for this substance, we might have a viable alternative to biopsy for diagnosing prostate cancer.

Automated cytology (study of cells) or cytogenetics (study of genetic material in cells), which are now available in research labs, can examine cells for the presence of abnormalities. Once such technology comes into more common use, it's conceivable that patients might be able to submit semen samples for staining and processing, and labs could search for malignant cells or analyze the cells' genetic profile to determine whether they harbor a malignancy.

Though PSA is not reliable enough to use in diagnosing cancer, we may be able to use sophisticated techniques from the molecular biology lab to search for telling traces of prostate cells in the bloodstream. One such recently developed approach, which is tongue-twistingly referred to as reverse transcriptase-polymerase chain reaction (RT-PCR), seeks out cells that are never found in men with normal prostates or BPH. Someday their presence might prove to be a reliable way to detect cancer. In fact, it takes a reasonable-sized cancer—one that poses some real life-and-health risks—to shed such cells into the circulation. The RT-PCR test could prove to be the discriminator we've long been hoping for, capable of finding serious cancers while avoiding the over-detection of trivial cancers that don't pose any significant threat and do not need to be treated.[30]

IN SUMMARY

A biopsy is the only means we currently have to diagnose prostate cancer, but the test is far from foolproof. Be sure to have a second, independent expert pathologist review your results. Always request a complete pathology report, including information on what was found in every sample core and whether there was any finding of high grade, poorly differentiated cancer.

10

■

Understanding
Your Cancer

READ THIS CHAPTER TO LEARN:

- How do we determine the clinical stage of a cancer, and what
  does it mean?
- How can you better understand how serious your cancer is by
  factoring in all the diagnostic information?
- What are nomograms, and how can they help you decide
  what to do about your prostate cancer?

often wish that we could find a different name for a malignant tumor
in the prostate than **cancer**. Few words carry a more explosive emotional charge, and few medical conditions provoke such overwhelming
distress and anxiety. In the minds of many people, cancer spells doom—
end of story. But that's far from the actual fact.

While it is true that all cancers share risky features, including the potential to spread to surrounding tissues and distant sites, the course of the
disease varies tremendously from organ to organ and from case to case.

Some malignancies, including certain forms of leukemia and pancreatic cancers, are overwhelmingly destructive, often causing death within a matter of months. But, thankfully, we can diagnose, treat, and arrest many cancers before they have the chance to do any serious or lasting harm. Slow-growing tumors, especially in older patients with a short remaining life expectancy, may not warrant any treatment at all.

Given current diagnostic and therapeutic tools, a huge and growing number of people get through a bout with cancer and go on to live out a normal life span. In fact, there are currently over 10 million cancer survivors in the United States alone, and nearly 2 million of them have survived prostate cancer.[1]

The outlook for prostate cancer patients has improved dramatically in the past twenty-five years. Before the advent of PSA testing, many of these tumors went undiscovered until they were well beyond any hope of a cure. Today, thanks to greater awareness and widespread screening, the vast majority of cases are diagnosed while the tumor is still small, contained, and curable. Most prostate cancers grow slowly and aren't likely to cause any problems or symptoms for many years. Still, having treatment now may prove to be an important investment in your future. I think of it as similar to a retirement fund. If you don't plan ahead, you could find yourself with a serious, irremediable problem down the road.

That said, prostate cancer *is not* a medical crisis that requires immediate or emergency intervention. The wisest approach is to weigh your options carefully and commit to a therapeutic strategy within about three to six months after you're diagnosed. (The exception is men whose tumors are large and high grade. They should aim to begin treatment sooner, in six weeks to two months, allowing time after the biopsy for the prostate to heal.) That should give you ample time to gather the information you'll need to make an informed decision about what course of action would be best in your particular case.

THE "STAGE" OR EXTENT OF THE CANCER

Suppose you were awakened by a sound in the middle of the night. Before you leapt into full combat mode, you would be wise to take a moment to consider the source of the noise. It might be perfectly innocent: the dog knocking something over or a child padding into the kitchen for a midnight refrigerator raid. Maybe you come fully awake and remember that you have a friend visiting or that one of the kids was expected home late. Waiting a beat to figure out what's really going on can help you to respond rationally and avoid doing something you might regret.

The same holds true when the diagnosis is prostate cancer. To arrive at a sensible plan of action, you need to learn as much as possible about your disease. How large and extensive is your cancer? How dangerous and aggressive is it? What risk, if any, does it pose to your life and health?

Clinical **stage** refers to the size and extent of your tumor. How big is it, and how much of the gland does it occupy? In most cases, the estimate is based on your digital rectal exam.

WHAT CAN YOU LEARN FROM THE DRE RESULTS?

While it's standard practice to base clinical stage on the digital rectal exam alone, the test has serious limitations. A doctor can only examine the rear portion of the prostate that rests against the front rectal wall. Tumors in other areas of the gland will not be detected, nor will cancers that are too small to feel.

Still, it's important to know whether your doctor detected any suspicious lumps or nodules during your DRE. If so, request a written report including significant details. How large was the affected area? In what part of the prostate was it located? Does the doctor believe that the lump

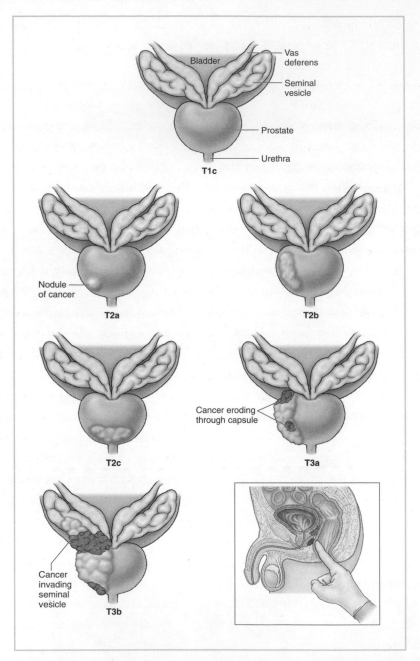

The TNM classification of prostate cancers is used to indicate the size and extent, or stage, of the cancer. "T" stands for "tumor," or the extent of the primary cancer in the prostate. Cancers are designated "T1" if they cannot be felt by DRE. T2 cancers are palpable but confined within the capsule of the prostate. T3 cancers extend through the capsule.

or nodule he felt was confined within the gland, or is there any reason to suspect that it may have escaped the prostate and spread?

It's useful to collect the results of all the DREs you've ever had. If you have been examined regularly, especially by the same physician, an abrupt change could signal that your tumor has suddenly become aggressive. On the other hand, if your last exam was a decade ago and your doctor finds a nodule now, it's impossible to know whether the tumor has been slowly, steadily increasing in size or has accelerated recently.

If more than one doctor examines you, be sure to note whether or not the DRE findings are consistent. It can happen that one physician feels a nodular thickening on the right base (top) of the prostate, while another reports an abnormality on the upper left. The DRE is a difficult test to learn, and accuracy depends on the doctor's sensitivity and training. Family doctors or internists who don't do these exams routinely often fail to pick up subtle abnormalities that an experienced urologist might detect. Findings are highly subjective, and even experts may disagree. Where results are discordant, I would rely on the opinion of the doctor who has the most experience in the field.

What is found on DRE should conform to what was seen on ultrasound during your biopsy. If the doctor felt something on the right base and that area appears abnormal on the ultrasound as well, I would have far more confidence that the results really reflect the cancer. I am less confident when the doctor feels something in the right base and that area appears normal on an MRI. In that case, I'd turn to the map of the cancer I can get from systematic biopsies to resolve the question (see page 179). If that still doesn't clear things up, a repeat biopsy may be required to determine exactly where the cancer is located and how large and serious it is.

WHAT OTHER TESTS CAN HELP TO CONFIRM THE TUMOR STAGE?

Generally speaking, your PSA reflects the volume of the tumor: larger cancer equals higher PSA. Since tumor size typically correlates with the seriousness of the disease, PSA provides a useful piece of the diagnostic puzzle.

As a rule, PSA levels lower than 2 are associated with a highly favorable outlook and a high probability that a cancer is contained in the prostate and curable with surgery or radiation. PSAs over 10 are progressively less favorable. The more elevated the level, the more likely the tumor is to spread.[2]

Interpreting PSA levels between 2 and 10 is tricky. Elevations in this range may stem from benign enlargement of the prostate, not prostate-cancer level.[3] As a result, it may not be so much worse to have a PSA level of 8 than 4, but a PSA level of 16 would be considerably worse than a level of 8.

Sophisticated imaging studies, along with a careful analysis of other test results, can shed additional light on the tumor's size and location. Though the prostate's particular anatomy and its obscure location deep in the pelvis make it difficult to visualize as clearly as we can a kidney or lung, dedicated prostate imaging specialists using state-of-the-art technology can make a valuable contribution to our understanding of a patient's particular disease.

Transrectal Ultrasound (TRUS)

Clinically significant prostate cancers respond differently to ultrasound waves than normal tissue does.[4] An expert can evaluate these visible areas of greater or lesser sound reflection to calculate where in the gland cancers lay and how big they are. Adding futuristic technology such as color Doppler effects (a name you may recognize from those vibrant weather maps on the Internet and TV) allows the imaging specialist to visualize the complex blood vessels that cancers require to grow.[5]

MAGNETIC RESONANCE IMAGING (MRI) WITH SPECTROSCOPY

This procedure, which measures the absorption and emission of light, is the best means we have today for looking at a cancer in the prostate.[6]

Diagram of the amount of cancer in systematic needle biopsy cores

Patient: Joe Smith (single, small cancer)

Part of the prostate	Left	Right
Apex	1 mm	
Middle		
Base		
Ruler 15mm	0 5 10 15	0 5 10 15

Patient: Bill Jones (large, multifocal cancer)

Part of the prostate	Left	Right
Apex	7 mm	5 mm
Middle	12 mm	
Base	9 mm	

Normal tissue   Cancer

Diagram used to represent the amount and location of cancer in systematic needle biopsy cores.

MRI wizards such as Dr. Hedvig Hricak at Memorial Sloan-Kettering, a radiologist who specializes in prostate imaging, can examine areas of the prostate that cannot be felt on DRE or seen on conventional imaging studies. The test also provides detail about the size and anatomy of the gland, which is useful in treatment planning.

Systematic Biopsy Results

We can use systematic biopsy results to create a virtual map of the tumor. If one core out of twelve or fourteen contains only a tiny amount of cancer, it's probable that we're dealing with small, early stage disease. On the other hand, if many of the biopsy samples turn up large amounts of malignant cells, the cancer has obviously progressed further, involving more of the gland and a greater risk of spread beyond its confines.

Mapping biopsy results is a simple matter of connecting the diagnostic dots. When a large percentage of several adjacent cores are positive for cancer, the tumor is likely to be large, bulky, and more serious. In contrast, if tiny clusters of malignant cells are scattered randomly throughout the gland, we're probably dealing with a number of smaller, less advanced, and lower-risk tumors.[7]

TNM STAGING

TNM Staging is the system most commonly used to stage all cancers (see the table on page 181). In addition to describing the extent of the primary or largest tumor (T stage), this approach notes whether a cancer has spread to lymph nodes (N stage) or if it has metastasized to distant organs (M stage).[8]

Stage T1 describes cancers that are either too small for the doctor to feel or located in the front (anterior) part of the gland, which cannot be reached during the digital rectal exam. Given early detection with PSA, this stage describes the majority of cases we diagnose today. Some prostate tumors are discovered incidentally when a pathologist examines

TNM STAGING SYSTEM FOR PROSTATE CANCER*	
STAGE	CHARACTERISTIC
T1	Can't be felt on DRE or seen by imaging
T1a	Incidental finding in <5% of tissue removed to treat BPH or bladder cancer
T1b	Incidental finding in >5% of tissue removed to treat BPH or bladder cancer
T1c	Tumor identified by needle biopsy, for any reason (e.g., elevated PSA level)
T2	Palpable or visible tumor, confined within the prostate
T2a	Less than half of one lobe
T2b	One lobe
T2c	Both lobes
T3	Tumor extends through the capsule
T3a	ECE, unilateral or bilateral
T3b	Seminal vesicle invasion
T4	Tumor is fixed or invades adjacent structures
T4a	Invades bladder neck, external sphincter, or rectum
T4b	Invades levator muscles or fixed to pelvic sidewalls
N0	No spread to regional lymph nodes
N1	Metastasis (spread) in a single lymph node, <2 cm in greatest dimension
N2	Metastasis in a single lymph node >2 cm but <5 cm, or in multiple lymph nodes, none >5 cm in greatest dimension
N3	Metastasis in a lymph node >5 cm in greatest dimension
M0	No distant metastasis
M1	Distant metastasis exists
M1a	Metastasis to lymph nodes beyond the prostate region
M1b	Bone metastasis
M1c	Metastasis to other sites

tissue that has been removed to treat the urinary obstruction caused by BPH. If less than 5 percent of the specimen is found to contain cancer, the clinical stage is set at T1a. When the cancer involves more than 5 percent of the excised overgrowth, the stage is reported as T1b. Clinical

*Source: Modified from Ohori, M., T. M. Wheeler, and P. T. Scardino. "The New American Joint Committee on Cancer and International Union Against Cancer TNM Classification of Prostate Cancer: Clinicopathologic Correlations." *Cancer* 74 (1994): 104–114. © 1994. Reprinted with permission from Wiley-Liss, Inc., a subsidiary of John Wiley & Sons, Inc.

stage T1c describes a tumor that cannot be felt on DRE but is discovered during a biopsy that was triggered by an elevated PSA.

If we feel a tumor on only one side of the gland, and it appears to be confined to the prostate, the clinical stage is T2a. A cancer involving both lobes but no evidence of spread beyond the gland is designated stage T2b. T3a cancers extend beyond the prostate's outer skin (capsule) on one or both sides, while T3b refers to tumors that have invaded the neighboring seminal vesicles. If the cancer has spread to other nearby structures such as the bladder neck, the external urinary sphincter, the rectum, or the pelvic wall, we classify it as stage T4 disease.

Where there is no evidence of lymph-node involvement, the node stage is recorded as N0. N1 refers to a cancer that has spread to nodes in the prostate area. The presence of cancer in lymph nodes can be determined by imaging studies such as CT scans or MRIs, but only if the nodes are enlarged. A negative CT or MRI is no guarantee that the nodes are not involved. These scans are not sensitive enough to detect tiny clusters of malignant cells in lymph nodes.

Stage M0 means there is no evidence of spread beyond the local area. If cancer is evident in lymph nodes beyond the pelvic region, we assign a stage of M1a. Where metastases to skeletal bones have been detected on a **bone scan**, the M stage is M1b. M1c describes spread to other distant sites such as the liver, lungs, or brain.

STAGE AND TREATMENT

Traditionally, clinical stage has dictated the kind of treatment we advise. Men with small, early stage TI or T2 cancers are seen as good candidates for curative radiation or surgery to remove the gland. Large, extensive T3b or T4 tumors are no longer curable with local therapy, so systemic treatments such as hormone therapy or chemotherapy would be more appropriate.

A major area of confusion and misunderstanding is what to do about T3a tumors, where the cancer has penetrated the capsule of the gland.

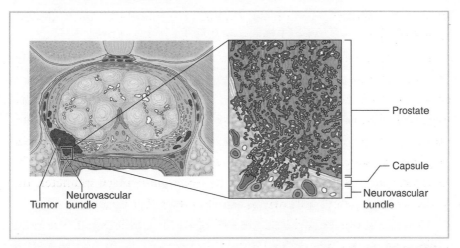

Extracapsular extension (ECE) of a prostate cancer refers to microscopic penetration through the capsule into the surrounding tissue. In most cases the cancer has not spread to distant sites and is still curable with surgery or radiation.

Extracapsular extension (ECE) means the disease is no longer organ-confined, but that *does not mean* it is no longer curable. Sticking your head out the window is not the same as leaving the house. You'd still be able to feel the air-conditioning and hear the radio, though you might have to turn both up to maintain the same effects.

In similar fashion, surgery or radiation can cure a tumor that has broken through the capsule of the gland, as long as it's contained in the local area. Radical prostatectomy can succeed as long as the surgeon operates widely enough to ensure that no cancer cells are left behind. Where there is extracapsular extension, we have to take extra care to remove sufficient tissue. If we leave cancer at the edge of what's removed (**positive surgical margins**), the risk of recurrence is far greater. Sometimes, getting safely around an area of ECE necessitates removing one or both erectile nerves, which can then be replaced with nerve grafts by a surgeon skilled in this procedure.

If radiation is the treatment choice, the area of ECE must be included in the target field. A careful assessment should be made of whether seed implants, which are normally recommended for only highly favorable cancers, are appropriate in this setting.

THE STAGING (PARTIN) TABLES

The **Partin tables** are mathematical models that predict what a pathologist would find if the prostate were surgically removed and examined under the microscope.[9] Pathological stage—the actual size and scope of the cancer—may turn out to be very different from the clinical stage we estimate from the DRE and other studies.

The Partin tables combine the Gleason grade, PSA, and T stage (based on the DRE) to assign a patient to one of four clinical states. Partin 1 is meant to suggest that the cancer is likely to be confined to the prostate (though this may not be the case); Partin 2 suggests that there has probably been extension of the tumor through the capsule of the gland but no seminal vesicle invasion or lymph node involvement has occurred; Partin 3 indicates that there is a high risk of seminal vesicle invasion, but no spread to lymph nodes; and Partin 4 describes a cancer that has probably metastasized to the lymph nodes or beyond.

Because they take several diagnostic factors into account, the Partin tables provide a more accurate estimate of the extent of the cancer than we can get from any single test result alone. They fail, however, to consider relevant data from imaging studies, systematic biopsy findings, the history of changes in the PSA, and the results of prior biopsies, all of which can give us an even clearer, more reliable picture.

Another limitation of the Partin tables is that many cancers fail to fit neatly into one of these categories. For example, a tumor may appear to be confined to the prostate despite the fact that some malignant cells we cannot detect have actually invaded the lymphatic system and spread to the lymph nodes. Though a man may have a favorable Partin score, local treatment with surgery or radiation would not cure the cancer in this case.

Partin tables can overgeneralize. For example, by clustering a broad range of PSA levels, the Partin tables suggest that a man with a PSA of 10.1 would have an equal risk that his cancer has spread to lymph nodes as would a man with a PSA of nearly 20. This is similar to suggesting that boxing any middleweight is the same, no matter if your opponent is at the very bottom or at the maximum for the weight class. In fact, higher PSA levels indicate an increased risk that cancer has spread beyond the prostate.[10]

Finally, the Partin tables predict mutually exclusive **disease states**. A patient expected to have extracapsular extension is placed in a different group from a man predicted to have seminal vesicle invasion, even though the latter would typically have ECE as well. Consequently, the risk of having extracapsular extension, which has important implications for treatment planning, can be underestimated by this system.

HOW IS STAGE DIFFERENT FROM PROGNOSIS?

Stage describes how large the cancer is and its location. But knowing the size of the enemy army, where the troops are encamped, and how much of your land they have infiltrated does not fully inform you about how fiercely they are going to fight or how likely they are to win the war. As a general rule, a larger, more extensive tumor poses a greater threat (as does a larger opposing army), but this is not universally true. What happens on the battlefield will ultimately depend on how well-armed, well-trained, deft, and determined the enemy forces prove to be, and how successful they are at defeating your efforts to thwart them. On the cancer front, some small prostate cancers are fiercely aggressive, while some large tumors, like slow, lumbering beasts, are not.

With cancer and other diseases, **prognosis** is an estimate of your outlook. How big a threat, if any, does the cancer pose to your long-term health and survival? Do you have a tumor that needs to be treated now, or can treatment be postponed until the cancer shows convincing signs of progression? How urgently should you begin therapy, and how forceful does your treatment need to be? What is the likelihood that any given treatment will cure or arrest the disease?

HOW AGGRESSIVE IS THE CANCER? THE GLEASON GRADE

Grade measures the cancer's aggressiveness and predicts how serious and dangerous it's likely to be. After your biopsy, a pathologist examines the sample cores that were taken under a microscope. Based on how closely the cancer cells resemble normal cells, each core is assigned a primary and secondary **Gleason pattern**. Those two patterns are then added together to arrive at your **Gleason sum**, **score**, or **grade** (for a full discussion of the Gleason grading system, see Chapter 9, Biopsy).

The more normal cancer cells appear to be, the more predictably and reasonably they behave. Poorly differentiated cancers with few remaining normal features are like wild animals that must be considered dangerous and erratic.

To gauge your prognosis, it's important to know the details of your Gleason grade. Like a rioting crowd, cancers tend to be driven by their worst elements. If your tumor has any poorly differentiated Gleason pattern 4 or 5 components, it will be more aggressive, grow more rapidly, and is more likely to spread.

If the pathologist reports any high grade cancer, be sure to find out how much. One tiny focus of poorly differentiated cells is far less ominous than biopsy results in which the predominant finding is high-risk Gleason pattern 4 or 5. Be sure to request a report of the Gleason grade of each biopsy core that was found to contain malignant disease. Having one core with a small amount of Gleason pattern 3 + 4 = 7 cancer is far less ominous than having multiple cores filled with Gleason grade 4 + 3 = 7.

PSA LEVEL AND PROGNOSIS

In addition to reflecting tumor size (volume) (see above), PSA can help us to understand how a cancer is likely to progress. A higher level carries a worse prognosis.[11] Faster increases in PSA (**PSA doubling time**, if they are genuine) indicate a more dangerous, aggressive tumor.[12]

Try to assemble every PSA you've had, going back to the very first time you were screened for prostate cancer. Given the long, slow evolution of this disease, we can learn far more from a historical time-lapse perspective than we can from a current snapshot. Even changes within so-called "normal" limits may be significant. Recent studies have shown that it's possible to observe telling changes in PSA ten, fifteen, or even twenty years before a man is diagnosed with prostate cancer.[13]

In evaluating PSA, it's important to focus on trends. Just as a one-day boost in the Dow Jones Industrial Average does not necessarily mean a bull market, a sudden spike in your PSA does not automatically spell serious trouble. Inflammation or any manipulation of the prostate, including a biopsy, can cause your level to soar. If your number has hovered in the 1 to 2 range over many years and it suddenly jumps to 6 or 26, something other than cancer is probably the cause. Retesting after a few weeks or months is certainly in order. This is true even after a biopsy has determined that you have prostate cancer. A follow-up test might confirm a lower PSA that is far more representative of the state of your disease.[14]

By looking at a series of PSA levels and their speed and direction of change, we can form reasonably valid opinions about which tumors are likely to be curable with local treatment and which will require systemic therapies, such as hormone ablation or chemotherapy. Still, though it can provide useful information, PSA is not a sure thing. It behaves more like a barometer reading, which may correlate strongly with the weather but certainly does not guarantee clear skies or rain.

To get the most accurate picture, you should continue monitoring your PSA until you begin treatment. Wait three to six weeks after the biopsy to be sure the inflammation has resolved, and then have your PSA tested periodically. Every six weeks is a reasonable interval to track changes, determine the true baseline, observe whether the cancer is growing slowly or quickly, and judge how great a risk there is of local or distant spread.

PSA DENSITY AND PROGNOSIS

To accurately interpret your PSA, you have to factor in the size of your prostate. A larger gland naturally produces more PSA, which registers as a higher number on the test. This does not suggest that any tumor present is likely to be large and aggressive. In fact, precisely the opposite is true. Our research has confirmed that the bigger the gland, the smaller and more favorable any cancers we find tend to be.[15]

A favorable ratio of PSA to prostate size is anything less than 1 to 10.[16] A 20-gram prostate can be expected to account for a PSA of up to 2. For a 100-gram prostate, the PSA would ideally be less than 10. Since most prostates in adult men weigh between 20 and 100 grams, much of the PSA between 2 and 10 may be due to benign enlargement of the gland (BPH). As a result, numbers in this range are less reliable in measuring the seriousness of a cancer than are numbers below 2 or above 10.

NOTE: PSA is far from a perfect measure. For one thing, cancer is not the only thing that causes PSA to rise. In addition to BPH, your level can be artificially elevated by inflammation, infection, vigorous manipulation, or a biopsy.

Also, while a higher PSA usually correlates with a larger, more aggressive cancer, there is an important exception. As malignant cells become wilder and more poorly differentiated, with a Gleason grade of $4 + 3 = 7$ or higher, they lose their capacity to behave like normal cells and may actually make less PSA per gram of tumor.[17]

Think of a factory where the machinery is neglected and gradually breaks down. As things deteriorate, fewer and fewer goods will roll off the line. In similar fashion, although a cancer may be far more advanced and dangerous, PSA output might be misleadingly low. Relying solely on your PSA to determine what is happening with a cancer could prove to be a serious mistake.

SHOULD YOU HAVE FURTHER TESTS TO TELL IF THE CANCER HAS SPREAD?

A prime worry with any cancer is whether the disease has spread. Many patients seek further testing in a quest for reassurance. It seems logical, in this age of futuristic scanning and imaging techniques, that there should be a way to determine the precise extent of your disease and predict its course with absolute certainty.

Unfortunately, there is no such crystal ball for prostate cancer. Scans that work well for other organs are unreliable in looking at the prostate. Results can be uncertain or yield false positives. The net effect may be to multiply your concerns unnecessarily. Worse, unclear findings might lead you down a treacherous path of ever more invasive and riskier diagnostic procedures.

To resolve this problem, the National Comprehensive Cancer Network (NCCN) has developed guidelines that patients and physicians can follow in deciding whether such tests are warranted.[18] These experts recommend that bone scans be reserved for men with stage T1 or T2 disease, who have a PSA greater than 10 or a Gleason grade of 8 or higher. Bone scans are also recommended for men with stage T3 or T4 disease, and for patients who have symptoms of advanced prostate cancer, such as bone pain. CT or MRI scans of the pelvis are seen as appropriate for all men with T3 or T4 disease, and for patients whose clinical stage is T1 or T2 if an analysis of their test results suggests a 20 percent probability of lymph-node involvement. To be absolutely safe, I'd advise that you have a CT scan or MRI to check your lymph nodes if the nomogram (see below) calculates that your risk of spread to the nodes is 10 percent or greater.

At Memorial Sloan-Kettering we've developed special mathematical models called **nomograms** to assess the risk that your disease would spread to lymph nodes.[19] Our entire suite of prostate nomograms is available at no charge. They're easy to use online at http://www.mskcc

.org/mskcc/html/10088.cfm. If you prefer, you can download them to a PDA that uses the Palm OS, or you can work them out in paper form. Input a few simple test results and you can get a much better notion of how serious your cancer appears to be. (See page 192 for more on nomograms.)

BONE SCAN

Since PSA screening came into wide use in the late '80s and we began to detect prostate cancer earlier and earlier, the value of a bone scan in most cases is highly questionable.

While it is common for advanced prostate cancer to spread to bones, it's very uncommon for cancer to register on a bone scan if the PSA is less than 20 and extremely rare with a PSA under 8.[20] Having a bone scan makes little sense unless you have a high risk of serious disease. Otherwise, you'd run a serious risk of false positives. Many things, including arthritis and old injuries, can register as suspicious on bone scans, especially to radiologists who are inexperienced in reading such scans. Making sure that such findings are benign requires further tests. While the bone scan itself is largely harmless and not invasive, follow-up studies to rule out metastases can be far riskier and more involved. Simple X-rays or even an MRI may not provide sufficient information. Even a bone biopsy, which can be difficult and painful, may not provide conclusive evidence of the presence or absence of cancer in the bone.

If your cancer puts you in the high-risk category for metastases (Gleason 8–10, PSA over 20, and stage T3 or greater), the test may provide some useful information for treatment planning and gives a baseline for comparison with future studies, but if that doesn't describe your situation, a bone scan offers little of value and has considerable potential to cause unnecessary problems.

CT Scan

The CT scan is not very good at detecting metastases or the presence of cancer in bone. Lymph nodes can only be seen on the scan if they are enlarged. Microscopic deposits of cancer cells won't show up at all.

Because of this general lack of sensitivity, CT scans have little use in the evaluation of prostate cancer, except for patients with aggressive disease and a high suspicion of lymph node involvement (see above).

Unless you are at high risk of having metastases, it's not worthwhile to have a CT scan to look for them.[21] The test is not totally harmless. It exposes you to radiation and to contrast agents, which, in rare cases, can cause serious allergic reactions.

TIPS ON INTERPRETING YOUR TEST RESULTS

In medical practice it's common to invoke general rules. Call the doctor if your fever hits 101 degrees. Have a flu shot if you're over 55. Start screening for colon cancer at age 50.

In similar fashion, it's neat, simple, and convenient to divide men with prostate cancer into risk groups. Low-risk disease is defined as a PSA under 10, a Gleason grade of 6 or less, and a stage T1 or T2a tumor. Intermediate-risk disease involves a PSA between 10 and 20, Gleason 7, and tumor stage T2b. A PSA over 20, Gleason grade of 8 to 10, and stage T3 or higher places a man in the high-risk group.[22]

Unfortunately, risk grouping carries risks of its own. Dealing with low-risk tumors is fairly straightforward. Very tiny cancers, which we refer to as indolent, might never cause any problems, especially in older men. The same is true for small, localized tumors with favorable characteristics (Gleason 6, PSA 10). Depending on a man's remaining life expectancy, it may be appropriate to monitor rather than treat the disease. If treatment is indicated, surgery or radiation would offer a high probability of cure. Seed implants, which are only appropriate for very favorable cancers, might be a reasonable treatment choice as well.

For men in the intermediate- and high-risk groups, the situation is much murkier. Someone with a small focus of Gleason $3 + 4 = 7$ cancer could be lumped as intermediate risk with patients who have extensive areas of pattern $4 + 3 = 7$ disease. Some patients whose numbers suggest high-risk cancer actually have a far more favorable prognosis when all of their diagnostic factors are considered. Risk groups do not provide us with the tools we need to make sound treatment decisions for an individual patient. What's right for men with similar test results might be completely the wrong approach for you.

NOMOGRAMS: THE KEY TO UNDERSTANDING YOUR RISK

Mathematical models that factor in all the relevant data are a much better way to gauge the current extent of your disease and what's likely to happen in the future. (See Chapter 12, Deciding How to Treat a Localized Prostate Cancer.) The Partin tables are staging nomograms. They predict how extensive your cancer would prove to be if the gland were examined after surgery. At Memorial Sloan-Kettering we've taken nomograms to the next level, developing models to predict the likelihood that your cancer will recur in the future if you opt for surgery, external beam therapy, or seed implants. You can find these online at http://www.mskcc.org/mskcc/html/10088.cfm.[23]

One of my patients with a Gleason sum of 8 despaired that his cancer must be incurable; but his PSA was only 4 and holding steady, and there was no clinical indication that the cancer had spread beyond the gland. Though the presence of poorly differentiated cancer cells was troubling, we were able to assess his chances of local cure using our nomogram. When all the diagnostic information was considered, his overall picture looked much brighter. With good modern surgery or radiation, he stood an excellent chance for a permanent cure.

IN SUMMARY

Prostate cancer is not a medical emergency. You can and should take time to size up your particular disease so you can make the soundest choice about treatment. To get the most accurate picture of what you're up against, consider all the relevant diagnostic factors. Mathematical models called nomograms can help you to evaluate the odds that you'll be cured with any given approach.

11

■

Understanding Yourself

READ THIS CHAPTER TO LEARN:

- Which emotional responses are common in prostate cancer patients and their partners?
- What can you do to cope with this disease effectively?

Few pieces of news are harder to hear than a cancer diagnosis. It's perfectly normal to feel angry, overwhelmed, disbelieving, horrified, or scared. People commonly equate cancer with a death sentence. On learning they have prostate cancer, many patients presume that what they need to do is get their affairs in order and await the worst. Even men who understand intellectually that prostate cancer is typically slow-growing and never an imminent threat often fear for their immediate survival. One patient described his initial shock and panic with poignant clarity: "Normally, I'm an optimist, but when I found out I had prostate cancer, I couldn't shake this image of an awful, gruesome death. I kept picturing crazy things like my bladder exploding. All I wanted to do was get this thing out—fast!" Another man recounted a similar sense of impending doom: "I started imagining that I might die of a heart attack or an accident first. I almost wanted those things to happen, so I wouldn't have to deal with this."

NORMAL STRESS
OR SERIOUS DISTRESS?

Denial is a protective response to highly disturbing news. Until we are psychologically prepared to confront an overwhelming reality, our minds try to blunt the situation with soothing doubts. How could I possibly be sick when I feel so well? Couldn't the pathologist be mistaken? What if my results were mixed up with someone else's? I bet I'll wake up tomorrow and find out this was all a bad dream.

Such thoughts help you to cope in the short run, but persistent denial poses a serious roadblock to rational decision making. Joe F., a 62-year-old commercial realtor, suffered from prolonged, paralyzing denial: "For almost a year, I honestly couldn't hear what the doctors were telling me. After every consultation, my wife would want to discuss whether I should choose surgery or radiation, and I'd argue that I didn't need treatment. I was fine. Nobody and nothing could get through to me. I was living in some sort of a bubble that protected me from what I couldn't face."

As denial yields to acceptance, men with prostate cancer must confront several disturbing unknowns. How serious is the tumor? What's the best way to treat it? What will it be like to go through surgery, radiation, or combination therapies? What's the chance that I'll have to deal with side effects like incontinence, impotence, or bowel problems? What, if anything, can be done about such things if they happen to me? How likely is my cancer to recur? What impact is all of this going to have on my life and my loved ones? "When I finally accepted that this was real, it was like opening Pandora's Box," Joe recalls. "I was so overwhelmed with the awful possibilities. I felt totally out of control."

This particular disease hits men right where they live. All approaches to treating prostate cancer, including watchful waiting, carry a risk of sexual dysfunction, urinary incontinence, and bowel problems. To some men this feels like a Hobson's choice—in other words, no real choice at all. Henry Ford famously declared that his 1914 Model T was available in any color, as long as it was black. As a prostate-cancer patient, you can elect surgery, brachytherapy, external beam radiation, combination treatments, or watchful waiting, as long as you accept that all of these involve some risk of harm to normal bodily functions.

Venturing into such alien, uncertain territory is bound to provoke anxiety, but the level of apprehension is highly individual. Your feelings might range from a mild undercurrent of edginess to unbearable, screaming-neon alarm. Anxiety can announce itself with physical symptoms, such as rapid heartbeat, tightness in the chest, shortness of breath, dizziness, stomachache, or the need to urinate with unusual frequency. Psychologically, extreme worry can leave you irritable, angry, or distractible. In severe cases of panic, you might feel as if you're losing touch with reality, having an out-of-body experience, going crazy, or even about to die. "I couldn't sleep, couldn't focus, couldn't function," Joe says. "I can't remember ever being so utterly lost and overwhelmed."

When you have a serious disease, some measure of anxiety is normal and possibly useful. There is some evidence that the accompanying jolt of extra adrenaline might enhance your mental or physical performance. But crushing or paralyzing anxiety is quite another story. If you suffer from overpowering fear, dwell obsessively on your disease, or feel the need to cling to others compulsively for reassurance, the problem is out of control and you should seek help (see page 201).

The same is true of depression. While sadness about being ill or grief over a possible loss of function is perfectly normal, having a disease should not throw your entire existence into total eclipse. Signs that your blue mood has crossed the line into major depression include severe lethargy, apathy, sudden changes in appetite or sleep patterns, or a loss of interest in things you previously found pleasurable. You might find it difficult to think, concentrate, or go about your normal routines. Severe depression can lead to suicidal thoughts or a preoccupation with death. "I had trouble with anxiety *and* depression," one patient explained. "When I first got the diagnosis, I honestly thought I'd sail through this thing with no problems at all. Instead, everything seemed worse than I expected. The slightest thing would set me off. I'd sink into a tailspin or fly off in a rage."

The stress of deciding what to do about your cancer can leave you feeling hopelessly ambivalent or utterly confused. Often there's no obvious best treatment choice with this disease. Experts and others may offer conflicting opinions, increasing your unease. Many men, in a quest to learn all they can and make the best decision, wind up suffering from information overload. They read everything they can find on the Internet, consult with everyone they can think of who might have any knowledge of this disease, and, unfortunately, wind up more uncertain than they were at the outset.

In times of extreme stress, some patients resort to self-medication with drugs or alcohol or become more deeply dependent on substances they already abuse. Such chemical coping can interfere with the clear thinking required to make a sensible treatment choice, alter the effectiveness of anesthetics and other medications, and stand in the way of an optimal recovery. If this applies to you, I urge you to seek help so you can develop other, healthier coping strategies (see page 201).

NOTE: It's very important to be honest with your doctor about any and all drugs you're taking, including the amount of alcohol you're drinking and any "recreational" drugs you use.

Many men find it difficult to discuss personal issues or admit to having emotional distress. Instead, they withdraw and let their feelings fester. If that describes your response to stressful situations, you might suffer a sense of isolation, and your close relationships may be placed under extra strain. "He keeps everything bottled up," one patient's wife said. "How can I help if he won't tell me what's going on?" Often, it's the partner who tells the physician that a patient is not coping well.

Men who are able to express what they're going through don't always get the desired response of support and understanding. Though we've come a long way, cancer still carries a degree of social stigma. Many people feel awkward around illness or are unclear about how to react. Such discomfort may be magnified when a patient expresses his own emotional problems in coping with the disease. At times, even the most well-intentioned comment can miss the mark and strike a raw sensitivity: "I love my sister, but she can drive me nuts," one patient told me. "In the car on the way to the hospital for my operation, she was still questioning why I wasn't getting seed implants. If seeds plus external radiation and hormones were good enough for Mayor Giuliani, why weren't they right for me? Though I was definitely not in the mood, I tried joking in the hopes that she'd give it up. I told her that particular combination therapy has only been proven effective on big-city politicians, but she just wouldn't stop. She had no idea how much I'd put into making this choice, how important it was for me to have my family's support."

Dr. Andrew Roth, a psychiatrist at Memorial Sloan-Kettering who specializes in treating patients with prostate cancer, says that many men he sees feel angry and betrayed. They've done everything right, watched their diet, exercised regularly, been religious about checking their PSA, and still their bodies had the audacity to develop this frightening disease.

Roth notes that for many men, the hardest part of having prostate cancer is a real or perceived loss of control. In dealing with the medical system, you may feel as if you're being forced to cede some of your power and autonomy to others. Specialists define what tests you should have and which therapeutic options are available to you. Those tests and treatments can involve embarrassing incursions into your intimate space. Prostate-cancer therapies can also make unwelcome demands on your time, not to mention your physical, financial, and emotional resources. "To me, having this disease was a major kick in the pants," one man confessed. "At work, I was accustomed to taking charge, putting my finger on a problem and finding the right solution. Suddenly, this cancer was at the very center of my world. Everything seemed to revolve around it, and I was stuck on the outside, looking in."

WHY IS PROSTATE CANCER PARTICULARLY STRESSFUL?

Many cultures prize stoicism, strength, and independence as the masculine ideal. From early childhood, boys are urged to avoid appearing needy or vulnerable. Those ingrained imperatives can be powerful enough to keep some men from seeking medical care, including potentially lifesaving checkups and tests.

The same masculine mystique can throw men diagnosed with an illness into serious conflict. They fear that being sick will mark them as weak. This can be especially true with a disease like prostate cancer that poses a threat to sexual potency and urinary continence. It's not unusual for prostate-cancer patients to expend a great deal of emotional capital on keeping their disease under wraps or agonizing over what might happen if they decided to disclose it. As one patient explained, "I couldn't stand the thought of people looking at me differently, feeling sorry for me. When I went for my radiation treatments, I'd put the newspaper over my face. I didn't want to see other patients or to have them see me."

Men often see prostate cancer as a direct assault on their virility. They worry about being able to perform sexually and satisfy their partner. They fear that they'll be diminished in the eyes of friends or colleagues. They are concerned about the effect this disease will have on their relationships, their earning capacity, their future plans. Men who are single or dating may feel particularly threatened by the potential loss of sexual function or fertility, and uncertain about whether, when, and how to discuss these issues with a potential new partner.

Prostate cancer often adds to the stress for older men, who are already burdened by ageist stereotypes and our society's obsession with eternal youth. The situation can seem even more intolerable if this is your first major run-in with illness. Living for many years without a serious disease can lull you into believing that you're going to dodge that bullet indefinitely. As one patient put it, "When the doctor said I had prostate cancer, I couldn't believe my ears. Suddenly, I felt like my own body—old faithful—was turning on me. It was as if all bets were off, and I couldn't count on anything anymore."

The average age at prostate cancer diagnosis is 69, a time when many men are grappling with major lifestyle changes such as retirement or the mounting independence of their grown children. Having this disease forces them to confront a possible reduction in sexual, urinary, and bowel functions as well. With advancing age, the risk of sexual and urinary side effects from prostate-cancer treatments increases. Though it's commonly believed, even among some health professionals, that older men are unconcerned about sexual decline, in fact, for many men it continues to matter a great deal.

Race can also pose a particular challenge. African-American men, who have the highest prostate-cancer incidence in the world, are far less likely than whites to undergo routine screening for this disease. For these men, cultural male values of strength and stoicism are often compounded by limited access to health care and inadequate awareness of their heightened vulnerability to this disease.

Sexual orientation may also increase the psychological burden. Many physicians lack awareness of the special sexual concerns of gay men with prostate cancer or feel uneasy addressing them. Some gay men find it difficult to be frank and open with their physicians as well. To make matters worse, prostate-cancer resources, including support groups, Web sites, articles, and books are overwhelmingly geared toward men in heterosexual relationships. Understandably, homosexual patients and their partners can feel excluded or poorly served. As one man put it, "The doctors simply had no idea about how all of this applied to me as a gay man. Here I was, struggling with what to do, and I had to explain things to them."

Being in a loving, supportive relationship can lessen the distress, but if the bond with your significant other is already frayed or tenuous, having a disease can make matters worse. Some shaky marriages crack under the strain of prostate-cancer diagnosis or treatment.

For many men with prostate cancer, PSA anxiety is the number-one source of emotional anguish.[1] They worry obsessively about their blood-test results, even to the point of needing sleeping aids or anti-anxiety medications. The slightest elevation in PSA level sends some patients spiraling into serious depression, though the result might be nothing more than normal variation or a laboratory error. Even in cases where a rising PSA signals that local treatment has failed to cure the disease, salvage treatments are sometimes effective, and therapies to control the cancer can keep most men active and symptom-free for many years, if not decades. Still, a morbid preoccupation with PSA can reduce a man's capacity to enjoy those years. "To me, waiting for PSA results is like hearing bullets flying overhead. You're constantly aware that the threat is out there, and you never know when you might get hit," one patient observed.

WAYS TO COPE

The National Comprehensive Cancer Network (NCCN) defines psychological distress as "an unpleasant experience of an emotional, psychological, social, or spiritual nature that interferes with the ability to cope with cancer treatment. It extends along a continuum, from common normal feelings of vulnerability, sadness, and fears to problems that are disabling, such as true depression, anxiety, panic, and feeling isolated or in a spiritual crisis."[2]

If having prostate cancer has tossed you into serious emotional turmoil, you're far from alone. Experts estimate that 25 percent of all cancer patients experience distress severe enough to interfere with their treatment, heighten the focus on physical symptoms, or hamper their recovery, and men with prostate cancer are no exception. In fact, at some prostate-cancer clinics, up to 31 percent of patients suffer sufficient psychological distress to warrant psychiatric evaluation. Anxiety accounts for the majority of these cases, with depression a close runner-up.

To manage the problem, the NCCN recommends that all cancer patients be screened to gauge their level of distress, followed by evaluation and treatment where appropriate. The call for universal screening acknowledges that doctors often believe that patients are faring better psychologically than they actually are. One study found that only 2 percent of cancer patients with serious psychological problems were referred for psychiatric evaluation. Other researchers found that oncologists missed signs of clinical depression in their patients more than half the time. Simple screening tests, readily available to medical personnel, such as the Hospital Anxiety and Depression Scale, the Distress Thermometer, or the Brief Symptom Inventory can signal that you might be in need of additional emotional support or the help of a mental-health professional.

If screening suggests that you're having significant coping problems, you should have a thorough evaluation to pinpoint the reason. The issue may be highly specific, like anxiety over losing time from work or difficulty arranging transportation to radiation treatments. In some instances, you might find that appropriate help is available within the cancer-treatment setting. Still, many patients, even those who are not having serious psychological problems, benefit from counseling or other forms of emotional support. Certainly, if you're having serious symptoms, such as disorientation or suicidal thoughts, you should seek psychiatric help without delay.

Depending on your individual needs and preferences, treatment might take the form of individual psychotherapy; group therapy; participation in support groups; complementary strategies to reduce mild to moderate anxiety, such as meditation, exercise, or massage; and/or medications to control psychiatric symptoms. Getting the right help can make all the difference in how well you'll fare in dealing with this disease.

For Joe, joining a local support group made all the difference. "It was such a relief to meet other men who'd been through this. Looking at them, I realized it was possible to have treatment and come out okay. Finally, I was able to face this thing with a clear head."[3]

MAKING WISE DECISIONS ABOUT TREATMENT

Try to identify and analyze emotional issues that may be driving your decision off the best possible course. Many men focus on one or two frightening things they've heard about treatment for prostate cancer. It may be impotence or incontinence or rectal bleeding or wound infection. Some patients are terrified of operations because someone close died unexpectedly after routine surgery, or they themselves had a difficult experience in the past. Others fear radiation because they heard a horror tale about a serious burn or saw something disturbing in a film.

There is an old dictum in psychiatry that the very thing you're most afraid to talk about may be the most crucial matter to discuss. This certainly holds true when deciding about prostate-cancer treatment, where your biggest fear might be a nonissue in your case or represent only a small, relatively insignificant piece of the puzzle. Perhaps in your mind "incontinence" evokes the specter of adult diapers or having to wear a catheter and leg bag, while the physician is actually referring to a slim possibility that you'll have some temporary, minor leakage that may require the use of a couple of small pads a day. Serious lasting incontinence is rare after prostate-cancer treatment, and even when problems persist, bulking injections or an artificial sphincter can typically restore urinary control (see Chapter 17, Urinary Side Effects).

While fear of erectile dysfunction is completely understandable, most men, given time, can enjoy a satisfying sex life following treatment. After nerve-sparing surgery, impotence is often transient. In many patients erections return after a few months, though others can take as long as three years to recover fully from the trauma radical prostatectomy inflicts on erectile nerves. Some men regain partial erections, which can be made fully functional with the aid of a pill like sildenafil or with penile injections or suppositories. Those who can't tolerate medications may achieve satisfactory erections using vacuum devices and penile rings that maintain rigidity. Where other methods fail, penile prostheses can restore function.

Unfortunately, some men reject such treatments, feeling that any erection that is not induced in the natural way is not okay with them. Worried about not being able to achieve satisfactory erections, they may avoid physical intimacy with their partners. This can place unnecessary strain on relationships.

"I realized that what I was terrified about, above all, was impotence,"

Joe said. "I thought having this cancer meant I'd never be able to have sex again. But then I talked to my doctor about what was likely to happen if I had my prostate removed. My tumor was small and nowhere near the erectile nerves, so they could almost certainly be spared. Since I was functioning well in that department before the operation, chances were I'd regain full or near normal function eventually. Regular arousal would help, and I certainly had no objection to that. Also, I found out that I'd have normal sensation in my penis and still be able to have orgasms, even though I wouldn't ejaculate. Suddenly, this didn't seem like such a major catastrophe after all."

Making a treatment choice for prostate cancer can resemble a game of chance. There is no crystal ball or absolute correct answer. You have to calculate probabilities, weigh risks against rewards, examine your risk tolerance, and, ultimately, go with your best instincts. However you decide to proceed involves some gamble. If you monitor the disease, you might miss the chance for a cure. If you treat it, you could suffer troubling side effects and require further treatment. You might choose surgery and afterward feel that radiation might have served you better, or vice versa. If you decide to start hormones early, you might later wish you'd waited. You might refuse systemic treatment and later wish you had not.

The fledgling field of medical informatics develops tools that are designed to optimize decision making and minimize regret. Instead of flying by the seat of your pants, you can use these tools to gauge the risks and benefits of treatment choices and get a clearer idea of your personal preferences.

An interesting and potentially illuminating informatics exercise challenges you to consider how large a risk you'd be willing to take to cure your disease, delay its progression, or avoid a certain side effect. The standard gamble asks the following: suppose there was a pill you could take tonight at bedtime that would make your prostate cancer disappear (or guarantee you would live an extra five years or that you would not be impotent), but there was a possibility that instead you would gently die in your sleep before morning.[4] Would you take that risk if your chance of death was 10 percent? How about 5 percent or 1 percent? Would you

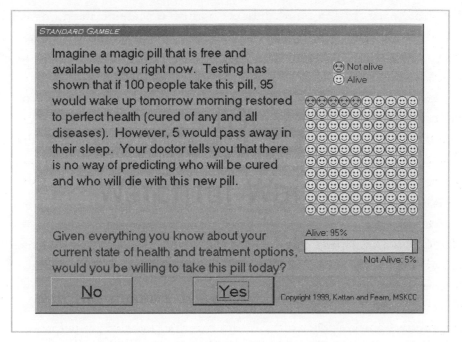

STANDARD GAMBLE

Imagine a magic pill that is free and available to you right now. Testing has shown that if 100 people take this pill, 95 would wake up tomorrow morning restored to perfect health (cured of any and all diseases). However, 5 would pass away in their sleep. Your doctor tells you that there is no way of predicting who will be cured and who will die with this new pill.

☹ Not alive
☺ Alive

Given everything you know about your current state of health and treatment options, would you be willing to take this pill today?

Alive: 95%

Not Alive: 5%

No   Yes   Copyright 1999, Kattan and Fearn, MSKCC

Screen shot of the standard gamble in computer form. The standard gamble is an exercise designed to help patients measure their tolerance for health-related risks.

risk treatment if instead of death, there was a chance you might go blind? By assessing how much you're willing to wager in order to avoid or achieve a given outcome, you can calculate how heavily specific factors are affecting your thinking or contributing to your psychological distress.

CONSIDERING YOUR PARTNER

Though you're the one who's been diagnosed with prostate cancer, the illness affects your loved ones, too. This is especially true of your significant other. Partners share the same worries. Can this illness be cured? What if it can't? What will treatment entail? How will he/I/we deal with side effects? What impact will all this have on our physical and emotional relationship? Our lifestyle? Our future?

Your partner's emotional distress could be as acute as yours, or even more so. In some ways it's easier to be squarely in the spotlight than waiting anxiously in the wings. You'll receive the care and attention. Your needs are far more likely to be noted and addressed. In stark contrast, your partner may be challenged to assume unaccustomed roles and responsibilities while subverting his or her own emotional needs.

Many men are uncomfortable expressing what they feel. If that describes you, be aware that bottled-up emotions can manifest in unfortunate ways. It's human to take out your fears and frustrations on the people you most love and trust. Unfortunately, this only magnifies their distress, while doing precious little to alleviate yours.

Millions of patients and their partners have weathered prostate cancer together and emerged with their relationships intact, or even strengthened. Other partnerships have unraveled. Based on numerous personal accounts, the key to success seems to be approaching this problem as a team, recognizing that you're in this together and that by pulling together, you'll have a far smoother, easier course.

STRATEGIES TO HELP YOU AND YOUR PARTNER TO COPE

WORK TOGETHER

Both of you should learn as much as is necessary to make rational decisions about this disease. Seek expert input together. Ask all the questions that are relevant to both of you. Do a comfortable amount of research, while avoiding information overload. Make sure you both understand the nature and possible consequences of the disease. Be sure to discuss your options as well as the pros and cons of each available approach with your partner before you settle on a treatment plan. "Once I read a few books and spent some time searching the Internet, I felt so much more on top of this thing," observed one patient's wife. "Once I calmed down a bit, he did, too."

Communicate

Tell your partner what's on your mind and encourage the same in return. Discussing sensitive issues like erectile dysfunction or incontinence can go a long way toward defusing such concerns. Explore together what can be done about sexual, urinary, or bowel side effects if they should happen to you. Keep in mind that prostate cancer treatment need not mean the end to pleasure, intimacy, or an active sex life. "I was afraid that I wouldn't know how to help him, and he was afraid that I wouldn't want to. When we finally got all that out in the open, I felt as if we'd come out from under a dark, giant cloud," one partner recalls.

Unspoken worries can loom larger than the ones you look hard in the eye. It's useful to discuss fears about survival or—from the partner's perspective—being left alone. It's positive to explore worries about what impact this disease and its aftermath could have on your relationship. If your foundation feels shaky or you think you might benefit from outside support, this is an excellent time to seek professional help.

Make Sure You're on the Same Page

Don't assume that you know what your partner wants or feels. One patient decided he was content with the size of his family and opted not to bank sperm before his radical prostatectomy. After the surgery, his wife admitted she regretted losing the possibility of having another child at some future time. "I should have told him how I felt, but I didn't want to make things even more difficult for him. Now it's too late," she says.

Take Appropriate Steps to Ease the Situation

Try not to take on too much. Get the rest and support you need. That goes for *both* you and partner. Don't be afraid to seek or accept help from friends, relatives, neighbors, colleagues, or professionals. Don't expect your partner to deftly take on responsibilities you may need to shelve for a time. If you normally pay the bills or cook dinner, maybe there's an alternative to asking your partner to take over if it feels too difficult. Watch for signs of serious anxiety or depression, and seek help if the situation seems out of control for either of you. Even if you're coping well, counseling or support groups may prove useful. There can be comfort in shared experience and in having a safe place to air difficult feelings.

REMEMBER, THIS IS TEMPORARY

Try to keep things in perspective. The trauma of diagnosis passes. The trials of decision making only continue for a short while. The rigors of treatment are temporary, and most side effects resolve on their own or can be overcome effectively. Chances are excellent that you will soon be able to put this disease behind you and get on with your lives.

IN SUMMARY

Dealing with prostate cancer can take a serious psychological toll on you and your partner. Getting the help you need will enable you to cope wisely and effectively with this disease.

12

■

Deciding How to Treat Localized Prostate Cancer

READ THIS CHAPTER TO LEARN:

- Which treatments are available, and what are the risks and benefits of each one?
- What factors should you consider in evaluating your treatment options?
- Is the type or quality of the treatment you get more important?

The patient, I'll call him Steve F., expected no problems when he went for his annual physical last year. Steve was 62, feeling fine, and his physical exams, including his DRE, had always been perfectly normal. When the doctor called a few days later to report that his PSA had risen from its usual low level to over 5, Steve was stunned. Still, he felt confident this had to be a false alarm. A close friend had recently been through just such an episode, and the cause had turned out to be a minor inflammation.

A few weeks later, when a biopsy found a Gleason 7 cancer on both sides of Steve's prostate, he was, in his words, "totally at sea." He and his wife spent well over an hour in the urologist's office, discussing his medical options. They talked about radiation, hormones, radical prostatectomy, and cryotherapy. But Steve had a hard time absorbing any of it.

The doctor explained the situation with the help of a brightly hued plastic model of the prostate. There it was—a small, irregular orb nestled deep in the pelvis amid a daunting tangle of erectile nerves, bladder, urinary sphincters, and bowel. In measured tones, he described Steve's prognosis. There was good news and worrisome news: Right now, the cancer appeared to be contained and curable, but, if left alone, it would eventually escape the prostate, spread to the hips and spine, and one day prove lethal. Suddenly, this obscure organ that Steve had barely ever given a passing thought loomed inside him like a ticking time bomb.

What I desperately wanted was the right answer—immediately! But the doctor refused to say, "This is what you should do." He told me there was no single correct response. He said I'd have to consider the possibilities and make the choice myself. So I talked to men I knew who'd had prostate cancer, did research online, read dozens of articles, and asked a doctor friend to help me interpret the medical jargon. I got tons of well-intentioned advice. But the more I found out, the more confused I felt. It took me weeks to reach the conclusion that in my case, surgery to remove the gland made the most sense. The surgeon could check my lymph nodes to tell whether the cancer had spread. If there was no spread, I had an excellent chance for a cure. And if I wasn't cured, I might have a second chance with radiation. Once I got past the initial terror, I was able to process what I'd learned and figure out the right way to go for me.

When it comes to prostate cancer, there is no magic bullet or sole acceptable response. To arrive at the action plan that's best for you, you have to balance the seriousness of your disease against the potential risks and benefits of available treatments.

For each man, the calculation is different. Prostate cancers vary enormously, as do the men who have the disease. Only you can decide what chances you're willing to take and which potential outcomes would have the greatest impact on your quality of life. Ultimately, the best measure of treatment success may be what is known as risk-adjusted quality of life. How long you live is important, but perhaps not as important as how long you live happily and well.[1]

Prostate cancer gives you the opportunity to make a deliberate, considered choice. In the overwhelming majority of cases, the disease is very slow-growing and is never a medical emergency. If you have a heart attack, medical personnel are trained to stabilize the situation quickly and then do what seems necessary to prevent or minimize damage. Some cancers grow with wildfire rapidity, and immediate intervention is essential. With prostate cancer, however, you have ample time to assess the situation, evaluate your particular needs and resources, and devise the most sensible, strategic plan of action.

When you're first diagnosed with a cancer, it's perfectly normal to be frightened and want to get rid of the tumor quickly, no matter the cost. But given the nature of this disease, you'll likely live with the consequences of your treatment decision for a long time. Taking some time to step back and think things through carefully is the best way to ensure that you will not be plagued by sorrowful regrets down the road.

You may be wondering why a doctor, the supposed expert in all this, can't simply make the decision for you. Some men view it as frustrating and immensely unfair to be burdened with such a difficult choice, especially at a time when they're feeling vulnerable, beleaguered, and scared. Unfortunately, medical science has no way to assess your very specific needs in all their striking complexity. Doctors can and should help you to understand the nuances of your medical situation, but only you can ultimately decide what trade-offs you can tolerate, what level of risk you find acceptable, and which potential sacrifices you're willing to make.

KEY FACTORS TO CONSIDER

How SERIOUS IS THE CANCER? This is a prime consideration. A high-risk, poorly differentiated tumor calls for faster, more aggressive intervention than does a small, moderately differentiated, or low-risk cancer.[2] Scientists in a major Swedish trial recently found that radical prostatectomy provided a clear advantage over watchful waiting in preventing metastatic spread, especially in men with localized tumors that were intermediate- or high grade.[3] Studies have also determined that **brachytherapy (seed implantation)** is less effective than surgery or external beam radiation for intermediate- (Gleason 7) or high-risk (Gleason 8 to 10) prostate cancers.[4]

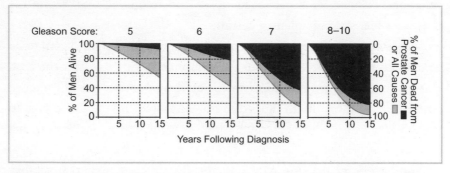

The lifetime risk of dying of prostate cancer versus some other cause, according to a man's age and Gleason score at the time of diagnosis, for men on a watchful waiting program.*

NOTE: In about a third of cases, the seriousness of prostate cancers is underestimated on biopsy. A tumor that appears to be a low-risk Gleason 6 or less turns out to be less favorable when a pathologist examines the prostate after it has been removed to treat the disease. Remember that a biopsy only samples a tiny amount of tissue. Prostate cancer tends to be multifocal, meaning it arises in several parts of the gland at once. Areas of aggressive, poorly differentiated cancer can be missed by a biopsy.

*Source: Modified from Albertsen, P. C., et al. "Competing Risk Analysis of Men Aged 55 to 74 Years at Diagnosis Managed Conservatively for Clinically Localized Prostate Cancer." *JAMA* 280, no. 11 (1998) : 975–980. © 1998, American Medical Association.

AGE (YEARS)	ALL MEN AND WOMEN	WHITE MEN	BLACK MEN
40	38.9	37.1	32.3
45	34.4	32.6	28.1
50	30.0	28.2	24.2
55	25.7	24.0	20.7
60	21.6	20.0	17.5
65	17.9	16.3	14.5
70	14.4	13.0	11.7
75	11.3	10.1	9.4
80	8.6	7.6	7.3
85	6.3	5.5	5.7

LIFE EXPECTANCY FOR MEN AGED 40 TO 85 YEARS (AVERAGE YEARS REMAINING)*

The risk posed by the cancer must be balanced against your life expectancy, which depends upon your age and state of health.[5] The shorter the time a patient has left to live, the less chance a tumor has to grow, spread, and cause harm. We rarely recommend a biopsy, much less treatment, for any man whose life expectancy is less than five years. Even a man who can be expected to live for a decade or more might reasonably elect to monitor, rather than treat, this disease, depending on how serious the cancer appears to be.

Calculating how this applies to you can be tricky. For one thing, no one likes to look his own mortality in the eye. Most people presume that they are going to live a long time, regardless of what the life expectancy tables suggest.

Such optimism is not necessarily unfounded. Expectations and outcomes are frequently at odds. Life expectancy tables are nothing more than statistical assessments of probability. They neither guarantee you a minimum number of years nor set a limit on your remaining lifetime. Many factors affect the estimate, including your general health, lifestyle, and family longevity, as well as a number of imponderables, including

---

*Source: Adapted from Arias, E. United States Life Tables, 2000. National Center for Health Statistics. National Vital Statistics Report, vol. 51, no. 3. 2002.

that most unscientific but undeniably key issue: luck. Despite a national median life expectancy for men in the United States of about 76, centenarians are one of the fastest-growing segments of our population, and an increasing number of the so-called "old old," over 75, remain capable of living vital, active, satisfying lives. Still, in consultation with your doctor, you should be able to make a reasonable assessment of whether active treatment in your particular case makes sense.

A key consideration is whether you have serious health issues other than prostate cancer, medically known as **comorbidities**. Depending on their severity, chronic problems with your heart, kidneys, liver, or other major organs can reduce your life expectancy by 20 percent or more. To gauge what this means in your case, your doctor can measure the current state of your health against a standardized comorbidity scale, such as the Charlson Comorbidity Index, the Cumulative Illness Rating Scale, or the Index of Coexisting Disease.[6]

The importance of having active treatment would be considerably different for a 70-year-old with serious medical conditions than for a healthy man of 50. Given a normal life span, the latter might be exposed to the risk of the cancer spreading over several decades. It seems a Faustian bargain to bet that you will die of something else before this disease causes severe problems. Whether putting off treatment is a smart bet or a sucker's gamble is a crucial piece of the decision you have to make.

Based on life expectancy tables and his excellent general health, Ralph R. realized that he was likely to live for another twenty years or more. "My prostate cancer was low-risk, with a Gleason 6, a PSA of 5.2, and only two biopsy cores positive, but I certainly didn't want to find myself dying of this disease with painful bone metastases at age 75. By taking a hard look at how long I was likely to live, I realized it was a pretty dumb idea to pass up treatment now that could get rid of this thing for good."

Once you've calculated the risk your disease poses, given your life expectancy, another important element to consider is:

HOW LIKELY IS YOUR CANCER TO METASTASIZE AND EVENTUALLY LEAD TO YOUR DEATH WITHOUT TREATMENT? If evidence points to a high probability that you would eventually suffer the bone pain and other symptoms of metastatic prostate cancer, treating the disease would make far more sense than watchful waiting.

If active treatment seems appropriate in your case, your next calculation should be to consider:

WHAT IS THE LIKELIHOOD THAT EACH AVAILABLE TREATMENT WOULD CURE YOUR CANCER? If your tumor extends beyond the prostate in a way that can be included in the radiation field, **external beam therapy** may offer you the best odds. On the other hand, a bulky tumor that's entirely contained within the gland may be difficult to irradiate successfully, and surgery might be preferable.

All medical treatments involve a mixed bag of effects and side effects. Before you settle on a course of action, it's wise to *consider both the potential short-term complications of the treatment and the risk it carries of long-term damage to urinary, sexual, and bowel function.*[7]

GENERAL GUIDELINES

Though we don't have definitive medical evidence yet, surgery to remove the prostate appears to confer a survival advantage in the long term (twenty, fifteen, or even as early as ten years after diagnosis). For this reason, radical prostatectomy is typically the preferred treatment choice for a young, healthy man in his 40s or 50s. Men over 70 are generally better served by radiation, though surgery may be a reasonable option for the occasional vigorous, healthy, older man with an aggressive cancer, who wants the tumor removed and accepts the increased risk of side effects that accompanies his age. For still older men in their late 70s or 80s, most doctors would advise watchful waiting or, if necessary, hormone therapy, though some healthy older men are reasonable candidates for external beam radiation or seed implants.

These general rules of thumb leave many men in a perplexing gray area. In the final analysis, some patients base their treatment choice on decidedly nonmedical issues, such as the amount of time they might lose from work or convenient access to specialists. Understandably, some men are mired in paralyzing confusion, unable to make a choice at all.

WHICH EXPERTS SHOULD YOU CONSULT?

One good way to resolve the treatment question is to seek opinions from doctors in different medical specialties. If the urologist who performed your biopsy and diagnosed your cancer recommended surgery, you may want to consult a medical oncologist or a radiation therapist, or even your primary care physician for another perspective (though keep in mind that not all doctors will have up-to-date, comprehensive knowledge of this complex disease). Most physicians are more than willing to help patients on a fact-finding mission. A doctor who is reluctant to cooperate with you as you seek further information is probably *not* someone you'd want to entrust with your care.

HOW TO EVALUATE EXPERT OPINIONS

Consider the advice you get in light of its source. Despite the best intentions, doctors tend to be biased in favor of what they do. As one patient advocate aptly observed, if you visit a Cadillac dealer, don't expect him to send you across the street to buy a Lincoln. In general, radiation therapists steer patients toward external beam therapy or seed implants, and surgeons advocate radical prostatectomy. Doctors who stake their professional futures and reputations on controversial treatments, such as cryotherapy or stringent diets, would be hard-pressed to recommend anything else.

Physicians are not immune from pressures that can cloud the purity of their advice. I'd be cautious about getting a second opinion from another doctor in the same office, who might be reluctant to contradict a colleague or close friend. Keep in mind that doctors in the same community may have social relationships or rely on one another for referrals. You might want to ask your doctor to disclose any financial relationship he has that might bias what he suggests. For example, does he own an interest in the brachytherapy center where you would have seed implants?

To get the most complete and balanced input, it's best to consult with unrelated specialists and challenge them to compare the advantages and disadvantages of available treatments in *your* case. Knowing that a given therapy leads to erectile dysfunction 30 percent of the time is not nearly as useful as finding out how that statistic is likely to apply to you. Your particular risk of losing erections may be dramatically higher or lower than average depending on your age, your level of sexual function before treatment, your anatomy, and the location and seriousness of your cancer.

Be sure to ask how likely each treatment is to eradicate your tumor, and seek a comparison of long-term results. For a typically slow-growing disease like prostate cancer, what happens in the short-term can be highly misleading. Virtually no one dies from this disease in the first five years after diagnosis. If we compared the death rate at five years for men who had surgery to that of those who ate spaghetti three times a week, pasta-eating would appear to be an equally effective treatment strategy.

Insist on scientific backup for claims that sound improbably optimistic

---

NOTE: Be careful about information you find on the Internet, where there is no control over what is posted and where many self-proclaimed "experts" are free to tout themselves, their practices, and their "miracle cures." You can find good information about studies, medical facilities, and other resources online, but healthy skepticism is in order. It's best to start with the most reliable sites (see the Resources section at the back of this book) such as the National Cancer Institute (www.nih.nci.gov), the American Cancer Society (www.cancer.org), the National Comprehensive Cancer Network (www.nccn.org), and the major NCI-designated cancer centers, such as Memorial Sloan-Kettering Cancer Center at the University of Texas, MD Anderson Cancer Center, and UCLA's Jonsson Comprehensive Cancer Center.

or simply too good to be true. Ask about the risks of immediate complications and long-term side effects that each option carries and what remedies are available for these problems, should they happen to you. I'd be wary of a specialist who offers you only one treatment choice and brushes off all the others. Such dogma ignores the enormous variability of this disease and the men who have it. Rarely is there only one rational way to go.

GETTING THE BEST ADVICE

QUESTIONS TO ASK, THINGS TO SAY, SAFEGUARDS

The answers you get can vary enormously, depending on the questions you pose. To elicit a doctor's most deeply felt conviction, try asking, "What would you do in my situation?" Or "What would you recommend to your brother or son?" Also, remember that a doctor's opinion is just that: an opinion. Often, it's based on his best judgment, not on proven medical facts.

LET THE DOCTOR KNOW WHAT'S ON YOUR MIND

It's important to be honest with your doctors and make them aware of central factors in your decision making. If fear of incontinence or impotence is driving your treatment choice, say so and challenge the doctor to put your mind at ease. If you have particular concerns about anesthesia, make sure you understand what kind the doctor prefers, the reasons for that preference, and what the alternatives might be in your case.

If a doctor fails to mention an issue that concerns you, don't hesitate to bring it up yourself. Physicians tend to focus on the questions they view as most medically significant, while patients understandably worry much more about possible effects of medical treatments on relationships, lifestyle, and career. Open dialogue is the best way to clear up troubling questions and get all the information you need.

THE X FACTOR

Some element of your response to a doctor and the advice he gives may have nothing to do with credentials, approaches, or results. A certain amount of gut instinct tends to factor into the mix. You may like the way a particular specialist smiles or answers questions or how much time she spends with you. Good chemistry is certainly a plus, but significant differences in medical expertise and experience should always take precedence over whether you happen to like a doctor or even know and trust her as a friend.

This is not to suggest that you should write off your instincts. Why would you put your trust in a doctor who is too arrogant, defensive, or dismissive to answer reasonable questions? The primary focus should be on you and your disease. You should feel that she's willing to put your best interests first and not be guided by issues of her own.

SECOND OPINIONS AND EXTRA EARS

A second opinion is always a good idea. If another doctor confirms what you've already heard, that's great. If the consultations are at odds, you'll want to ask more questions or seek someone in another specialty that can help you sort things out.

It's a good idea to bring your partner along when you meet with specialists. Prostate cancer affects you both, and so will the outcome and effects of treatment. Collaborating in the information-gathering and decision-making process is important. If you don't have a significant other, ask a trusted friend or relative to back you up. Negotiating the medical maze can be frightening and stressful, and a second pair of ears will help you to keep advice and information straight. You may also want to take notes or bring a tape recorder, so you can review the conversation and confirm that your impressions of what was said are correct.

DECISION-MAKING TOOLS

Medical recommendations boil down to simple predictions. When a doctor sets your fractured arm in a cast, she's predicting that that's the best way to promote healing and avoid long-term damage to the limb. When a physician advises increased exercise or a cholesterol-lowering drug, the guess is that these changes will reduce your risk of heart disease. Such estimates are based on current scientific understanding in the field. Emerging studies lead to constant shifts in our thinking and practice.

While a doctor may appear to pluck recommendations from thin air, in fact, deciding what to do in any given case for any given patient actually involves a multi-branched and often knotty decision tree (not to mention the occasional foray onto a shaky limb). The human organism and human diseases are extraordinarily complex, and many issues must be factored into a medical calculation. How old is the patient? What are his central values and concerns? What other medical conditions does he have? How aggressive is this particular cancer? How likely is it to spread over time, if left untreated? How successful is each available treatment likely to be in arresting this disease?[8]

USING NOMOGRAMS

More accurate predictions naturally lead to better decision making. But increasing accuracy is no simple feat. As Yogi Berra once famously opined, "It's hard to make predictions, especially about the future."

Nomograms are mathematical tools designed to predict medical outcomes (see Chapter 10, Understanding Your Cancer).[9] These graphic models can gauge your odds of disease progression or cure, depending on the treatment course you choose. One man electing to undergo radical prostatectomy might lower his ten-year risk of metastatic spread by 20 percent, while another patient could have a 25 percent better shot at a cure with hormones and radiation. Prostate-treatment nomograms can help you to answer crucial questions.[10] If your tumor is confined to the prostate and you choose watchful waiting, what is the risk that the cancer would spread in the next ten years? What are the chances that you have extracapsular extension (ECE) or seminal vesicle invasion (SVI)? How great a threat would there be of spread to the lymph nodes? How likely would your PSA be to rise within five years after radiation therapy, indicating that the cancer was not cured?[11] If you choose radical prostatectomy, what are the odds that you'd have a recurrence within five years?[12]

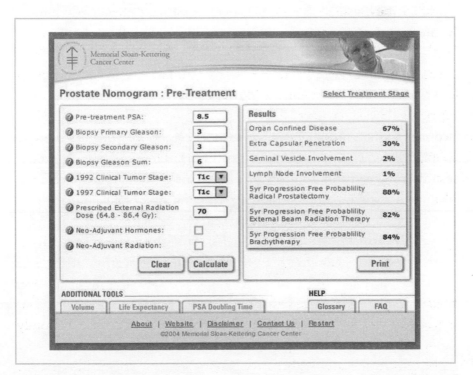

Screen shot of Memorial Sloan-Kettering nomogram Web site showing predicted pathological stage and prognosis for each treatment alternative. Note that five-year progression-free probability percentages are approximate and vary by plus or minus 10 percent.

By combining all your relevant diagnostic features and weighting them appropriately, nomograms offer more solid predictions than we could make by looking at specific factors like your PSA, clinical stage, general health, age, family history, or tumor grade alone. Nomograms also help us to avoid undue reliance on broad generalizations or such vague and often misleading categories as "risk groups."[13] You want to know what's likely to happen to you, not what generally happens to someone who— like you—has an intermediate- or high-risk cancer. Nuances of your diagnostic profile can make a tremendous difference in your prognosis. A man with a negative DRE, a small focus of cancer, and a PSA of 4 would have a far more favorable outlook than someone with a large, palpable nodule, extensive cancer on both sides of the gland, and a PSA of 12, even though both of these patients have been assigned a "high risk" Gleason grade of 8.

These nomograms can be used in paper form and can also be accessed online or downloaded to a PDA that uses the Palm OS operating system. You can find them at http://www.mskcc.org/mskcc/html/10088.cfm.

The Bottom Line

Nomograms are not intended to make a decision for you, and they are not infallible. The findings were based on limited numbers of centers and doctors, and validated on large, but not universally representative, groups of patients. Any particular prediction has a built-in error rate, usually plus or minus 10 percent, so differences of less than 10 percent between treatments may be meaningless. Still, these tools can be useful in the process of choosing between competing alternatives. If external beam therapy offers you a 20 percent long-term survival advantage over seed implants, you might well choose the former.

WHY THERE ARE FEW CLEAR ANSWERS: PROSTATE CANCER AND CLINICAL TRIALS

If you're grappling with the question of what to do about your prostate cancer, you may wonder why we don't have definitive studies that prove conclusively which treatment works best. It's tempting to imagine how much easier decision making would be if we had the results of head-to-head trials comparing surgery, brachytherapy, external beam radiation, and watchful waiting. You could simply weigh the survival benefits against the risks of side effects and choose the option that offered the most favorable odds.

In fact, it's unlikely that comprehensive treatment comparison studies will be done in the near future. One major obstacle is the staggering expense. A single trial comparing one of the four major approaches to another would cost about $100 million in 2004 dollars. Such trials would not lead to the development of a major new profitable drug for a pharmaceutical company to market, so there's no incentive for drug companies to sponsor them. The sole remaining funding source for an expense of this magnitude is the federal government, and, given the other stumbling blocks such a study would face, it's highly unlikely that our tax dollars will be committed to such a cause.

Even if we had the funding, finding men to take part in treatment comparison trials would be a major hurdle. Patients are typically willing to accept being randomly assigned to take one drug versus another (or a placebo), but ceding control about major treatments such as surgery versus radiation is quite another story. Multiple centers have tried to enroll patients in the SPIRIT (Surgical Prostatectomy versus Interstitial Radiation Intervention Trial) study, which proposes to randomly assign patients with favorable cancers (a PSA level less than 10 and a Gleason sum of 6 or lower) to radical prostatectomy or brachytherapy. To go forward, this trial must enroll 2,000 patients, but in the first full year of recruitment, only 30 men agreed to take part. Even if the investigators are successful in mustering the required 2,000 subjects, given the slow course of prostate cancers, it could take ten years or longer to determine whether one of these approaches offers a significant long-term survival advantage. At that point we would face yet another, and perhaps insurmountable, problem. Technology in prostate-cancer treatment changes constantly, but to yield valid results, the treatment protocol in a study must remain constant. By the time the SPIRIT trial reached a conclusion, state-of-the-art brachytherapy techniques and surgical procedures would be strikingly different from what they are today. The outcome of a trial using today's methods would not be all that relevant to a man's treatment choices a decade from now.

Another barrier to studies comparing prostate-cancer treatments is the large number of men that must be enrolled to yield meaningful results. Prostate cancer typically strikes older men, and, given the slow progress of the disease, many patients die of other causes before their prostate tumors prove lethal. A successful trial must follow enough men to demonstrate a significant survival benefit, as well as enough subjects to expose any significant problems that might arise from the treatment itself. After all, if you have a fatal complication from a treatment, you are just as dead as if you succumbed to the cancer. A clinical trial must demonstrate both effectiveness and safety.

Finally, one can argue, as we did during the Prostate Cancer Progress Review Group (PRG), which I cochaired at the National Cancer Institute in 1999, that the various treatment approaches all work reasonably well, and the differences between them are small enough to render these long, large, expensive studies unnecessary. This group of scientists and physicians concluded that we're better off expending our energy and resources to develop new curative treatments for advanced cancer and to identify better ways to characterize the cancers we diagnose, so we can tell which ones require active treatment and which need more than local therapy to offer a chance at a cure.

HOW TO COMPARE
THE TREATMENT OPTIONS

Watchful Waiting (expectant management, **active monitoring**, deferred therapy)

This treatment option involves no disruption in your normal activities and causes no immediate side effects. By opting for this approach, patients (especially older men who are in poor health) can avoid the complications of treatment for a disease that is unlikely to cause any problems in their remaining lifetime.

Is it for you? On the downside, you risk having the tumor spread while you're monitoring the disease. Vigilance cannot guarantee that we won't miss the window of opportunity for a cure. For young, healthy men, this is not a wise way to go. Many older men who might be well served by a wait-and-see approach can't bear the anxiety and opt to treat the cancer instead. (See Chapter 13, Watchful Waiting, for a full discussion.)

Brachytherapy (seeds, seed implants)

Logistically, this is the simplest of local treatment options. After a single treatment-planning session, the implant can often be done on an outpatient basis. Recovery is rapid, and men soon return to normal activities.

Is it for you? Brachytherapy is most appropriate for a very narrow spectrum of cases. Seed implants are not recommended for someone with a large prostate (over 50 grams) or a man with **obstructive voiding symptoms** such as hesitancy, intermittent stream, dribbling, decreased urinary flow rate, and straining to urinate. All of these indicate that the urinary channel is partially blocked, and swelling from the needles used to implant the radioactive seeds could shut down the flow altogether. Acute urinary retention requires emergency catheterization and often surgery to relieve the blockage.

A prior TURP (transurethural resection of the prostate) to alleviate the symptoms of benign prostate enlargement leaves you with inadequate tissue for proper seed placement and greatly increases the risk of incontinence after brachytherapy. If your prostate lies behind a high pubic bone, proper seed placement may be far more difficult or even impossible. Pretreatment tests can determine this and other significant aspects of your anatomy and disease.

Because they offer the least powerful form of cancer therapy, permanent iodine or palladium seed implants are only recommended for men with the most favorable, least risky tumors (a PSA level less than 10 and a Gleason sum of 6 or less, stage T2a or lower). The track record for long-term cancer control is not as good for brachytherapy as it is for good modern external beam radiation or radical prostatectomy. This is a particularly important consideration for young men who are likely to live for several decades, during which time their cancer could spread and cause serious harm.

While serious short-term side effects are minimal, seed implants can cause a variety of vexing problems in the long term. Brachytherapy results in more erectile dysfunction and more urinary side effects, though fewer bowel problems, than external beam radiation. Seed implants cause as much urinary and erectile dysfunction (ED) as surgery, though these side effects kick in and worsen over time with seeds as radiation damage accumulates, while they improve over time after radical prostatectomy as the trauma from surgery resolves.

Following brachytherapy, the PSA does not go to zero, and there's often a temporary, meaningless rise in PSA level, called a PSA bounce, which makes it difficult to diagnose recurrences promptly. By the time

NOTE: A temporary high-dose-rate implant (HDR) is sometimes recommended for men with aggressive, high-risk disease. This is a far more effective, aggressive therapy and should not be confused with permanent, low-dose iodine or palladium implants. (See Chapter 15, Radiation Therapy, for a full discussion.)

we are able to confirm that the cancer has started to grow again, the chance to cure the disease with salvage surgery might be lost.

External Beam Therapy

Radiation treatment with high-dose **3-D conformal radiation**—or, better yet, 3-D conformal therapy with IMRT—offers a good chance at a cure for localized cancer (see description of 3-D conformal radiation on page 302). Standard therapy using a conventional linear accelerator is far less successful at curing the disease and increases the probability that you'll develop serious urinary, sexual, and/or bowel problems. I don't recommend that you go this route. If you opt for external beam therapy, choose a center that offers a good, modern approach. (See Chapter 15, Radiation Therapy.)

Is it for you? Since this treatment involves about nine weeks of daily weekday therapy, the logistics can be difficult. If you don't live near a center that offers modern 3-D conformal radiation therapy, you might have to relocate for the duration or deal with a cumbersome daily commute to get the care that offers the best outcome with the lowest risk of side effects. On the other hand, if you have easy access to good modern radiation, the procedure involves little disruption to your normal schedule. Also, unlike surgery and seed implants, external beam radiation does not require anesthesia.

Though modern treatment has reduced the risks of serious side effects, any external beam treatment still carries some risk of bowel injury, urinary problems, and erectile dysfunction, all of which tend to worsen over time as the effects of radiation damage accumulate.

Because the urethra cannot be totally eliminated from the radiation field, men with obstructive voiding symptoms and those with large prostates would be at high risk for acute urinary retention (see description of brachytherapy on page 225). Since the rectal wall lies perilously close to the prostate, patients with colitis or inflammatory bowel disease may not be good candidates for radiation treatment. Prior radiation to the area for any reason probably means you've had your lifetime limit and you cannot be irradiated again.

After any form of radiation, patients may feel insecure about whether or not the cancer has been eradicated, since the prostate remains in place.

The PSA goes down but rarely becomes undetectable. As discussed above, there is often a bounce, or meaningless, transient rise in PSA, which can cause extreme anxiety or a critical delay in detecting a recurrence. (See Chapter 15, Radiation Therapy, for a full discussion.)

Radical Prostatectomy

With surgery, the PSA does go to zero, and recurrences can be detected early, but the treatment is disruptive. Patients lose time from work and require hospitalization and anesthesia, and full recovery can take several weeks or even months. Still, radical prostatectomy can offer a significant benefit in terms of peace of mind. Many men feel better knowing that their cancerous prostate is no longer in their body. Also, though surgery is the most difficult treatment in the short run, it offers excellent cancer control in the long term. For a young, healthy man, this is an especially important consideration.

While incontinence and erectile dysfunction are common right after surgery, only 1 to 2 percent of men operated on by top specialists still have any urinary control problems a year after the procedure. The average time before regaining partial erections is four months, and a return to full function generally takes a year or two, though recovery can continue for three years or even longer. For men who do not recover erections sufficient for intercourse, even with oral medications like sildenafil, several other therapies, including injections, suppositories, and penile implants, are available.

Is it for you? Radical prostatectomy is major surgery and carries all the attendant risks. If you have serious medical conditions aside from prostate cancer or have had serious adverse reactions to anesthesia in the past, you may not be a good surgical candidate. (See Chapter 14, Surgery, for a full discussion.)

HOW TO MAKE THE CHOICE

You are not simply a pile of reports or a collection of diagnostic numbers, and your situation, in all its complexity, is unique. Try to ignore

NOTE: *The quality of treatment may be more critical than which treatment you choose.* The success of all prostate-cancer therapies hinges on the expertise of the person delivering them and the quality of the technology and facilities available to that expert. If you can gain access to equally excellent surgeons and radiation programs, you should opt for the treatment that offers you the best chance for a long-term cure with the lowest risk of side effects. On the other hand, if you can get excellent brachytherapy but only mediocre surgery or external beam radiation, seed implants may well be your best option. Bad surgery may be worse than good radiation, even though good surgery might be better than good radiation for your particular tumor, or vice versa.

For cancer care in general, expertise can make an enormous difference in the outcome. More experienced hospitals and more experienced surgeons and radiation oncologists have fewer complications and better cure rates. *Always strive to put yourself in the best possible hands!*

ALSO: You want to be cared for by a busy, experienced doctor, but high volume alone does not guarantee optimal treatment. One highly disturbing study found that in some cases, doctors who did a procedure all the time continued to do it poorly.[14] The best defense is to seek a highly experienced expert with a wonderful reputation and an excellent track record.

both the grisly horror tales and the stellar success stories you're bound to hear. Avoid being seduced by what a celebrity does or what worked, or didn't work, for a friend or relative. Don't succumb to a compelling sales pitch or strong-arm tactics. Your best choice will be based on your particular medical situation, preferences, and concerns.

Three years after his radical prostatectomy, Steve F. is content with his choice. "If I had it to do over again, I would do the same thing," he says. "I'm back to functioning mostly as I was before. And I can't tell you how nice it is to speak of the cancer in the past tense."

IN SUMMARY

All treatments for prostate cancer carry a risk of side effects. To decide what's best for you, you have to weigh the risks and benefits of available options against the seriousness of your disease and several other factors, including your life expectancy, lifestyle, general health, and personal values. In the final analysis, the quality of the treatment you receive may be more important than which option you choose. Be sure you place yourself in the care of a highly experienced expert with an excellent track record!

13

◼

Watchful Waiting

READ THIS CHAPTER TO LEARN:

- What does it mean to monitor prostate cancer rather than treat it right away?
- Does this approach make sense for you?

Among the many long-standing questions and controversies surrounding prostate cancer is whether it makes sense to treat the disease at all. Those who argue against active intervention point to the fact that countless men have cancer cells or minuscule tumors in their prostate glands that would never cause problems or symptoms if left alone. For every man who dies of prostate cancer, four to five are diagnosed with the disease. For every man diagnosed, two or three others have some cancer cells in the gland that would never be detected unless their prostates were removed for some other reason, such as bladder cancer or benign prostate enlargement, and examined in the lab. Put another way, a 50-year-old man has a 16 percent chance of being diagnosed with prostate cancer in his remaining lifetime, but only a 3 to 4 percent risk of dying of the disease. Forty-two percent of men in their 70s have some tiny clusters of cancer cells in their prostates, though the vast majority will never be discovered, much less cause any problems or harm.[1]

Most prostate tumors grow very slowly. On average, it takes two years for a cancer in the prostate to double in size. That's two years to grow from two cells to four, and another two years for those four cells to become eight, which gives you a good idea of why these cancers can take decades to become detectable (though some develop at a far slower rate, and advanced, metastatic prostate cancers can double in as little as a month or two).[2] Often, the disease is diagnosed in older men who, as is commonly stated, are more likely to die *with* their prostate cancer than *of* it.

Unfortunately, it is difficult to predict with absolute certainty which cancers will remain small and harmless and which will spread, become incurable, and ultimately prove lethal, without active treatment. We don't want to hit a fly with a sledgehammer, but what if the insect that appears at first to be harmless turns out to be capable of delivering a deadly sting?

TRADITIONAL WATCHFUL WAITING

In the traditional sense, **watchful waiting** meant do nothing. Proponents claimed that it spared patients the side effects of needless treatment. They argued that men who left their prostate cancers alone lived as long and did as well as men who had radiation or surgery.[3]

Recent studies have proven that posture wrong for all but the most favorable, lowest-risk cancers. A landmark Swedish trial reported in 2002 clearly demonstrated that eight years after diagnosis, patients on traditional watchful waiting were twice as likely to have metastases as were men who'd had their prostates removed.[4] Ironically, this finding came out of the very country where traditional do-nothing watchful waiting had been most ardently and universally embraced. Some critics point out that the overall survival rate was no different at eight years between men who had surgery and those who had no treatment, but that observation is highly misleading. Because localized prostate cancer takes so long to

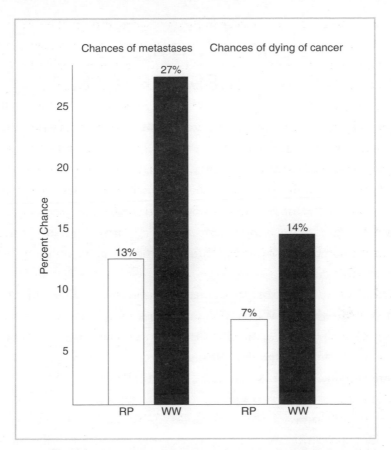

In a randomized clinical trial comparing radical prostatectomy (RP) to watchful waiting (WW) in Sweden, men who had their prostate surgically removed were much less likely to develop metastases or to die of their cancer.

progress, 90 percent of all men diagnosed with the disease survive for ten years regardless of what they do. Demonstrating that watchful waiting confers the same survival advantage as surgery or radiation at eight years after diagnosis is not meaningful. You could show a similar survival rate for men who played poker, watched football, or read *People* magazine.[5]

DO ALL MEN WITH PROSTATE CANCER NEED TREATMENT?

Historically, advocates of watchful waiting in lieu of surgery or radiation have based their argument on a lack of hard evidence that treating prostate cancer had any significant impact on the course of the disease. Fortunately, we now have good data to show that early intervention significantly lowers your risk of developing metastases or dying of prostate cancer. The groundbreaking Swedish study confirmed the superiority of radical prostatectomy over watchful waiting in preventing metastatic spread of this disease.

This *does not* mean that every man with prostate cancer should have immediate treatment. Watchful waiting goes by a number of aliases—deferred therapy, active monitoring, and expectant management—all designed to acknowledge that prostate cancers can change and that they require vigilance. Tumors that seem very nonthreatening when first detected may eventually turn aggressive and dangerous. Instead of deciding at the time of diagnosis that you will never have radiation or surgery, the right idea is to monitor the progress of the cancer carefully and start definitive treatment when and if it seems necessary.[6]

Why would a rational person go through a painstaking biopsy to find a cancer and then choose not to treat it? In fact, this often makes sense, and I've become a strong advocate of deferred therapy for many patients. Every once in a while—about 1 in 100 cases—we perform a radical prostatectomy and find no cancer in the prostate at all! Far more often—1 in 4 cases—the cancer turns out to be so tiny and insignificant when examined under the microscope that I question whether it was worth removing.[7]

With prostate-cancer screening so widespread, we are finding many cancers so small and so early in the course of the disease that they pose virtually no threat. In fact, the risks of treatment may far outstrip the risk posed by the disease.

Why then do most doctors recommend treatment for almost every-one—at least men younger than 75? Simple insecurity is part of the rea-son. It's impossible to be absolutely, unequivocally positive that any given cancer is insignificant in fact. When in doubt, most physicians prefer to treat rather than risk misdiagnosing aggressive disease.

Nevertheless, for many men, deferring therapy is a sound option. Monitoring rather than treating the disease certainly makes sense for pa-tients with a life expectancy of less than five years. I would find it diffi-cult to justify recommending aggressive intervention for an 80-year-old with other serious medical conditions, such as heart disease or diabetes. Chances are slim that the prostate cancer would cause any problems in his remaining lifetime. If symptoms arose, they could almost always be managed effectively with hormones.

On the other hand, few doctors would be comfortable deferring treatment for a healthy 50-year-old, in which even a small, highly favorable cancer might have thirty years or more to progress and become deadly. There is always some risk that the cancer will spread and become incur-able despite careful monitoring. When a young, healthy man insists on putting off treatment indefinitely, I'm reminded of a cartoon that shows someone who has jumped off the roof of a skyscraper. When he reaches the thirtieth floor, he's still smiling and feeling fine. The question is what happens later.

If you're between those age extremes, the decision about whether to opt for active intervention now or wait and monitor the situation closely may be much cloudier. Screening with PSA allows us to detect these cancers five to ten years earlier than was previously possible when diag-nosis relied on DRE or symptoms. In many cases, we find prostate can-cers twelve to eighteen years before they are likely to spread and become incurable. Men aged 60 to 75 who are diagnosed with a very tiny, early cancer could opt rationally to follow the disease for a while before decid-ing whether to have treatment. If the tumor is tiny and has very favor-able characteristics—I like to refer to these as **indolent cancers**[8]—it might take fifteen to twenty years to spread instead of the six to eight years it took for the more serious cancers studied in the Swedish trial to

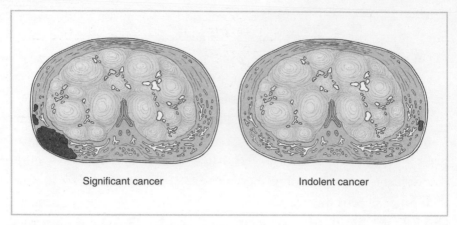

Significant cancer   Indolent cancer

Indolent cancers, which are much smaller than significant cancers, are confined within the prostate and contain no poorly differentiated (Gleason pattern 4 or 5) components.

progress.[9] Realistically, many men in this age group would die of other causes before their prostate cancers presented any problem. In the meantime, regularly monitoring changes in the PSA, free PSA, and DRE, along with periodic repeat biopsies, would usually give us ample warning that the cancer is beginning to change and that treatment should be started. But there's always the possibility, however small, that the disease will spread no matter how vigilantly we monitor it. Many men are unable to live with that uncertainty and opt for immediate treatment instead.

The general rule of thumb is that deferred treatment is a reasonable approach for someone whose remaining life expectancy is less than ten years, unless he has an aggressive cancer with a Gleason sum of 7 or above. But assessing how long you are likely to live is far from an exact science. A good starting point is the life expectancy tables available from the U.S. Vital Statistics Bureau or your life insurance company.[10] Most financial management software quickly calculates your life expectancy from your gender and your present age. Still, this is no more than a ballpark figure. The state of your health, family longevity, lifestyle, and several other factors can affect the number of remaining years you actually have. (See Chapter 12, Deciding How to Treat Localized Prostate Cancer.)

Many people think that having a life expectancy of less than ten years means there's no chance that you'll live longer, but the estimate actually

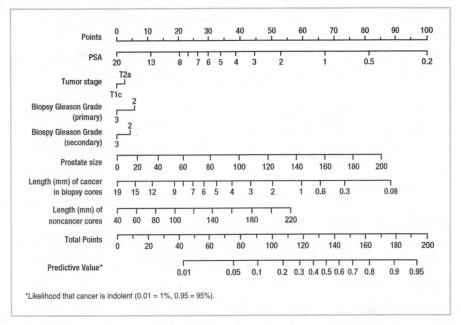

Nomogram to determine the likelihood that you have an indolent (tiny, insignificant) cancer. To use the nomogram, drop a line straight down from the "points" line to the value of each factor (PSA, tumor stage, etc.) to determine the points for each factor. Add the sum of points for each, then drop a line from the "Total Points" line to determine the "predictive value" or probability that the cancer is indolent.[†]

indicates a fifty/fifty chance that you will live that long. Some men in this group will die far sooner, and others will survive considerably longer.

Another factor in deciding whether or not to defer treatment is the size and seriousness of your tumor. A man in his mid-60s who has a favorable cancer (no palpable nodule, a PSA less than 10, and a Gleason sum of 6 or less in only one or two biopsy cores) may be as reasonable a candidate for deferred therapy as a patient in his mid-70s to 80s whose tumor is more aggressive.

Sixty-six-year-old Ray F., a Massachusetts importer, chose to monitor rather than treat his favorable tumor. "My business involves a lot of travel, and it would be difficult at this point to take time off. Also, I'm

[†]Source: Modified from Ohori, M. T., et al. "Counseling Men with Prostate Cancer (PCA): A Nomogram for Predicting the Presence of Indolent (Small, Well–Moderately Differentiated, Confined) Tumors." *Journal of Urology* 170, no. 5 (2003): 1792–1797. Reprinted with permission from Lippincott Williams & Wilkins.

hoping for advances in the field that may make treatment easier. I have a great doctor, and I'm confident waiting with him in my corner. But I must admit that living with a cancer in my body takes a psychological toll."

DEFERRED THERAPY
(ACTIVE MONITORING)

Watchful waiting, in the traditional do-nothing sense, has largely been abandoned in favor of deferred therapy, which calls for regular, rigorous monitoring. The protocol includes regular blood tests for PSA and free PSA, periodic digital rectal examinations, other imaging studies where indicated, and repeat biopsies.[11]

The prevailing current philosophy is to be on guard and prepared to intervene as soon as the disease shows any clear signs of progression. If the cancer proves to be more extensive or higher grade on a subsequent biopsy, if it is seen to grow on ultrasound or MRI, or felt to enlarge by DRE, it's time to begin treatment. Changes in PSA are harder to interpret. The PSA normally fluctuates day to day by as much as 36 percent,[12] so we have to see a steady, persistent rise, involving at least three consecutive new peaks, to be sure that a change is significant. The rate at which PSA level increases, expressed as **PSA doubling time**,[13] may give us some indication of what the tumor is doing, but a large Canadian study showed that this measure alone is far from completely reliable.[14] (The patients in the study were not monitored with regular, periodic prostate biopsies, which might have picked up signs of advanced disease. Some patients developed aggressive cancers or metastases despite a PSA that did not change at all or rose slowly.)

If your tumor appears to be small, confined to the prostate, and highly favorable (a PSA level of less than 10, nothing palpable on DRE, and only one or two biopsy cores positive with a Gleason sum of 6 or lower and no poorly differentiated Gleason pattern 4 or 5 cancers) and you opt to monitor rather than treat, a repeat biopsy is the next essential step. This should involve taking at least six, and preferably ten to four-

NOTE: Some tumors will grow, spread, and become incurable despite the most scrupulous, state-of-the-art monitoring. This is the major risk in deferred treatment: Once the horse is out of the barn, locking the door won't bring it back inside.

teen, sample cores. If this second biopsy shows a much more extensive tumor or any poorly differentiated Gleason pattern 4 or 5 cancer, treatment should not be delayed. On the other hand, if the second biopsy finds no cancer, as happens in 40 to 50 percent of cases, chances are much lower that the cancer will require treatment.[15] Because a biopsy samples only about 1 percent of prostate tissue, very tiny cancers may not be picked up. This does not mean that the gland is cancer-free, but generally a negative repeat biopsy indicates that the tumor is small and low risk. In fact, studies done at Memorial Sloan-Kettering have found that 85 percent of patients whose repeat biopsy was cancer-free showed no signs of disease progression within ten years.[16]

But hopefully ten years is not the rest of your life. Monitoring will have to continue as long as you are healthy and expected to live more than five years longer. There is always a risk that the cancer has been underestimated, even with a repeat biopsy. Despite our best vigilance, even two or three biopsies cannot provide an iron-clad guarantee that a tumor poses little risk and won't progress. Biopsies can miss signs of serious disease.

If you decide to continue on a deferred therapy protocol, you should be checked every three months in the first year with a digital rectal exam and a blood test to measure your PSA and free PSA and make sure the cancer is not growing rapidly. At one year, you should have imaging studies of the prostate with transrectal ultrasound or, better yet, an endorectal MRI. If the biopsy at one year shows no cancer or only a small amount of Gleason 3 + 3 or less, and there has been no change in the digital rectal exam or PSA level, patients are followed every six months with a DRE and PSA. The free PSA should be checked as well, and another biopsy done at the end of the second or third year. Assuming that everything remains stable, we continue to watch the PSA and free PSA levels and do a digital rectal examination every six months. At the end of five years, we do another set of biopsies and continue this program indefinitely, with six-month checkups and a biopsy every two to three years as long as your remaining life expectancy is greater than five years and active treatment would be realistic if we found evidence that the tumor was progressing.

The Advantages

The obvious advantage of deferring treatment is that you avoid the side effects of treating a cancer that currently poses little threat. For a man over 70, especially one with serious medical problems, or for a younger man with a very low-risk tumor, this may be a sound approach.

The Risks

Some men would like to believe that their cancer is static and never going to change, but, in fact, cancer cells are dynamic. They double periodically and grow exponentially, even though they may start as a tumor so tiny we refer to it as indolent or clinically insignificant. Like a hibernating bear, an indolent cancer is not dangerous, but, given enough time, hibernating bears and indolent cancers may awaken and bare their claws.

The question with any malignant tumor is not whether it will ever grow but when it will become incurable. Virtually all cancers large enough to be detected on biopsy constantly shed cells into the bloodstream and lymphatic system. Early on, these cells are like solitary scouts armed with meager provisions, setting off tentatively to explore the terrain. At this stage, they lack the capacity to establish a viable outpost in the bone marrow or lymph nodes and form metastases. But with time—like more knowledgeable, better-equipped scouting parties—cancer cells develop the ability to gain a foothold and flourish in distant sites. Once they're entrenched, they grow, causing serious symptoms and, ultimately, death.

By nature, cancer tends to be somewhat unpredictable, and we can't rely on it to behave in logical or linear ways. You probably remember the common math problem that goes like this: If a train leaving New York City heads west at 60 miles per hour, and another train leaving San Francisco heads east at 45 miles per hour, at what point will they pass each other? Imagine trying to answer that question without knowing how fast the trains were traveling or whether their speeds would remain constant. In similar fashion, cancer sometimes defies our most cautious expectations.

Deferring treatment poses other risks as well. If the tumor grows larger or invades adjacent structures, a wider operation or higher dose radiation and hormone treatment may be required to stop it. You would face an increased likelihood of serious side effects for treatments that are less likely to cure your disease. At Memorial Sloan-Kettering, we followed a group of eighty-eight patients on watchful waiting[17] and found that, on average, the probability that their cancers would remain curable was reduced by about 1 percent per year. Results varied widely. Some men showed no change at all, while others lost as much as 3 to 4 percent for every year they deferred treatment. Put another way, if you are 50 and decide to monitor rather than have treatment, your chance of a cure will likely go down by about 10 percent by age 60.

While you are monitoring the disease, a change in your health could limit your treatment options. If your prostate enlarges, radiation can pose greater risks. If you develop diabetes or heart disease, you may no longer be a good candidate for surgery. Even if your health remains the same, aging alone can diminish your tolerance for treatment and increase the risk and severity of side effects.

Over time, there is a tendency to let down your guard. If you go for six to eight years with no signs that the cancer has spread, it's easy to lose sight of the fact that the tumor continues to double in size, no matter how slowly, and may eventually progress out of control.[18] The best candidates for deferred therapy are those men whose age, health, and tumor characteristics suggest that they will never need treatment.

CAN DIET AND SUPPLEMENTS STOP PROSTATE CANCER?

While deferred therapy is a logical choice for the right patients, many men with potentially dangerous cancers shun proven therapies in fear of side effects and instead turn to diet, supplements, mind/body work, or alternative medicine. It's tempting to imagine that by maintaining a healthy lifestyle or following an ascetic regime, we can alter the course of this disease.

Unfortunately, though there are some factors that show promise as possibly preventing prostate cancer, such as a low-fat diet, an active exercise program, and supplements such as selenium, vitamin E, lycopene, soy, and related substances, none of these has a demonstrated ability to change the course of this disease once it has been established.

In a recent large study of men with colon polyps, strict adherence to a low-fat, high-fiber diet had no effect on recurrence of the polyps and no impact on PSA levels, which were also monitored during the five-year trial.[19] Dietary effects on developing cancers are probably exerted over many, many years. Once a man has been diagnosed with prostate cancer, nothing short of active treatment with surgery or radiation will make it go away.

While some supplements and herbal remedies do lower PSA levels, not one has been shown to eliminate cancer. Powerful hormone therapy that shuts down and blocks male hormones drops the PSA to undetectable levels, but it cannot get rid of a cancer completely.

DO ANY OF THE "MIRACLE" PROSTATE CANCER CURES REALLY WORK?

When it comes to prostate cancer, claims for curative miracles abound. A brief Internet search will unearth numerous extravagant, unproven, and often absurd claims that everything from diet to self-hypnosis, taking performance-boosting hormones, or even drinking one's own urine can arrest, shrink, or eradicate an established prostate cancer.

During more than three decades of reading the literature, conferring with colleagues, and practicing in the field, I have never heard of a single case in which a prostate cancer disappeared spontaneously. Though rare, instances of malignancies vanishing without treatment have been reported with certain other cancers, such as melanomas and kidney cancers, which are highly vulnerable to the body's own immune response.

Once you have been diagnosed with a clinically significant prostate cancer, only radiation therapy or surgery to remove the gland holds the hope of a cure. While it's true that not every prostate cancer warrants active intervention—especially tiny cancers in older men—you would do yourself a far better service to evaluate and weigh your options carefully with established experts than to put your faith in people who prey on men's fears and profit from the sale of empty promises.

THE FEAR·FACTOR

I have had patients say that they would rather risk death from their cancer than the loss of erections or urinary control that sometimes results from surgery or the bowel, urinary, or sexual complications of radiation—even though these side effects only affect a fraction of patients, are often temporary, and are generally treatable when they do occur. When a cancer is small and poses little danger, deferring treatment may be the best response. In the face of a life-threatening cancer, fear of side effects can be paralyzing and stand in the way of a rational choice.

If concerns about side effects are behind your decision to defer treatment, keep in mind that incurable prostate cancer causes considerable side effects of its own. **Hormone therapy**, which we use to alleviate symptoms of advanced disease, can cause a loss of erections, libido, body hair, and muscle mass as well as osteoporosis, hot flashes, breast enlargement, and depression. As it progresses, the cancer itself can lead to erectile dysfunction and serious urinary problems, not to mention severe bone pain, a host of other systemic problems from metastases, and, eventually, death.

WHY SOME MEN SWITCH FROM ACTIVE MONITORING TO TREATMENT

In our study of eighty-eight men who started on a deferred therapy program, about 10 percent per year dropped out and sought treatment during the first five years, even though some of the tumors showed no sign of growth. These men simply found the anxiety of living with a cancer intolerable.[20]

About one-third of the men showed signs that the cancer was changing for the worse and were referred for surgery or radiation therapy. Still, though two-thirds could have continued to monitor their disease, almost half of the patients decided to have their cancers treated within the first five years.[21] Several other studies, enrolling hundreds of patients, have shown similar rates of change from expectant to active treatment.[22]

Our study has now followed these patients for ten years. Two-thirds of the men have switched to active treatment, despite the fact that many of their cancers showed no signs of progressing. To date, all of those who were eventually treated with radical prostatectomy remain cancer-free. No patient has yet developed metastases or died of prostate cancer. More studies are needed to document what happens in the longer term, since the risk of developing metastases increases over time for patients who defer treatment.

THE FUTURE

To help men make wise choices about active monitoring versus deferred treatment, we need more accurate ways to size up prostate cancers and separate the tigers from the pussycats. In one highly promising approach, scientists are studying the activity patterns of thousands of genes in minute biopsy specimens. Someday, analysis of these "high throughput DNA arrays" may enable us to predict the behavior of individual prostate cancers with far greater certainty. Researchers are also exploring protein patterns in the blood or tissue (proteomics) and analyzing cancer cells circulating in the bloodstream to develop a means of predicting which cancers pose a serious threat.

Another investigational focus is on better imaging. In the future, optical imaging, or "Micro" PET (positron emission tomography) images, fused with MRI may be able to measure small cancers and chart their growth rate, as we can do now for lung cancers.

Finally, some chemical cousins of PSA appear to change ten to twenty years before tumors become biologically active and start to grow quickly. Studies are in progress to isolate and examine these factors. Someday we hope to have a constellation of serum markers that we can track through a simple blood test. This would provide a crucial early-warning system so we'll know which men can safely continue to defer treatment and which should switch to active intervention while we can still cure the disease. Especially promising is a recently developed test, reverse transcription–polymerase chain reaction (RT-PCR), which can pick up tiny clusters of cancer cells circulating in the blood. RT-PCR may be able to alert us to the presence of cancers far earlier than we can detect them now.

IN SUMMARY

For many men, especially those with tiny indolent cancers and a short life expectancy, carefully monitoring prostate cancer rather than treating it makes sense. Nevertheless, living with the anxiety of having an untreated cancer often leads patients to seek active treatment. Also, no matter how cautious and vigilant we may be, there is no guarantee that the disease won't progress while we're monitoring it.

14

■

Surgery

READ THIS CHAPTER TO LEARN:

• Does surgery to remove the gland make sense for you?
• How has radical prostatectomy changed, and which type of procedure should you seek?
• How can you choose the best surgeon?

Given widespread screening with the PSA test, we now detect most prostate cancers while they are still small, contained, and highly curable. When we find those cancers in healthy men who have many years of life ahead of them, surgery is an excellent way to be rid of the cancer for good.

In fact, when performed by a skilled, experienced urologic surgeon using modern techniques, surgical removal of the entire prostate may offer the *best* chance for a permanent cure. Surgical failures usually result because a cancer we had thought curable actually was not—tiny imperceptible metastases in distant sites already existed at the time the prostate was removed, so an operation could not arrest the disease. Recurrences in such cases tend to show up in the first several years after radical prosta-tectomy. In my experience, if PSA remains undetectable in your blood-stream for five to seven years after surgery, the chance that you'll ever have metastases is remote. This is an especially important consideration for young men, whose tumors—if not cured—have many years to spread and become deadly.

Surgical treatment for prostate cancer entails complete (radical) exci-sion of the gland (prostatectomy). During a **radical prostatectomy**, we also take out surrounding tissue, including the seminal vesicles. Removing only the tumor, a common practice in breast cancer, is not an option, for several important reasons. Prostate cancer tends to be multifocal, meaning it arises in several areas at once. A pathologist examining a cancerous prostate after surgery will find an average of five to six separate malignan-cies, distributed in an unpredictable pattern throughout the gland.

Modern diagnostic tests are not accurate enough to determine pre-cisely where these tumors lie. Most are too small to feel on digital rectal examination, and they may not be discovered on biopsy, which only samples a tiny fraction of prostate tissue. Even modern imaging tools, like color Doppler ultrasound or MRI with spectroscopy cannot detect a malignant tumor within the prostate in the way that a mammogram can pinpoint a cancer in the breast or a CT scan can localize a lung tu-mor whereby the surgeon knows exactly what to target and remove.

Even if we were able to identify and remove the major focus of can-cer in the prostate, the other small tumors would eventually grow and spread. While tumor size does correlate with the seriousness of a cancer[1]—i.e., the bigger the cancer, the worse it behaves—the relationship is far from perfect.[2] Ironically, some large prostate tumors are relatively slow-growing with little capacity to metastasize, while a much smaller malig-nancy can be aggressive and pose a real threat of lethal spread.[3] At this point, we have no way to determine precisely how many small cancers there are in a man's prostate. We can't predict with certainty which of them would turn out to be harmless if left alone and which might even-tually prove deadly, even if we deployed the mightiest medical and sur-gical weapons in our arsenal against them.

Given the location of the prostate deep in the pelvis, any attempt to remove the obvious cancer without excising the entire gland would still risk serious complications—including heavy bleeding, damage to erectile nerves, and acute urinary retention. Basically, you'd risk the side effects of prostatectomy without reaping any of the benefits. If we are going to operate, removing the entire prostate is the only logical approach.

For many men, radical prostatectomy is a safe and highly effective treatment choice. If you choose surgery and all goes well, you'll be able to live out the rest of your life with no sign of prostate cancer and no life-altering side effects.

A SHORT HISTORY OF PROSTATE-CANCER SURGERY

Compared to many types of surgery, radical prostatectomy is a decidedly new kid on the block. Evidence from Neolithic sites confirms that trepanning, a procedure in which a hole was bored in the skull (some say to release demons) was practiced 40,000 years ago. Amputations date to the Cro-magnon era. Skeletal remains of a 45,000-year-old male whose arm had been amputated are on display at the Smithsonian Institution.

In striking contrast, Theodor Billroth, a renowned German surgeon, reportedly made the first attempt to remove a cancerous prostate in 1867.[4] Billroth also performed the first surgical procedures for rectal, esophageal, and laryngeal cancers; developed a new way to resect (remove) part of the stomach for gastric cancer; and devised novel methods for educating surgical residents that remain in use today. This remarkable innovator was a close friend of Johannes Brahms and an accomplished musician in his own right. Despite copious other commitments, Billroth found time to serve on occasion as a guest conductor for the Zurich Symphony Orchestra.

In the United States, removal of the prostate for cancer was not attempted until 1904, when Hugh Hampton Young, the "Father of American Urology," operated on an elderly preacher. When that patient died years later of an unrelated cause, the autopsy showed no evidence of cancer.[5]

These early surgical procedures used the **perineal** approach, in which the patient was placed in an odd, head-down position and the incision was made behind the scrotal sac. The method held blood loss to a minimum, and patients recovered quickly. Nevertheless, the surgeon's view of crucial structures was highly restricted, providing more of a meager porthole than an open window to the surgical field. Incontinence after surgery was common, and impotence was seen as inevitable.

In 1945, a British surgeon named Terence Millin pioneered a new technique involving a vertical abdominal incision to remove the prostate from its perch behind the pubic bone. Millin's procedure resulted in more blood loss, but it provided surgeons with a much better view of the operative field and far better access to critical organs. After many important refinements, radical retropubic prostatectomy, or open prostatectomy, remains the most popular and effective technique for surgical treatment of prostate cancer today.

NOTE: Though some surgeons continue to prefer it, I see little reason to use the perineal approach today. The prostate can be removed, but given the limited visibility, the surgeon has no flexibility to excise surrounding tissues that might harbor cancer. Even advocates of this procedure only support its use for small-volume, favorable-risk cancers (a PSA level of less than 10, a Gleason sum of less than 7, no more than two biopsy cores containing cancer). For more serious cancers, the risk of incomplete removal with positive surgical margins is just too great.

Also, while some surgeons have performed nerve-sparing perineal prostatectomy, in actual practice both nerves are almost never spared. Consequently, this procedure results in an unacceptably high rate of impotence. I consider the perineal operation reasonable only for men over 65 with no erectile function, who have a small, favorable cancer.

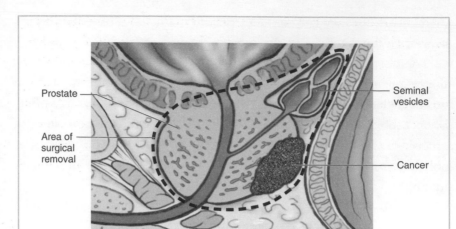

The dotted line indicates the tissue removed in a radical prostatectomy.

Many men are terrified of radical prostatectomy because of horror stories that stem from the bad old days of prostate-cancer surgery. Until the early 1980s, removing the prostate was virtually synonymous with serious and sometimes catastrophic side effects. Often, the operation caused severe bleeding that, in the worst cases, could be life-threatening. The surgery left 15 to 25 percent of men incontinent, and the great majority lost their ability to have erections. Bowel injuries and urinary strictures (narrowing of the urethra by scar tissue) occurred with troubling frequency. Understandably, few patients elected to have the procedure, and most doctors were reluctant to recommend it. By the 1960s, following the development of the linear accelerator that could deliver X-rays to a targeted organ, external beam radiation became the prostate-cancer treatment of choice. Radiation remained the dominant option for nearly thirty years, even though irradiating the gland before the discovery of modern conformal therapy caused serious side effects and often failed to arrest the disease.

As in real estate, the central issue in prostate operations is location, location, location. The prostate lies deep in the abdomen, where it is difficult to access or examine. Several critical structures, including the rectum and bladder, lie perilously close to the gland. The urethra, which carries urine from the bladder and sperm from the testes through the penis, tunnels directly through the prostate. To perform a radical prostatectomy, a surgeon must sever the urethra near the bladder neck and then, after removing the gland, carefully connect the cut ends to form an anastomosis, which is basically what you'd need to do if you wanted to reconnect the severed ends of a rubber hose. Little more than two decades ago, doctors performing this highly complex, delicate surgery were seriously handicapped by incomplete and often erroneous ideas about prostate anatomy.

MODERN RADICAL PROSTATECTOMY

Nerve Sparing

Beginning in the 1970s, surgeons began to develop a far better understanding of the anatomy of the prostate and nearby organs: the bladder, rectum, seminal vesicles, and urinary sphincter. Techniques were developed to control bleeding from the many blood vessels that surround the gland. Working in a bloodless field, surgeons could take time to appreciate the subtle nuances of pelvic anatomy and avoid injury to the nearby urinary sphincter and rectum. The rate of serious side effects began to decline. But the most important step—one which established radical prostatectomy as the major treatment for prostate cancer—was the development of the technique called **nerve sparing**.

Men first strolled on the moon in 1969, but astonishing and unimaginable though it may seem, we did not figure out the exact anatomy of the nerves responsible for penile erections until 1981. Credit for that monumental discovery goes to Pieter Donker, a Dutch urologist, who identified the **cavernous (erectile) nerves** in a stillborn baby boy. Donker proved that these nerves ran along the outside of the prostate, not *through* the gland, as experts in urology had believed.

Donker shared his findings with Patrick Walsh of the Brady Urological Institute at Johns Hopkins, who realized that it was therefore possible to preserve erectile nerves during radical prostatectomy and leave prostate-

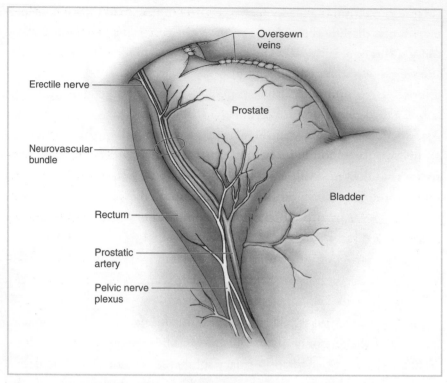

View of the surgical field from the perspective of the surgeon. The feet are at the top of the field, and the head at the bottom. The neurovascular bundle (NVB) containing the cavernous (erectile) nerves runs alongside the rectum and passes along the prostate and the urinary sphincter, into the penis.

cancer patients with their potency intact.[6] Walsh performed the first nerve-sparing radical prostatectomy in 1982. Today, most surgeons routinely strive to preserve erectile nerves when removing the prostate. Doing so allows most men who were previously potent to regain erections after surgery and reduces the incidence of urinary incontinence, which also appears to depend to some degree on preserving these nerves.[7]

Unfortunately, sparing erectile nerves is not always possible. The primary goal of radical prostatectomy is cancer cure, which depends on removing the entire tumor and leaving no malignant cells behind. If a pathologist finds cancer at the border of the excised gland (positive surgical margins), there is an increased risk that the tumor will spread and eventually become incurable. Sometimes, prostate cancer extends through the capsule of the gland and grows into the erectile nerves, necessitating their removal. In other cases, a patient's cancer may make it impossible to excise the gland successfully without damaging or destroying these nerves.[8]

Nerve Grafts

If, in your particular situation, sparing one or both erectile nerve bundles would risk incomplete removal of the cancer, **nerve grafts** can improve your chances of recovering sexual function. We use a nerve from the side of the foot (sural nerve) or within the pelvis (genitofemoral nerve) to replace a nerve that needs to be removed.[9]

Today, many top medical centers offer nerve grafts for radical prostatectomy patients whose erectile nerves cannot be spared, and the results

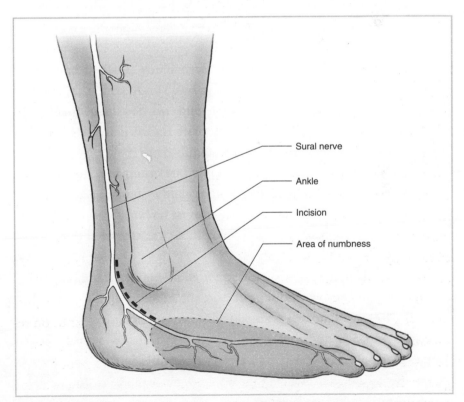

Incision used to obtain the sural nerve for use as a nerve graft. Removing the nerve leaves a numb area on the foot that shrinks over time.

Historical Note

In the early 1990s, a patient of mine developed a very aggressive, high-grade cancer. After studying his case, I told him I thought there was little chance that we could excise the tumor completely without removing both of his erectile nerves. Dr. Noel Mills, a friend and cardiovascular surgeon knowledgeable about nerve grafts in other surgical procedures, suggested that we try to replace the nerves with grafts.[10] In fact, prostate cancer surgeons had considered the idea, but nobody had developed a technique for doing it. With my patient in mind, I set out in earnest to explore the possibility of finding an effective stand-in for lost or damaged erectile nerves.

I broached the idea to neurosurgeons and plastic surgeons, several of whom suspected it might not be feasible. They were concerned that the erectile nerves are autonomic (involuntary), different from the sensory or motor nerves that were being successfully grafted in other parts of the body. Also, cavernous nerves are actually a network of nerves (plexus), not a single discreet fiber, so any replacement would have to be quite large.

In 1996, I finally found a wonderful expert in nerve grafting. Dr. Rahul Nath, a plastic surgeon at Baylor College of Medicine, worked with me to perform the first single-sided nerve graft in a radical prostatectomy patient in January 1997. In March of that year, we grafted nerves on both sides in a man whose cancer made nerve-sparing impossible. Ten months after surgery, this patient reported no erectile function; but by fourteen months, he had recovered erections adequate for intercourse with the use of sildenafil, and some erectile function, though not as strong, without medication. Without the grafts, his potency would have been lost.

By 1999, results were in on the first twelve patients who had received bilateral nerve grafts. Nine (75 percent) recovered partial erectile function, and 50 percent had full recovery of erections (two with the use of erection-inducing medication), an outcome in the range that many surgeons were reporting for nerve-sparing operations.[11]

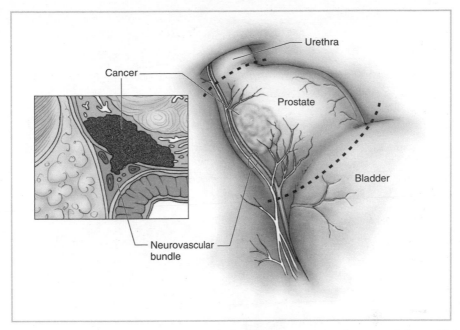

When a large cancer grows into a neurovascular bundle, the nerve must be removed along with the prostate to cure the cancer. Dotted lines show what is removed during the operation.

have been highly encouraging. Without grafts, men who lose both nerves during surgery almost never recover erectile function. With grafts, 30 to 40 percent of patients recover (50 percent with erection-promoting drugs). Removing one nerve substantially reduces the chances of recovering potency, depending on a person's age. In my experience with 60-year-old men, only 30 percent recover when one nerve is removed, compared to 70 percent who do so when both nerves are spared.[12] When one nerve is resected and then replaced by a graft, 50 percent recover. This is not quite as good as when both nerves are spared, but twice as good as the outcome without grafts.[13] Operating on seven out of eight cylinders is far better than trying to run on only four or—in a truly futile enterprise—none at all. If erectile function is important to you, you may want to consider finding a surgeon who can do a nerve graft if it proves necessary to remove one or both of your erectile nerves in order to cure the cancer.

Some doctors are skeptical about nerve grafting, arguing that a can-

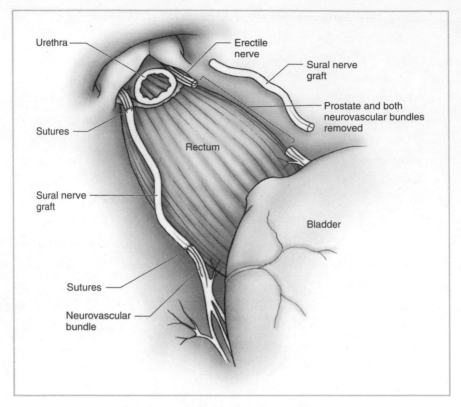

Bilateral nerve grafts to replace the erectile nerves.*

cer large enough to invade the erectile nerves is not curable and surgery should not be done. I disagree. Even a large tumor that has grown into the nerves can sometimes be cured as long as it is completely removed. Even if the cancer eventually recurs, there's a benefit to removing the primary tumor, which would otherwise be left to grow and cause symptoms. Incurable prostate cancer does *not* mean you're going to die soon or spend all of your remaining years debilitated by the disease. Most men live symptom-free for many years, and there's no reason they shouldn't

*Modified from Kim, Edward D., et al., "Interposition of Sural Nerve Restores Function of Cavernous Nerves Resected During Radical Prostatectomy." *Journal of Urology* 161, no. 1 (1999): 188–192. Reprinted with permission from Lippincott Williams & Wilkins.

be offered the chance for good erectile function and a satisfying sex life during that time.

The Downside of Nerve Grafts

Nerve grafting does involve a bit more operating time, and it can add the cost of a plastic or neurosurgeon, though in some cases the urologist performs the graft himself. Some patients experience inflammation or a wound infection at the donor site on the foot. In 1 to 2 percent of cases, men develop pain in the area from which the nerve has been taken. If this persists, it may be necessary to operate again to reposition the cut end of the nerve. Borrowing your sural nerve will leave a small area of numbness on the top of your foot, but this does not interfere with walking or running and shrinks over time. If we use the genitofemoral nerve for a graft, there may be a small area of numbness on your scrotum and inner thigh. Most patients don't notice this except at the time of an examination, and again, the numb area gradually gets smaller in size.[14]

RESULTS TODAY

The technique we currently use for modern radical prostatectomy is quite different from the nerve-sparing procedure of the early 1980s. After

NOTE: While nerve grafts mark an important step forward in reducing sexual problems after radical prostatectomy, nerve sparing—when possible—is always the better choice. Doctors should not use the possibility of a graft to justify removing nerves unnecessarily. In most cases both nerves can be safely preserved. Only 10 to 20 percent of surgical patients have a real risk of cancer penetrating through the capsule close enough to jeopardize an erectile nerve. Even then, many times we can dissect a bit wider, remove the cancer completely, and still preserve most or all of the nerve.[15]

analyzing the long-term results of thousands of cases, we have learned how to excise the cancer completely in almost all cases, while preserving both neurovascular bundles in over 90 percent of patients. By recognizing the wide variation in prostate cancers and appreciating subtle variations in the size and shape of individual prostate glands, expert surgeons have learned to tailor the operation to each patient's anatomy and tumor. We have also discovered how to minimize trauma to the **external urinary sphincter**, reducing the risk of serious, long-term urinary incontinence to 1 percent. Serious blood loss is rare today, hospital stays are no longer than two to three days, and the urinary catheter is typically removed in seven to ten days. Most patients regain continence in a few days or weeks, and sexual function typically begins to return in a few weeks or months, though full recovery can take as long as three years.[16]

To measure success, we consider how likely a man is to be cured of cancer and to recover completely normal urinary and sexual function after surgery. At Memorial Sloan-Kettering Cancer Center, the answer is 60 percent. Six of every ten patients live out their lives after the surgery, cured of cancer and functioning exactly as they did before the operation. Many more return to near normal with only minimal effects on urinary or sexual function. Often, these problems can be overcome with modern treatments. (See Chapter 17, Urinary Side Effects, and Chapter 18, Sexual Side Effects.)

Nevertheless, radical prostatectomy remains one of the most challenging procedures in oncology, and national results reflect the struggle that most surgeons have with this operation. Among all surgeons nationwide, positive surgical margins are reported in 25 percent of patients, serious incontinence in 8 percent, and 55 percent of men fail to recover erections.[17] The difference in outcomes between top experts and surgeons who rarely perform this operation can be enormous.[18]

LAPAROSCOPIC SURGERY

A promising young player on the surgical stage is **laparoscopic prostatectomy**. Since 1998, surgeons at the Institut Mutualist Montsouris in

Paris have removed over 1,000 cancerous prostates using this approach. In a marvel of high-tech instrumentation, a magnifying, lighted, robotically controlled scope inserted through the navel transmits a magnified image of the surgical field to a monitor in the operating room. Despite the lack of a large "window" through the skin, the laparoscopic surgeon has an excellent view of internal structures at twelve- to fifteenfold magnification, so the procedure can be tailored to suit each man's prostate anatomy and disease.[19]

The abdomen is inflated with gas to make room for insertion of the surgical instruments. Microsurgical instruments are threaded through four or five other tiny incisions, each only ¼- to ½-inch long as compared to the typical 3- to 4-inch incision that runs from below the navel to the pubic bone for open prostatectomy. Because the scars are tiny, laparoscopic procedures have been dubbed "band-aid" surgeries. Laparoscopic prostatectomy is also referred to as minimally invasive, though, in fact, removing the prostate requires deep invasion of the abdomen no matter what technique is used.

In addition to the robotic arm that holds the camera, many laparoscopic surgeons rely on the da Vinci Surgical System, which uses computer technology to translate and stabilize the doctor's hand and finger motions, allowing control of the microsurgical instruments inside the patient by remote. Theoretically, the surgeon and patient need not even be in the same room during the procedure.[20]

The Advantages of Laparoscopic Surgery

Compared to open prostatectomy, the laparoscopic technique promises shorter hospital stays, more rapid recovery, reduced blood loss, less postoperative pain, and a speedier return to normal activities. The most common complaint after this surgery is bloating from the carbon dioxide gas that is introduced into the abdomen to facilitate the procedure.

Thanks to the pioneering work of Dr. Bertrand Guillonneau, head of the Section of Minimally Invasive Surgery in Urology at Memorial Sloan-Kettering, we know that it is possible to achieve the same results

NOTE: The world's leading laparoscopic prostate cancer surgeons agree that the Aesop robotic arm, which holds and directs the scope used to visualize the surgical field, is very helpful, but they are skeptical about the value of the da Vinci system. They note that the surgical robot adds nothing to their ability to do the operation and might even slow down the procedure. Still, many less experienced laparoscopic surgeons turn to the da Vinci system as a means to circumvent the long learning curve required to master this challenging operation without robotic assistance.

The debate about the surgical robot remains unresolved, but I'd be wary about a physician who believes he can compensate for a lack of expertise by using robotics. While it may be possible to remove the prostate with the robot, I'd reserve judgment until surgeons using the da Vinci system demonstrate a low rate of positive margins, excellent urinary continence, and recovery of erections in most men. Today, there are no such results.

with a laparoscopic procedure that the best open surgeons report. Dr. Guillonneau has performed over 1,000 laparoscopic radical prostatectomies. Of his 250 most recent cases, the rate of positive margins was less than 10 percent, social continence (wearing two or fewer small pads per day) at three months was 75 percent, and 53 percent recovered erections adequate for intercourse at three months with or without sildenafil or similar medications. While we do not yet have definite data, recovery rates for urinary continence and erectile function a year after the operation appear to be comparable to the rates achieved by open surgeons at Memorial Sloan-Kettering.

THE DOWNSIDE OF LAPAROSCOPIC SURGERY

For surgeons performing laparoscopic radical prostatectomy nationwide, the outcomes are not nearly as promising. Because the procedure is rela-

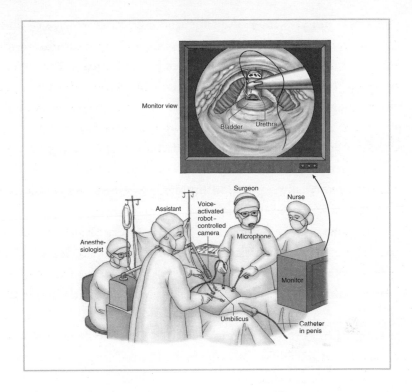

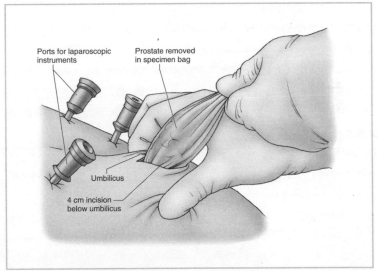

(top) Scene in the operating room during laparoscopic radical prostatectomy. Monitor view shows the urethra being sewn to the bladder after the prostate is removed.

(bottom) In laparoscopic radical prostatectomy, the prostate is removed through a small incision below the belly button.

tively new, it is not yet widely available, and most doctors have very limited experience. Inexperienced surgeons can have catastrophic results, with the need to convert to an open procedure midstream to stop blood loss or repair an injured organ. There have been unfortunate disasters with inexperienced surgeons struggling for six to eight hours to remove the prostate. Not only is the rate of positive surgical margins high, but recovery of erections is poor because of damage to the erectile nerves by surgeons still on the "learning curve." For radical prostatectomy, surgeons must perform the operation hundreds of times before mastering the procedure after being properly taught. This is an operation in which self-learning may take a decade! Also, no long-term follow-up studies are available, so we can't be certain that laparoscopic procedures offer the same rate of cancer control as open surgery.

Lymph nodes in the prostate area are a common site of prostate-cancer spread. For patients with aggressive tumors, we remove these pelvic lymph nodes during surgery, a procedure called **pelvic lymph node dissection (PLND)**,[21] to assess whether the cancer has spread beyond the gland. If it has, chemotherapy, hormone therapy, or experimental therapies may be necessary to control the disease. While PLND has been performed through the laparoscope, it is not clear that node dissection can be done as thoroughly as it can with the conventional procedure. At this point, I would favor open radical prostatectomy for a patient with an aggressive tumor who needs a pelvic lymph node dissection to assess whether the cancer has spread. Open surgery is also preferable for a man with high-grade cancer (a Gleason sum of 7 or greater) overlying the neurovascular bundle. The crucial decision in such cases is not whether to preserve the nerves entirely or to remove them, but whether it is feasible to dissect widely enough around the cancer without removing some or all of the nearby nerve. With loupes (small magnifiers) and a headlamp, the open surgeon can manipulate the prostate, expose the nerves, feel any cancerous nodules, and decide exactly how widely to dissect to completely remove the cancer while maintaining normal urinary function and preserving the nerves to promote the recovery of sexual function to the maximal possible extent.

For any man, I would *only* recommend laparoscopic radical prosta-tectomy if it can be performed by a highly skilled surgeon who has a great deal of experience with this procedure and is capable of achiev-ing the same low rate of positive surgical margins, incontinence, and erectile dysfunction as the best open surgeon. To date, very few surgeons have mastered this approach, and only one, Dr. Bertrand Guillonneau, has reported long-term results comparable to those of experienced open surgeons.[22]

Still, many patients are understandably drawn to the laparoscopic ap-proach. To meet rising demand, many surgeons have taken up this new technique. Keep in mind that what sounds like a kinder, gentler opera-tion may in fact turn out to be quite the contrary in the hands of some-one who lacks the appropriate skill. The potential advantages of a small incision, less blood loss, and a slightly quicker recovery are not worth the risk of incomplete excision of cancer, long-term incontinence, or per-manent problems with erectile dysfunction.

IS SURGERY RIGHT FOR YOU?

Radical prostatectomy may be the right treatment choice if your cancer is localized to the prostate or the immediate surrounding tissues (which can include clinical stages T1, T2, or a small T3 tumor) with no evi-dence of distant spread. If the cancer is, in fact, confined to the prostate, 90 percent of patients will live out their lives with no further sign of prostate cancer and no need for further treatment.[23] Even if the cancer is highly aggressive (with a Gleason sum of 7 or more in the biopsy), over 80 percent of men are cured with surgery as long as the cancer is still confined. If your test results raise the possibility of local spread of the cancer, radical prostatectomy may still be a good treatment option, but the surgeon will have to modify the operation to make sure all of the cancer is removed. In long-term results from my own patients and from other surgeons at Memorial Sloan-Kettering, seven of ten men whose cancer extends through the prostate into the surrounding tissue (extracapsular extension) and one of three with seminal vesicle invasion remain free of cancer recurrence ten years after surgery, if they've had the proper operation. Occasionally, a tumor that has spread to a lymph node can be cured by removal of the prostate and lymph nodes. The common suggestion that surgery is only effective for men with cancer that is confined to the prostate underestimates the real power of radical prostatectomy to stop this disease. In fact, more than 50 percent of men with a cancer that has spread locally can be cured with radical prostatectomy. On the other hand, 10 percent of radical prostatectomy patients whose cancer appears to be confined actually have microscopic metastases that were not detected, and the PSA eventually rises again. The important question is not whether a man's cancer is confined to the gland but whether the tumor is *contained* in the prostate area and can be removed completely.[24]

Few men treated surgically die of their cancer. In my radical prostatectomy patients, whose average age at the time of surgery was 62, the risk of death from any cause fifteen years later, at the average age of 77, was 46 percent. This is exactly what one would expect in any group of men, including those who never had prostate cancer. Only 7 percent of my surgery patients eventually died of prostate cancer. Even men with seminal vesicle invasion or lymph node metastases—the most aggressive tumors—had only a 30 percent risk of dying of their cancer in the next fifteen years.[25]

Realistically, radical prostatectomy will not remove an extensive T3 or T4 cancer with obvious seminal vesicle invasion. Hormone therapy followed by radiation or participation in a clinical trial of new chemotherapeutic agents (see Chapter 21, Treating Metastatic Prostate Cancer) would be better treatment choices.

Except in the rare case of a localized but very aggressive tumor that might spread soon and cause serious symptoms, I would not recommend radical prostatectomy for a man whose life expectancy is less than a decade. In cases of typical, slow-growing prostate cancer, radiation can control the disease for years. Some of the side effects of surgery are age-related. The rate of incontinence increases in men over age 70,[26] and the risk of erectile dysfunction is higher after age 60.[27] For surgery to make sense, you need to be young and healthy enough to come through the operation well and benefit from the long-term survival advantage that removing the gland may provide.

Serious medical conditions, such as active heart or lung disease, uncontrolled high blood pressure or diabetes, or a prior history of thrombophlebitis (blood clot in the legs) or pulmonary embolism (blood clot in the lungs), put you at increased risk for major surgical complications. So does the presence of urinary incontinence, which strongly predicts more serious incontinence after surgery. Diabetes, high blood pressure, smoking, and heart disease increase the incidence of postoperative erectile dysfunction. You may not be a good surgical candidate if you've had a serious adverse reaction to anesthesia during a previous operation.

DISADVANTAGES OF SURGERY

Radical prostatectomy is major surgery and requires a hospital stay of two to three days. Full recovery of your normal energy level can take as long as two to three months, though most men can return to work and most normal activities after a few weeks (except heavy physical labor, which should be avoided for up to six weeks).

Blood loss during this operation has been greatly reduced by modern surgical techniques,[28] but many patients still lose enough blood to require transfusion. This does not mean your doctor has done a bad job. In fact, doing the *best* procedure can involve more blood loss than one aimed at minimizing the need for transfusion at all costs. Clamping or cauterizing every tiny bleeder near the neurovascular bundles can increase the risk of damage to these exquisitely sensitive erectile nerves. If your surgeon believes that you may need blood during or after surgery, you might want to bank your own for maximum safety (see full discussion on page 277). Typically, you should plan to bank two pints. One is not enough to stimulate your body to make more red blood cells, and three requires an extra week or two to get your blood count back up to baseline before surgery. There is no good evidence that blood stimulators such as erythropoietin (Epo) or Procrit reduce the need for transfusions, except in men who are chronically anemic.[29]

SURGICAL COMPLICATIONS

Any surgery carries a small risk of lethal complications, which can result from either the procedure itself or the anesthesia. Radical prostatectomy is no exception, though thankfully the instance of surgically related deaths is very rare.[30] According to a Medicare database from the 1990s, the mortality rate for prostate-cancer patients ages 65 to 79 was about 1 in 200.[31] Widespread statistics are hard to find for younger men, but reported outcomes from several Centers of Excellence worldwide suggest that for men below age 65, the risk of death from radical prostatectomy is about 1 in 1,000. The death rate for all surgical procedures in this country is about 1 in 3,000. The risk is greatest for older men and those with serious medical conditions (**comorbidities**) aside from prostate cancer. Severe complications within the first thirty days after surgery, called the perioperative period, are uncommon. The ones we watch for are thrombophlebitis, pulmonary embolism, arrhythmia (abnormal heart rhythm), and myocardial infarction (heart attack). Pneumonia is a concern after general anesthesia and a major reason that patients are encouraged to breathe deeply and to get up and walk as soon as possible after surgery.

Other potential problems that may occur soon after this operation include wound infections (which affect 1 to 2 percent of patients), urinary tract infections (3 to 4 percent), and bleeding (2 to 3 percent). Some men also experience urethral stricture (narrowing of the tube by scar tissue) at the site of the anastomosis (where the urethra is rejoined). Repairing a stricture may require dilation in the office or incision through a cystoscope under anesthesia.

NOTE: On average, strictures occur in 15 percent of men, but the incidence ranges from 1 to 75 percent, depending on the skill of the surgeon.[32] This is another important reason to find an experienced—and busy (see, however, the caveat to this on page 272)—specialist to perform your radical prostatectomy.

SIDE EFFECTS OF RADICAL PROSTATECTOMY

INFERTILITY

When you have an orgasm after your prostate is removed, no seminal fluid will be released. The orgasm will be "dry," with no ejaculation. Consequently, you will no longer be able to father children through sexual intercourse. If this is an issue for you, make arrangements to bank sperm before your operation. The more you bank, the better, but you should not contribute more than once every three days or the sperm will be too dilute. Give yourself ample time to bank six to twelve deposits before surgery.

Sperm are still produced after radical prostatectomy, but, as happens after vasectomy, they are no longer released. Instead, they migrate as far as the **epididymis** (the ducts that drain the testicles), where they slowly deteriorate and are reabsorbed with no negative effects.

INCONTINENCE

Many men facing prostate cancer surgery worry about losing urinary control. Fortunately, severe, permanent incontinence is largely a thing of the past.[33] Most men are dry within a few days or weeks after the catheter is removed. (See Chapter 17, Urinary Side Effects.)

It's a good idea to bring a few absorbent pads when your catheter is removed. About half of our patients stop wearing pads after a day or two. By six weeks after surgery, three out of four patients no longer need pads for leakage. By one year, nine out of ten men never need them, and the other one out of ten wear a pad a day at work or while engaged in intense physical activity. Only about one man in a hundred has troublesome urinary leakage a year or more after the operation serious enough to warrant medical intervention. And there are ways to correct the problems that do arise. With modern treatment, men are not doomed to live with severe incontinence after radical prostatectomy.

Many doctors advocate **Kegel (pelvic floor) exercises** once the catheter is removed. One clinical trial showed better continence with regular use of these exercises,[34] but I suggest waiting to see if you quickly regain control on your own, which most men do, before starting them.

The probability of incontinence after radical prostatectomy varies. Men over 70 are at increased risk, as are those who had any stress incontinence prior to surgery. Incontinence rates are higher in patients with large cancers, whose neurovascular bundles have to be removed. Intact erectile nerves appear to play some significant role in urinary control. The single greatest predictor of urinary continence, however, is the skill of the surgeon performing the operation.[35]

ERECTILE DYSFUNCTION

Along with the fear of incontinence, prostate-cancer patients worry most about a loss of erections. Today, in my practice, the vast majority of patients who were potent before surgery eventually recover erections sufficient for intercourse.[36] As with incontinence, the outcome hinges heavily on the skill of the surgeon, so make sure you're in the best possible hands. Recovery of erectile function also depends on your age, the quality of your erections before the operation, and the preservation of erectile nerves during the operation. (See Chapter 18, Sexual Side Effects, for a full discussion.)

Erections typically take longer to recover than urinary control. The average man experiences his first workable erection about four months after surgery, and erections can take two to three years to recover fully. If both nerves are spared, about 85 percent of men will recover erections sufficient for intercourse, and about 55 percent say they are functioning as they were before surgery by three years after a radical prostatectomy.[37]

Ejaculation and Orgasm after Surgery

Erection, **ejaculation**, and orgasm are independent—though interrelated—sexual functions. **Infertility** (the inability to conceive children) is not synonymous with erectile dysfunction, and a loss or lessening of erections does not mean you can no longer have sexual pleasure. Even men who can't have erections continue to have normal sensation in the penis and can experience orgasms, though they no longer ejaculate. (See Chapter 18, Sexual Side Effects.)

NOTE: If left untreated, prostate cancer can cause erectile dysfunction and much worse, not only by growing directly into the nerves that lie close to the prostate but also by requiring further treatment—radiation or hormone therapy—that can cause loss of erections and (in the case of hormones) decreased libido as well.

The Bottom Line

The discomfort and negative effects of radical prostatectomy are typically temporary. The immediate interruption in your normal activities usually lasts a week or two, your energy level may be reduced for a month or two, incontinence usually resolves in a few weeks or months, and erections begin to return within the first year. Recovery is simply a matter of time, and the chances that your cancer will be cured are excellent!

CHOOSING A SURGEON

Radical prostatectomy is a delicate, complex, and technically challenging surgical procedure that should *only* be undertaken by an experienced, board-certified urologist. Ideally, you'll want to be in the hands of a surgeon who specializes in the procedure, has done it many times, still performs it routinely, works in a top-notch facility with the latest medical technology and techniques, and has a proven track record of successful results.

While the risk of fatal complications from radical prostatectomy is uniformly low, regardless of the surgeon's skill level, expertise can have a huge impact on major postoperative complications, including blood clots, pneumonia, and cardiac arrhythmias.[38] A highly skilled surgeon knows how to reduce the risk of urethral strictures, incontinence, erectile dysfunction, and positive surgical margins.[39] The **surgical margin** is the outer surface of the tissue—that is, the very edge—of what a surgeon removes. A **positive surgical margin** means the pathologist found cancer cells right at that cut border. When that happens, chances are the surgeon has not taken out enough tissue to excise all the cancer. Positive margins greatly reduce the probability that the tumor has been cured and increase the risk that you'll need further treatment, such as hormone therapy, down the road.

Getting to the right doctor can require homework, legwork, and persistence. Thankfully, prostate cancer is almost always slow-growing and poses no imminent threat. Once you decide to have surgery, you have ample time to evaluate surgeons carefully and make a thoughtful, considered choice. Waiting a few months to have the operation will not make a significant difference in your chance for a cure.

To start the process, you might ask your primary doctor and any specialists you see to recommend top surgeons in the field. To get the most heartfelt response, try asking who they would go to if they had prostate cancer, or who they would trust to operate on someone in their family.

Many men seek recommendations from family, friends, or acquaintances. It's comforting to know someone or, better yet, several people who have had a good experience with the doctor you plan to use. If you lack such contacts, you can ask the surgeon(s) you're considering for referrals to patients who might be willing to talk with you about their radical prostatectomies.

Several magazines and books publish annual lists of "best doctors" by location and specialty.[40] Generally, these selections are based on the opinion of other physicians in the field (akin to a Zagat guide for doctors). These listings can be useful, though they may be biased somewhat by issues such as familiarity or popularity, which have nothing to do with professional skill. I would not rule out a surgeon solely because he is absent from such a list, but it can be reassuring to confirm that the doctor you're considering is highly regarded by his peers.

Finding out which surgeons have a negative record can be much trickier. State medical boards keep records of complaints against physicians, but this information is generally not available to consumers. You can find out about serious disciplinary action that's been taken against a doctor by contacting the state medical board, but such records may not alert you to major infractions that occurred years ago or in another jurisdiction the doctor may have left under a cloud. Rules governing disclosure of such matters vary from state to state, and as yet there is no national registry of medical complaints or misconduct by doctors.

Because of the intricacy and complexity of radical prostatectomy, you might want to seek a physician who has a regional, national, or even international reputation as an expert in the field. Staying close to home and dealing with doctors and hospitals you know might offer a measure of comfort and ease, but getting the best available procedure with the fewest side effects will have a far greater long-term impact on your quality, and possibly quantity, of life. I'd urge you to consider carefully what price you're willing to pay to avoid some temporary inconvenience.

Be sure to interview surgeons you're considering, and check their credentials. Though it doesn't guarantee expertise, it's fair to assume that a doctor who has trained at a Center of Excellence for prostate cancer has been exposed to good surgical technique. Board certified means the surgeon has achieved a level of professional training in his chosen specialty, but being a board-certified urologist does not necessarily mean that a doctor has the training and experience required to remove a prostate well. Some urologists specialize in kidney stones or benign prostatic enlargement and rarely perform prostate-cancer surgery. Others have a more general practice and highly limited experience with radical prostatectomy, though given the opportunity they may be willing, or even eager, to do the procedure.

Be sure to ask how many radical prostatectomies the doctor has done and how often he does them. I'd avoid someone who performs this operation less than once a month, which is not often enough to develop or maintain a high level of skill. Twenty to fifty radical prostatectomies a year should be the minimum acceptable number, and busier, more experienced surgeons are likely to have better results. Gaining competence in the modern, anatomical, nerve-sparing approach requires considerable experience and regular practice. Ideally, you should seek someone who specializes in radical prostatectomy and performs the procedure several times a week.

Few surgeons track their own results. Collecting information about the rates of positive surgical margins, incontinence, and erectile dysfunction is laborious and expensive. Outside of major medical centers, few doctors can afford the resources to collect this data. So when they are asked about side effects and surgical successes, most doctors quote statistics from textbooks or medical journals. The best physicians, whose professional reputations depend on a candid analysis of their own outcomes, carefully monitor how their patients fare and report those outcomes in respected professional journals. If you are eager to find a recognized expert, you might ask whether the doctor you're considering can steer you to papers he has published on his radical prostatectomy results.

NOTE: While it's generally true that busier surgeons have better outcomes, this is not universally the case. In a study of over 10,000 patients across the country, we made the startling and disquieting discovery that some surgeons continue to do the same procedure badly, even though they do it all the time.[41]

In considering surgical outcomes, be sure you're comparing apples to apples. Some doctors define incontinence as having to wear any pads on a regular basis, while others deem a patient continent unless urinary leakage has a serious impact on quality of life.

Some surgeons are rigorous about patient follow-up, using standardized interviews and questionnaires, while others report success rates based on very limited data. It's important to know where the quoted numbers come from and how they are likely to apply to you. Is your risk of side effects greater or less than this doctor's average patient? Hearing that a surgeon's patients have an 80 percent potency rate doesn't mean much if you're destined to be in the unfortunate minority. If your cancer is large and one nerve must be removed, your chances of recovering erections can drop to less than 30 percent, depending on your age. If both nerves need to be excised, return of erectile function is virtually zero. Given that a nerve graft or grafts could increase your odds considerably, you might want to consider a doctor who does grafting when nerves must be excised.

NOTE: Even the best reported results are not an absolute guarantee of surgical skill. Some surgeons limit their caseloads to only the most favorable patients, artificially inflating their record of good outcomes. Adequate due diligence and several credible recommendations are your best route to a good surgeon.

PERINEAL VERSUS RETROPUBIC

Ask whether the surgeon uses the more widely accepted retropubic approach or performs radical prostatectomy through the perineum, which lies between the scrotum and the rectum. Perineal prostatectomy makes it far more difficult to spare erectile nerves, customize the procedure to suit the individual cancer, or do a thorough pelvic lymph node dissection (PLND).

OPEN VERSUS LAPAROSCOPIC

If the doctor's approach is laparoscopic, ask how long he's been practicing this technique and how many cases he has done. I'd be skeptical of someone who has less than a hundred of these operations under his belt. The learning curve for this very challenging procedure is long and slow. You don't want to be a guinea pig.

I'd also question whether the doctor was experienced in open radical prostatectomy before he began doing laparoscopic prostatectomy. Most laparoscopic surgeons were trained as endourologists, experts in treating kidney stones, not cancer, and they may not appreciate important principles of cancer surgery, the techniques required to remove a cancer completely, and the best uses and limitations of adjuvant therapies such as hormones and radiation, which may or may not be necessary, depending on the nature of your disease.

If you're considering a laparoscopic prostatectomy, be sure to get details about the surgeon's record with this approach. How often does he need to convert to an open procedure midstream, meaning he was unable to complete the procedure successfully through the laparoscope? The answer should be almost never, definitely less than 1 percent of the time. How long does the operation typically take? What is his rate of positive surgical margins? How much blood loss does his average procedure involve? What percent of patients develop urethral strictures? How quickly do his patients regain sexual potency and urinary continence? You'll want to find a surgeon who can offer outcomes at least as good as you could expect with an open procedure, which has a longer, stronger track record.

I'd be skeptical of anyone who dodges questions about his results. Doctors are ethically bound to keep careful records about new procedures like laparoscopic radical prostatectomy. If the program is too new to have statistics about recovery of erections, which can take years, the doctor should be able to tell you about his rates of urinary continence and positive surgical margins, which are available soon after each man's operation. Finally, you might ask if he would choose his laparoscopic procedure over open surgery for himself or his close family.

Be aware that surgeons can be susceptible to marketplace issues. When a new approach like laparoscopic radical prostatectomy comes along, there's pressure to offer the procedure in response to patient demand. To get a new program up and running, doctors may place an overly optimistic spin on results.

NOTE: In the final analysis, the quality of the surgical procedure is the most critical issue, and this depends on the quality of the surgeon. Shop for the *surgeon,* not the approach. In the best hands, both laparoscopic and open surgery can offer excellent results.

NERVE SPARING

You'll want to know whether you're a good candidate for nerve-sparing surgery and how often the surgeon you're considering actually spares the erectile nerves. Does he offer nerve grafts when these nerves must be removed to cure the cancer? Even if sexual potency is not an issue for you, nerve-sparing surgery can help you recover urinary continence.[42]

NOTE: Some surgeons *always* remove the nerves on the side of a positive biopsy. Others *never* remove the nerves and recommend radiation therapy later if the surgical margins turn out to be positive. I would avoid anyone who espouses either of these all-or-nothing approaches. What you want is a surgeon whose guiding principles, in order of importance, are: first, to cure the cancer; second, to preserve urinary control; and third, to do everything possible to preserve sexual function within the limits necessary for cancer cure.

PREPARING FOR SURGERY

It's generally wise to wait about six weeks after your biopsy for the prostate area to heal before having surgery. While you may be understandably anxious to get rid of the cancer quickly and put the operation behind you, the delay will not endanger your life or reduce your chance for a cure.

It's important to stay as active as possible before radical prostatectomy. Being in good shape facilitates recovery, so exercise is valuable. If you've been involved in a regular fitness program, keep it up. If not, get the go-ahead from your doctor, and then try to get more physical activity in the weeks before surgery.

Maintaining a healthy weight is always desirable, but I don't recommend crash diets to slim down or beef up before the operation. Dietary imbalances can have a negative effect on healing, so you don't want to be depleted of essential nutrients. Strive to maintain a normal, well-balanced diet, but don't make drastic changes. If you're overweight, you can aim for a moderate reduction in your overall caloric intake and increase your exercise with the goal of losing about a pound a week.

Be sure to tell your surgeon and anesthesiologist about any medications you're taking. This includes over-the-counter drugs, nutritional supplements, and herbal, homeopathic, and so-called "natural" remedies. A recent study found that some seemingly innocent substances, including vitamin E and saw palmetto, may interfere with commonly used anesthetics and increase the risk of operative bleeding.[43]

You'll be told to stop taking vitamin E and anything containing aspirin ten days before the operation. Blood platelets take ten days to turn over, and if you use these substances, every platelet in your body becomes less sticky and takes longer to coagulate. This increases your risk for serious bleeding during and after surgery. Forty-eight hours before the operation, stop taking nonsteroidal anti-inflammatory agents (NSAIDs), such as ibuprofen (Advil, Motrin) or naproxen.

Make sure your surgeon knows about any previous surgery or major injury you've had to the penis, prostate, or pelvic area—including a hernia operation; appendectomy; bladder, colon, or rectal surgery; or a penile prosthesis. Scarring and fibrosis from such operations or injuries, even if they happened long ago, could make a radical prostatectomy more difficult. This may not be a contraindication to surgery, but you don't want your doctor to be surprised.

The same holds true for minor procedures. Tell your doctor if you've ever had a Foley catheter placed in your penis, or if you had surgery for hypospadias (small penile opening) as a little boy. Also, indicate if you've had gonorrhea or other sexually transmitted diseases. Any of these could increase the chance that you have a urethral stricture. If the surgeon is aware of this, he can arrange to view the area with a cystoscope and dilate or treat any stricture that exists (which can hinder the return of urinary continence after surgery).

Radiation effects last a lifetime, so be sure your surgeon knows about radiation treatments you have had to the pelvic area for any reason, no matter how long ago. Irradiated tissue could substantially increase the difficulty of the procedure and slow the healing process.

If your surgeon recommends it, the next step would be to bank your own blood (autologous donation). You will not be able to do so if you have active hepatitis or other infectious conditions, or if you are anemic or have a cardiovascular problem that could be worsened by anemia. Blood banked by patients for their own use is discarded if transfusion proves unnecessary. If you're unable to give blood, you may want to ask friends or relatives to donate for you. If you don't need blood that's been banked in your name (directed donation), it will be used for somebody else. There is always a chronic shortage and critical need.

The day before radical prostatectomy, most patients are put on a clear liquid diet. You will probably be told to take a self-administered Fleet enema at home on the night before surgery. It's not necessary to go through rigorous bowel preparation involving strong laxatives and multiple enemas, because bowel injuries are so rare nowadays. They occur in less than 1 percent of patients, and when they do, they can be closed uneventfully and treated with antibiotics to prevent infection.

For the two weeks before surgery, keep alcohol intake to no more than one to two glasses of wine (or the equivalent) per day. Heavy alco-

hol ingestion makes you relatively resistant to the effects of some anesthetic agents and pain medications. It's essential to stop smoking two
weeks before the operation. Smoking is associated with a substantially
increased risk of pneumonia, partial lung collapse, and prolonged coughing, which can be painful postoperatively.

Typically, preoperative testing will include a blood hemoglobin test
(to anticipate your need for a blood transfusion) and a urinalysis (to make
sure you don't have an active urinary tract infection). Other blood levels
will be checked if you're taking medications for conditions such as high
blood pressure or diabetes. The specific tests you get will depend on your
age, general health, and the kind of anesthesia your doctor uses. If you're
scheduled to have spinal or epidural anesthesia, pre-op tests will include
coagulation studies and a careful history of any bleeding problems. If
you're over 50, you'll probably have a chest X-ray and electrocardiogram. The exam will also include a careful medical history, and you will
be asked to sign an informed consent giving permission for the surgery.
These forms tend to detail every conceivable dire possibility, no matter
how improbable or rare, so they can be frightening. (If you read the
package insert that comes with any over-the-counter drug, including aspirin, you'd find similarly hair-raising, worst-case scenarios.)

Try to get a good night's sleep before your operation so you don't feel
sleep-deprived. On the night after surgery, a nurse will awaken you every
two to four hours to check vital signs and make sure you're doing well.

THE OPERATION

Typically, you'll be admitted to the hospital on the day of your surgery.
You should not eat or drink anything within six hours of your operation. Anything in your stomach can cause vomiting and aspiration when
you are given anesthesia. If you're taking medications for high blood
pressure, diabetes, heart disease, or other serious medical problems, be
sure to ask your doctor or anesthesiologist whether you should continue
them on the morning of your operation. Some medicines should be
stopped (e.g., drugs to treat diabetes can drastically lower your blood

sugar if you are not eating), while others, such as medicines for a heart arrhythmia, should be continued.

Make sure to see your surgeon briefly before the operation. It's comforting to know that the doctor you've chosen is actually there. Also, it's important to make sure that you are properly identified and scheduled for the right procedure. Serious mistakes happen rarely, but extra vigilance can help to ensure that they won't happen to you.

Choose your anesthesiologist carefully. At a minimum, you should have your surgeon's reassurance about the anesthesiologist who is going to take care of you. If you meet an anesthesiologist as part of your pre-op checkup, it's not likely to be the same person who will be with you during surgery. Most anesthesiologists work in groups and rotate in the operating room, but you can seek your surgeon's recommendation and request a particular doctor. Ask if your surgeon would be comfortable using this particular anesthesiologist personally or for close family. Most patients put a great deal more stock in choosing the person who will perform the operation than the one in charge of anesthesia, but, in fact, the anesthesiologist, not the surgeon, has the responsibility for vital functions that could be a matter of life and death.

NOTE: Anesthesia for radical prostatectomy can be general, spinal, epidural, or a combination. All are safe and effective. I'd advise that you go along with the protocol regularly used by your surgical team. They'll be most adept at what they do routinely.

Radical prostatectomy can take anywhere from one and a half hours to as long as five, depending on the surgeon's technique, your anatomy, and the nature of your cancer. A pelvic lymph node dissection adds time to the procedure, but it can also provide valuable information for planning future treatments if they prove necessary in your case. Patients tend to presume that a longer procedure is undesirable, but that is not necessarily the case. Modern radical prostatectomy is more like brain surgery than traditional urology: the erectile nerves must be handled with exquisite delicacy, and that requires cautious deliberation, not speed. The procedure should take as long as necessary to ensure optimal results.

DURING SURGERY

I begin by making a 3- to 4-inch vertical incision in the abdomen, starting just above the pubic bone to a point about two-thirds of the way to the belly button. A surgical retractor holds the tissues apart, allowing a good view of the bladder and the pelvic lymph nodes. At this point, I remove the nodes in the prostate drainage area to check for spread of the cancer if diagnostic signs point to that possibility. There are thousands of lymph nodes in the body, so you won't miss these few, and removing these nodes rarely causes swelling or other side effects.

The next step is to isolate the prostate from surrounding tissues, taking care to dissect widely enough to excise all the cancer and leave no malignant cells at the edge (surgical margin) of what is removed. At this

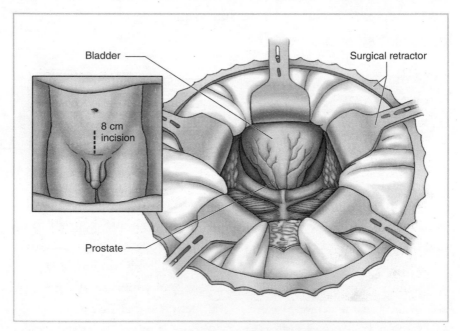

The incision used for open radical prostatectomy and the exposure of the bladder and prostate as seen by the surgeon. A surgical retractor holds the incision open.

point, I can see the urethra and the neurovascular bundles and determine where I must dissect to get safely around the cancer, while preserving the erectile nerves to the maximum possible extent. First, I tease the nerves away from the prostate along the apex (bottom), divide the urethra, and then tease the nerves away from the prostate. Next, I remove the prostate and the seminal vesicles and reconnect the bladder to the cut end of the urethra. Done properly, the removal of the seminal vesicles does not increase the risk of incontinence or erectile dysfunction. Since 5 to 10 percent of patients have seminal vesicle invasion and more have extension of cancer cells around the seminal vesicles, these sacks should always be removed. Some surgeons mistakenly believe they need to preserve the bladder neck to retain urinary control. But, in fact, continence does not depend on sparing the bladder neck. It's far more crucial to divide the bladder neck well away from the prostate to avoid leaving cancer cells (or normal prostate tissue that could later grow or develop cancer) behind.

Next, I test the erectile nerves with a neurostimulator called the CaverMap to be sure they are functional and intact. If they aren't, or if I've had to remove one or both nerves to control the cancer, I do a nerve graft.

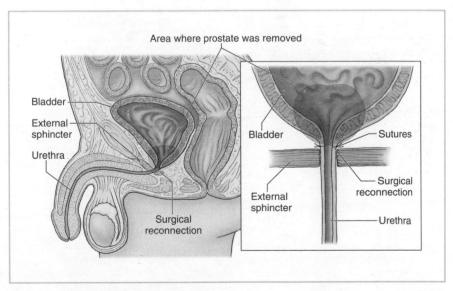

After a radical prostatectomy, the bladder is brought down and reconnected to the urethra just above the external urinary sphincter.

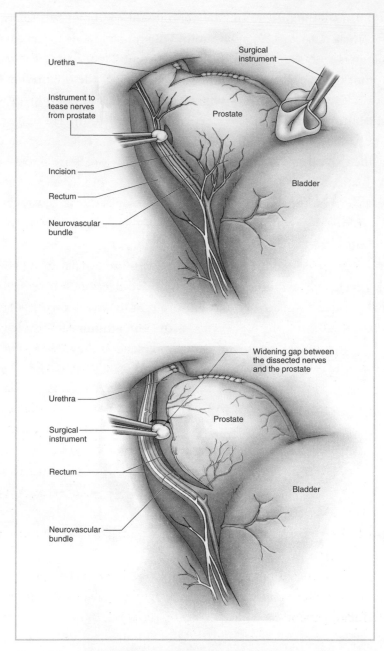

View of the surgical field from the perspective of the surgeon. The feet are at the top of the field, and the head at the bottom. The surgical technique for dissecting the neurovascular bundles (NVB) away from the prostate is the most delicate phase of the operation, where the surgeon must dissect widely enough to completely remove the prostate and the cancer without damaging the erectile nerves in the neurovascular bundle.

I then make sure the new end-to-end connection (anastomosis) be-tween the urethra and bladder is watertight.

Finally, I close the wound with internal absorbable sutures that do not need to be removed and I insert the Foley catheter. A balloon the size of a large marble in the bladder holds the catheter in place until the urethra heals around it.

After Surgery: Common Problems, Removing the Catheter, Recovering

You'll remain in the recovery room for a few hours after the operation, where you'll be monitored closely to make sure that you recover fully from the anesthesia and that your blood pressure is stable, your breathing and heart rate are regular, and you show no sign of bleeding. Hospital policy varies, but at Memorial Sloan-Kettering Cancer Center, close family can visit with you briefly while you're in recovery.

You should expect to awaken from the operation without severe pain. Most hospitals today have a pain-management service, which sets the standards for postoperative pain control. The goal is to relieve discomfort while still keeping you alert. Overmedication can lower your blood pres-sure, reduce your respiratory rate, increase the risk of postsurgical com-plications, and make it harder for you to get up and around (which is important for healing). This does *not* mean you have to suffer a lot of dis-comfort. Patients do better and return to normal activities sooner when postsurgical pain is well controlled.

Pain tolerance and perception vary widely. Some men experience lit-tle or no pain after radical prostatectomy, while others require more pain relief. Today, patient-controlled analgesia (PCA) is common. By pressing a button, you can administer exactly the amount of pain medicine you need. Studies have shown that patients actually require less medication with these systems, and there is no risk of accidental overdose. I opt for epidural anesthesia because it provides a great deal of comfort in the im-mediate postoperative period without making patients groggy. Other surgeons prefer to prescribe powerful anti-inflammatory drugs such as ketorolac (Toradol), which also acts as a effective, non-narcotic pain reliever.

From recovery, you'll be sent to your room. Most men are awake and alert the evening of the operation. A family member or close friend can stay with you if you like and if the facility allows. Having somebody around to help you do simple things, like reach for the water, can be reassuring at first, and I encourage this. Rarely would your medical condition warrant a full-time private-duty nurse.

As soon as possible after the procedure, hospital personnel will get you to sit up on the side of the bed and, shortly afterward, in a chair. Depending on the time of your operation, this could happen later the same day or the following morning. This may seem difficult at first, but it's important. Pain medication will help reduce any serious discomfort. Be sure to tell your doctor if you're not getting sufficient relief.

By the second or third day after surgery, most men no longer need any strong injectable or narcotic pain medication. Simple oral analgesics like acetaminophen with hydrocodone (Vicodin or Percocet) are usually sufficient.

Your intravenous line will stay in for a day or two, until you're able to take liquids and solid foods. You'll have one or two small plastic drains in the side(s) of your abdomen for two to three days, until the wound drainage decreases, to avoid the accumulation of fluid that could become infected. You may also have compression boots or elastic stockings on your legs to encourage blood circulation and reduce the risk of clots, though the best prevention is leg exercise and walking. If you've had epidural anesthesia, the line may be kept in for a couple of days for continued pain management. I leave the Foley catheter in for about ten days, until the new connection between the bladder and urethra is well healed.

You may have a few strips of sterile tape across the incision, and a gauze dressing for the first day or two to catch any seepage. If your doctor uses metal clips or conventional stitches instead of absorbable sutures, you'll need to have them removed about a week after surgery.

By the second day, you should be up and about, able to walk the halls with little support or assistance. Physical activity will lower the risk of blood

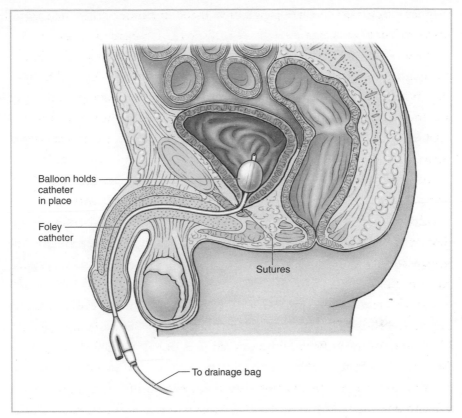

Balloon holds
catheter
in place

Foley
catheter

Sutures

To drainage bag

A Foley catheter through the urethra is held in place by a balloon in the bladder. The catheter allows the urine to drain into a drainage bag until the reconnection heals.

clots and pneumonia and help you to recover intestinal function. To prevent blood clots, it's important to keep the circulation moving in your
legs. Avoid standing still for more than a few minutes, and keep your feet
elevated when you sit. The more you move around, the sooner you'll be
able to eat, pass gas, and have a bowel movement—all part of normal
recovery.

You can start most regular oral medications the morning after surgery,
but some drugs are best avoided at first. Your blood pressure will likely
be lowered by bed rest in the hospital, so blood-pressure medication
should not be necessary for the first couple of days. If you take aspirin

regularly to prevent heart disease, you can start this again by the second or third day after surgery.

Once your lines are out (except the catheter), there's no danger in showering. Soap, water, and exposure to air will help the wound to heal. A tub bath, which could allow water to seep in and increase the risk of infection, is *not* recommended until after the catheter is removed.

Generally, it takes four to five days after surgery to have a bowel movement and a week to ten days to regain your normal regularity. I recommend a stool softener such as Colace for six weeks after the operation. If you're constipated, don't hesitate to take a mild laxative, such as Dulcolax or milk of magnesia, at bedtime, until your bowel movements are regular. Because a prostatectomy is performed in close proximity to the rectal wall, you shouldn't take an enema for three weeks after surgery, but suppositories are safe. In any event, avoid straining at stool, which exerts pressure on the wound and could increase your risk of a pulmonary embolism.

Early activity soon after the operation is not dangerous. Given modern wound-closure techniques, you needn't worry about pulling out your sutures or tearing the incision. I discovered one of my patients, a marathon runner, running up and down twelve flights of stairs in the hospital two days after surgery without doing himself any harm (though I didn't and wouldn't recommend this). Moderate exertion and regular activity, like climbing stairs or walking a few miles, are not risky after the surgery and are likely to be beneficial. The only things you'll need to avoid are extreme abdominal straining and dangerous physical activities, like playing tackle football or mountain climbing, for at least three to six weeks after the operation. You should not drive until the catheter is out; you are off all strong analgesics such as Percodan, Percocet, and Vicodin; and you have no pain that would limit your ability to move your legs or react quickly. If you need to fly soon after surgery, remember to drink a lot of fluids, avoid dehydrating substances such as caffeine and alcohol, walk around frequently during the flight, and keep your legs elevated when you sit. Short of these restrictions, regular activity is good for you once all your tubes have been removed.

Walking is good exercise while the catheter is in place. During the day, you'll attach the catheter to a small leg bag, which won't be noticeable under loose-fitting trousers.

The catheter requires some care and attention. Twice a day, clean the tip of the penis with soap and water. Half-strength hydrogen peroxide diluted with water can remove any crusting or blood. Placing medicated, antibacterial ointments like bacitracin or K-Y Jelly around the penile opening (**meatus**) will keep the skin lubricated and reduce irritation.

It's not unusual or dangerous to have some blood pass around the catheter or in the urine. Small clots in the catheter bag are perfectly normal and nothing to worry about. If you see clots, or if your urine looks dark or cloudy, increase your fluid intake until the urine returns to normal.

Some patients experience bladder spasms, typically caused by irritation from the balloon in the bladder, which holds the catheter in place. But a spasm could also mean that the catheter is twisted or blocked. To keep the tubing straight, it's useful to anchor the tube loosely to your leg with a piece of tape. Bladder spasms that persist can be treated with anticholinergic medications, such as long-acting tolteradine (Detrol LA) or oxybutynin (Ditropan), after a blockage has been ruled out.

At night, be sure to switch to a large drainage bag. The volume of urine will be too much for a small leg bag to accommodate, and the urine will back up, causing a distended bladder, painful urinary retention, and a greater risk of urinary tract infection.

COMMON PROBLEMS

IN THE TESTICLES

Some men have pain or aching in their testicles after the operation. This can last for four to six weeks or, in rare cases, a few months. Often, testicular pain will respond well to anti-inflammatory medicines such as ibuprofen (Motrin) or to scrotal support with a loose jockstrap. Some men also find soaking in a hot tub bath helpful, which is fine once the catheter is removed. Most often, this discomfort goes away on its own. Rarely, it's a bona fide infection, requiring antibiotics. Signs of infection include increasing swelling and pain, exquisite tenderness, and fever.

IN THE PENIS AND SCROTUM

Swelling and discoloration of the skin over the penis and scrotum are common after radical prostatectomy. While alarming, this is usually caused by a harmless accumulation of wound fluid that makes its way by gravity to the lowest point—the genitalia. Mild swelling can be relieved by elevating the area with a rolled washcloth under the scrotum while sitting or lying in bed and by the use of a loose scrotal support or jockey shorts when standing. Severe scrotal or penile swelling is fairly uncommon and usually results from the intravenous fluids you were given during and right after the operation to increase blood volume and reduce the need for blood transfusions.

WEIGHT GAIN

While most patients weigh a few pounds more the day after surgery, some gain ten, fifteen, or even twenty pounds of fluid weight. This excess salt water, administered intravenously to keep you hydrated during the operation, can show up as swelling in your genitals, feet, and ankles. Since gravity carries fluid to the lowest point, the swelling often increases on the second or third day as you spend more time up and about. I ask my patients to weigh themselves every day while they're in the hospital. If I detect troublesome swelling and a man's weight is up ten pounds or more compared to his preoperative level, I'll recommend a daily diuretic such as spironolactone (Aldactone), which promotes the excretion of water without washing away the potassium that is essential for regular heart rhythm and bowel function. Because of the fluid weight gain and abdominal soreness from the incision, be sure to bring boxer shorts and sweatpants or other loose-fitting pants without a belt or zip-per to wear home from the hospital.

REMOVING THE CATHETER

Many men dread having the catheter removed, imagining a painful trauma. In fact, it's a simple maneuver, usually done in the nurse's office, and most men are so tired of the catheter that having it out is a tremen-dous relief. I ask patients to start a short course of antibiotics the day be-fore to reduce the risk of a urinary tract infection. An effective way to take out the catheter and immediately test whether a patient can urinate is called a fill-pull-flow test. The nurse fills the bladder with water through the catheter until you feel the need to urinate, the balloon hold-ing the catheter in place is deflated, and the catheter slides out while you are standing. Then you void into a container, so the nurse can measure how much you have eliminated.

Bring a pad along to wear home. Most men experience some leakage at first. Small absorptive pads such as Depend Guards for Men are avail-able at most drugstores.

RECOVERING

ACTIVITY

It's important to keep active after you go home from the hospital. For the first two to three weeks, get up every hour or so to walk and keep the circulation flowing in your legs. Being active will help you heal and re-gain a normal energy level sooner.

That said, you are likely to feel some fatigue, which will worsen late in the day. Get the extra rest you need, and take a nap in the afternoon, if necessary.

Diet

You can eat a normal diet, but try to get extra iron from foods such as beef and spinach for the first few weeks to make up for any blood loss during surgery. Iron supplements can make you constipated, so I rarely recommend them unless a man has a measured iron deficiency.

THE PATHOLOGY REPORT: WAS THE CANCER CURED?

The Surgical Pathology Report

A pathologist will examine the tissue removed during surgery, and you should have the report in one to ten days. One of the advantages of re-moving the gland is that we can get more detailed and accurate infor-

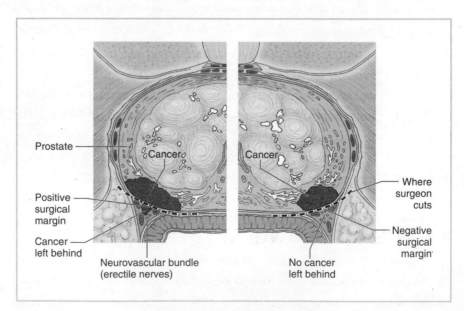

The dotted line indicates where the surgeon cuts between the cancerous prostate and the normal surrounding tissue. In the panel on the left, the surgeon cuts too close to the prostate, leaving cancer cells behind (positive surgical margin).

mation about the nature of your cancer. One-third of the time the Glea-son grade in the surgical specimen turns out to be higher than it ap-peared to be on biopsy. In 5 percent of cases, the grade is lower. In some instances, a tiny focus of more serious cancer is found.

After surgery, the Gleason sum will be reported as a single number between 6 and 10. This represents the Gleason patterns of the two most common tumor cells present, not necessarily the worst ones. It's impor-tant to know whether the pathologist found any poorly differentiated tissue (Gleason pattern 4 or 5) in the gland. If such aggressive elements were found, you should ask about their size and extent.

From the pathology report, you can also learn whether your cancer was confined to the prostate. If you had extracapsular extension, was it focal (small) or established (more than two microscopic high-power fields)? Was there seminal vesicle invasion? If so, did this grow directly from the prostate tumor—as happens in 80 percent of cases—or did you have a microscopic amount of cancer in the seminal vesicles that grew separately and has a more favorable prognosis? Did the cancer spread to the lymph nodes? If so, how many were involved? How many were re-moved? Did the cancer grow through the capsule of the lymph nodes (extranodal), or was it contained? Was there a possible surgical margin, meaning that some cancer was likely left behind and you may need fur-ther treatment to cure the disease?

All of these factors will determine whether you need further treatment and, if so, what kind. By plugging the specifics into our postopera-tive nomogram (decision-making tool), you can estimate your prognosis. (The prostate nomograms are available online at http://www.mskcc.org/mskcc/html/10088.cfm.)

PSA TESTING AFTER SURGERY

Six to eight weeks after surgery, you should have your PSA level checked. If the cancer has been completely removed, the PSA will be *undetectable*. Since it is impossible to measure zero PSA, the laboratory will report your PSA level as "less than" some very low level. This is less than 0.05

in our laboratory at MSKCC, though other labs count less than 0.1 as undetectable. A measurable PSA at this point is a sign that cancer is still present or that normal prostate tissue has been left behind, and further treatment may be indicated (see Adjuvant Therapy, below).

If the PSA is undetectable, you should have your level measured every three months for the first year, every six months during the second to fifth year, and then annually for the rest of your life. I see patients every six months for a checkup during the first year and annually after that. Further tests, such as bone scans, are not necessary unless your PSA rises (see Chapter 20, Rising PSA after Surgery or Radiation Therapy).

ADJUVANT THERAPY: WILL YOU NEED ANY OTHER TREATMENT?

Adjuvant therapy is defined as additional treatment required because you are at high risk for cancer recurrence though no clear evidence exists that some tumor remains. Deciding whether you should have such treatment depends on a careful analysis of the potential benefits weighed against the risk of side effects from the treatment.

The two most common forms of adjuvant therapy after surgery are external beam radiation and hormone therapy. Chemotherapy, which is commonly used after surgery for breast cancer, was not traditionally a standard part of therapy for prostate cancer. This may change, as recent studies have shown that certain combinations of chemotherapeutic drugs confer a survival advantage for men with advanced prostate cancer.

Bicalutamide (Casodex), a drug that inhibits the action of male hormones, has been shown to delay progression of the disease, and studies are under way to determine whether that will translate into a prolonged survival advantage. I would be cautious for now, since this drug actually shortened survival in a study of watchful-waiting patients.

Adjuvant External Beam Radiation

If you have positive surgical margins, adjuvant radiation therapy may make sense. Some doctors recommend adjuvant radiation for patients with extracapsular extension or seminal vesicle invasion, but if the surgical margins are negative, it's much less likely that cancer cells have been left behind, and radiation is less likely to help. If your lymph nodes were positive, radiation will not reduce the high probability that the cancer has already spread elsewhere.[44] There have been no properly performed trials proving that adjuvant radiation prolongs life, so many doctors recommend waiting until the PSA level rises before giving radiation. I turn to the postoperative nomogram to determine the risk of recurrence without adjuvant radiation. If the surgical margins are positive and the risk of recurrence is greater than 30 to 40 percent, early radiation makes sense rather than waiting for the PSA to rise (see www.nomogram.org).

Adjuvant radiation would begin three to six months after the operation, when the incision has healed and you've regained urinary control. If return of urinary continence takes longer, therapy can be delayed until nine months to a year after surgery. Because the treatment is meant to eradicate microscopic clusters of cancer cells rather than a large tumor, a low radiation dose of 64–68 Gy (see Chapter 15, Radiation Therapy, for a full discussion) is delivered to the prostate area only, not the full pelvis, and no hormones are required. According to data from Memorial Sloan-Kettering and Baylor College of Medicine, radiation given in this setting markedly reduces the chance that you will develop a rising PSA. Seventy-five percent of our patients with positive margins treated with adjuvant radiation remained recurrence-free at seven years, compared to only 25 percent without radiation.[45] Though not a randomized controlled trial, these results suggest a real potential benefit for adjuvant radiation in selected men with positive surgical margins.

THE FUTURE

Neuroprotective agents currently under investigation may reduce the incidence of erectile dysfunction after radical prostatectomy.[46] Regular nightly use of Viagra or a similar oral medication enhanced recovery of spontaneous erections a year later in one study. Open surgery is constantly being refined with an eye toward minimizing side effects and maximizing cancer cure. Many surgeons are striving to master the complex techniques required to perform top-notch laparoscopic radical prostatectomy. As they do, this "minimally invasive" approach holds the promise to minimize recovery times and reduce the disruption in patients' lives.

IN SUMMARY

For a healthy man who likely has many more years to live, radical prostatectomy, which offers the best proven long-term durable results, can be an excellent treatment choice for localized prostate cancer. Though this is the most disruptive approach in the short run, with modern nerve-sparing surgery most men soon regain normal urinary control and recover normal sexual function over time. The quality of the surgery is critical, far more important in the long run than the type of procedure you have. Be sure to put yourself in the hands of an experienced specialist with an excellent track record.

15

■

Radiation Therapy

READ THIS CHAPTER TO LEARN:

- How does radiation work, and what does radiation therapy for prostate cancer entail?
- What are the types of radiation, their advantages and disadvantages, and which might be best for you?
- What should you look for in a radiation program?

Simply put, radiation kills cells. Exposure to enough radioactivity damages the cell's genetic blueprint, DNA. Lacking these critical instructions, irradiated cells die off when they try to divide. As a result, rapidly dividing cells are eradicated sooner than those which multiply slowly.

Radiation can also control cancer by cutting off the blood supply a tumor requires to survive and grow. The cells lining blood vessels are extremely vulnerable to high-energy X-rays. Even with relatively low-dose therapy, a tumor's blood supply can be destroyed, leading to the cancer's demise.

Recent experiments at MSKCC indicate that radiation can induce programmed cell death (**apoptosis**), effectively causing cells to commit suicide.[1] Normal cells regularly die off, and new ones arise to take their place. Lacking this innate control, untreated cancer cells multiply and spread in a mounting swath of destruction. By robbing the tumor cells of their immortality, radiation heads off this dangerous overgrowth.

Radiation effects are fractional, meaning the tumor is killed by degrees. With each day's dose, a small proportion of the cancer is destroyed, and then a portion of what remains is killed, and so on. If we get the number low enough, the body can naturally eliminate the remaining malignant cells on its own. Treatment failures in radiation do not usually represent growth of a new cancer. More often, the original tumor has been dealt a stunning blow but not knocked out. Over time, the remaining cancer cells regroup and multiply until they are large enough to cause a rising PSA, which signals that the cancer has returned.

If you douse a lawn with powerful herbicides, you'll kill both the weeds and the grass. Radiation oncologists face a similar conundrum. They need to administer enough destructive rays to eradicate the cancer without inflicting unacceptable damage on normal surrounding tissues. When the therapeutic target is the prostate, which lies perilously close to the bladder, urethra, erectile nerves, and the bowel, the challenge is especially daunting.

To make matters worse, tissues in the body have widely varied radiation tolerance. The intense therapy required to kill prostate cancers would destroy the adjacent rectal wall, where the normal cells divide far more rapidly and are, consequently, exquisitely susceptible to radiation effects.

Modern radiotherapy can be administered via **external beam therapy** or **seed implants (brachytherapy)**. Some doctors advocate a combination of the two. Since radiation works best and is safest for a small tumor in a small prostate, hormones are sometimes recommended to shrink a large cancer or a large gland before treatment.

The amount of radiation energy received by the target organ is expressed in **Gray (Gy)**, named for Louis Gray, an English radiologist and physician. The **rad**, an earlier way of describing dose level, was shorthand for radiation absorbed dose (100 rads equal 1 Gy). Treating prostate

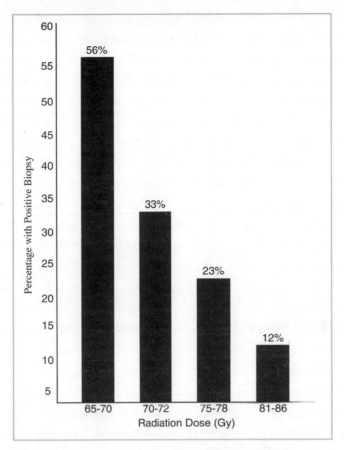

The higher the radiation dose, the lower the chance that the cancer will recur, as indicated by a biopsy of the prostate three years after radiation therapy.

cancer requires a minimum of 70 Gy, sometimes expressed as 7,000 centigray (cGy). The cancer cure rate increases with the strength of the dose.[2]

Some patients ask why all the radiation can't be given at once. In fact, early on, some radiation therapists advocated saturation, with one large exposure of the tumor to a radioactive source, over fractionation (many smaller doses). They found that delivering the treatment over time markedly improved results and reduced side effects. This is comparable to the difference between brief regular exposures to northern sunlight and many hours spent baking under a blazing tropical sun. Minimal sun exposure in the first case provides some important, cumulative benefits, such as helping the body to synthesize vitamin D. In more intense, concentrated doses, the sun's rays can cause serious burns and permanent cell damage.

> NOTE: Some researchers are now investigating the possibility that, given highly precise modern techniques, saturating the tumor with one large radiation dose may prove valuable.

A BRIEF HISTORY OF RADIATION THERAPY

In 1895, William Roentgen, a German physicist, discovered a strange greenish light that could pass through soft tissues in the body but not through most metals or bones. He dubbed his discovery the X-ray, with X meant to indicate that the source of this astonishing phenomenon was unknown.

News of Roentgen's breakthrough spread quickly and fueled the imaginations of scientists around the world. In little over a year, the mysterious rays earned a place in medical treatment and diagnosis. For the first time, doctors had a way to visualize some of the body's internal structures without having to operate. In recognition of this landmark achievement, Roentgen was awarded the first Nobel Prize in physics in 1901.

Inspired by the X-ray and the accidental finding of uranium rays soon afterward, Marie Curie, then a young graduate student in Paris, resolved to study a variety of chemical compounds and to find ways to unleash their radiation. The research she did with her husband, Pierre, led to the discovery of radium and its potential use in the destruction of cancer cells. Mme. Curie went on to become France's first female university professor and the first person to be named a Nobel laureate twice.

Unfortunately, the Curies' pioneering research brought them more than accolades. As a result of their frequent, unprotected exposure to radioactive materials, the couple suffered chronic, debilitating health problems, including skin lesions, weakness, and intractable pain. The Curies not only helped introduce the world to the potential positive power of radioactivity, they were also among the first to demonstrate its alarming side effects.[3]

Studies in the early twentieth century confirmed that radiation could kill rapidly dividing organisms, such as bacteria, and could slow the growth of rapidly dividing cancer cells. Investigators inserted radioactive pellets into tumors in test tubes or animals. As they had hoped, the treatment caused cancers to shrink.

The first radiation therapy for prostate cancer in humans was performed at Johns Hopkins University by Dr. Hugh Hampton Young.[4] Young (who also pioneered surgery for prostate cancer) implanted very high-intensity radium or radon pellets in patients with prostate and bladder cancers. These primitive attempts at brachytherapy did yield some temporary remissions, but they came at a considerable cost of radiation injuries to patients and medical personnel. Until work was done on the atom bomb during World War II, the dangers of handling radioactive materials were not fully appreciated, and shielding techniques were woefully inadequate.

Early on, seed placement was freehand and imprecise. Doctors would operate to implant six to eight radioactive pellets in a cancerous prostate. Typically, certain areas of the gland received inadequate radiation to kill the tumor (**cold spots**), while other sites received too large a dose (**hot spots**), causing an unacceptable incidence of serious side effects, especially damage to the rectum and bladder.

The first external beam therapy, developed in the 1940s, involved taking radioactive cobalt, putting it in a machine fitted with lead shields, and then opening a shield like a camera shutter to expose the target to destructive gamma rays. Cobalt radiation worked well for highly sensitive cancers such as testicular seminomas that could be killed off with a very small amount of radiation, but it proved too diffuse and hard to control to give in the much higher doses needed to wipe out prostate cancers.

Severe side effects, including bladder damage and dramatic injury to the rectum, overwhelmed the limited benefits of the treatment. Because of constraints on the dose that could be given safely, most tumors soon recurred.

The development of the linear accelerator in the late 1950s allowed radiation oncologists to deliver external radiation with greater safety and precision than was possible with cobalt. Dr. Malcolm Bagshaw at Stanford University championed the new approach, treating thousands of patients. Bagshaw proved that radiation could cure some prostate cancers, though, by modern standards, cancer control remained woefully inadequate and side effects unacceptably high.[5]

As a result, the 1970s saw a renewed interest in seed implants. Radiation effects from an implanted seed fall off quickly as you move away from the source of the energy rays. Brachytherapy appeared promising as a way to concentrate high doses in the prostate while minimizing damage to surrounding tissues.[6] Theoretically, it seemed possible to administer 120 to 180 Gy of radiation using iodine-125 seeds, instead of the standard 65 to 70 Gy being given at the time by external beam therapy.

People were seduced by those higher numbers, but despite highly optimistic expectations, seed implants did a dismal job of curing cancers.[7] In fact, studies showed that cancer control with brachytherapy was hardly better than that for patients on watchful waiting, who received no treatment at all.

Further study turned up two wild cards. One was cold spots. With brachytherapy, some areas of the cancer were simply missed or received too low a radiation dose to kill the malignant cells. Also, the high expected overall dose failed to materialize. When 140 Gy was delivered over six months with iodine seeds, the biological effect on cancer cells proved to be no greater than giving 70 Gy of external beam treatment over seven weeks. Seed implants acted like a time-release capsule that delivered the medication slowly but didn't increase its overall strength or effectiveness.

RADIATION TODAY

Given the best modern equipment in the hands of the best practitioners, it's now possible to give powerful, effective radiation therapy with a slim risk of serious side effects. For many men with prostate cancer, radiation is an excellent treatment choice, but, as with surgery, it's important to understand the particulars and make sure you're in the best possible hands. All radiation is definitely *not* created equal.

For prostate cancer, treatment can be administered by external beam, seed implants, or a combination of the two. For each strategy, different centers offer a wide range of technology and expertise.

EXTERNAL BEAM
RADIATION THERAPY

CONVENTIONAL THERAPY

In this approach, a linear accelerator (a machine that produces high-energy radiation) administers the minimum acceptable dose of 70 Gy over about seven weeks of daily weekday therapy sessions. Treatment targets the prostate, seminal vesicles, and frequently the pelvic lymph nodes. Depending upon the precision with which the radiation physicist calibrates these complex machines, the actual dose a patient receives can vary, affecting cure rates and the risk of complications.[8]

Conventional radiation therapy irradiates a box-shaped area around the plum-shaped prostate. Parts of surrounding organs—the rectum, bladder, and urethra—are in the radiation field. Some of these tissues, especially the rectal wall, are extremely vulnerable to radiation damage. As a result, one-third of men suffer immediate side effects such as rectal bleeding, diarrhea, bowel urgency, and urinary urgency and frequency.

The prostate is a notoriously difficult organ to target accurately within the radiation beam. Varying amounts of gas or stool in the rectum, the amount of urine in the bladder, even the act of breathing can alter the position of the prostate during treatment, diverting radiation from the intended target. Some areas of the gland can receive too small a dose to kill the tumor (cold spots), and the local recurrence rate, especially for moderate- or high-risk cancers, is high.

Conventional radiation packs an insufficient wallop for any but the most favorable cancers. We now know that 70 Gy is too small a dose for any patient with a Gleason sum of 7 or more.[9]

3-D Conformal Radiation Therapy (3D-CRT)

The development of three-dimensional (3-D) conformal radiation therapy (3D-CRT) in the late 1980s took a giant step toward solving these problems. A computer program, aided by a CT scan or MRI, accurately measures the gland in three dimensions and computes how the intended dose of radiation should be delivered. Radiation to surrounding organs and damage to normal tissues are markedly reduced. Using 3-D conformal radiation therapy, the risk of serious side effects at 70 Gy went down to less than 1 percent, allowing some radiation oncologists to safely increase the dose to a more effective 75 or 76 Gy.[10]

As the dosage level increases, so does the probability that the cancer will be completely wiped out. In a study by MSKCC radiation oncolo-

> NOTE: Better local cancer control translates into better cure rates. Increasing the dose to 75 Gy left 81 percent of men cancer-free in the long term, as opposed to a 59 percent success rate at 70 Gy. Similar gains were seen for men with intermediate- and high-risk cancers. Simply put, bigger guns pack more firepower and can bring down bigger game. A little .22 might be fine for hunting rabbits, but you'd need a high-powered .3006-caliber rifle if you were out for big bear.

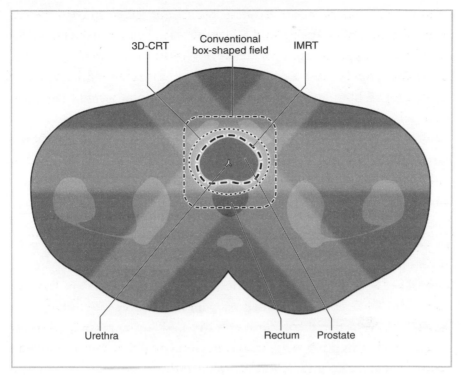

More of the surrounding tissue receives a full dose of radiation with conventional (box-shaped) radiation therapy than with 3-D conformal radiation therapy (3D-CRT). In intensity modulated radiation therapy (IMRT), even less tissue is exposed to the full dose.

gists, nearly half of men given a low 64.5 Gy dose had a cancer in their biopsy two to three years after treatment. At the minimum acceptable dose for prostate cancer (70 Gy), 30 percent of men had a positive biopsy after therapy. After 81 Gy, less than 10 percent of men tested positive for cancer.

The software required for 3-D conformal radiation is widely available, affordable, and compatible with any modern linear accelerator. No one in a developed country should be treated with radiation for prostate cancer without 3-D conformal technology.

Intensity Modulated Radiation Therapy (IMRT)

Intensity modulated radiation therapy (IMRT) fine-tunes 3-D conformal technology even further. By using sophisticated computerized algorithms, this technique delivers the treatment dose at varying intensities throughout the targeted field. Cancer cells in the prostate and surrounding area (within 1 centimeter of the edge of the gland) can be zapped with more damaging rays, while delicate adjacent tissues are spared. The extraordinary precision of IMRT allows radiation therapists to further increase the treatment dose to 81, 86, or even 91 Gy, while holding serious side effects to a minimum. Pioneering this technology, the radiation oncology team at MSKCC—Zvi Fuks, Steven Leibel, and Michael Zelefsky—were able to reduce serious intestinal complications from 17 percent to 2 percent while substantially increasing cure rates. These high doses are so effective that most men can avoid adjuvant hormone therapy, with all of its side effects, which are often used to enhance cure with conventional doses of radiation (see page 297).[11]

In addition to software, IMRT requires the addition of sophisticated hardware, involving slim tungsten plates that open and close to control the radiation intensity. The technology is relatively expensive and only available at a limited number of centers. While not yet the required standard of care, in my view, 3-D conformal radiation with IMRT is today's best option for any man choosing radiation for prostate cancer.

Proton Beam Radiation

Proton beam radiation was developed shortly after World War II as an outgrowth of research into particle accelerators and first used experimentally in cancer therapy in the mid-1950s. The approach was popularized in a small number of centers where it was touted as a means to treat aggressive tumors in deep internal organs, including the prostate and brain.

Proton beams can be delivered to the precise contours of the target, where they abruptly deposit their energy, avoiding spillover into adjacent tissues. Because damage to surrounding organs is minimized, proponents claim that high, extraordinarily effective treatment doses can be administered. Extravagant claims have been made that the therapy can boast a 100 percent success rate without complications or side effects, but we lack credible studies and long-term data to support this.[12] Experts question whether proton beam therapy is superior to modern high-dose 3-D conformal radiation with IMRT.

The technology is extraordinarily cumbersome and expensive and rarely available. If you happen to live near one of the twenty or so centers worldwide that has a proton beam unit, it can provide good state-of-the-art therapy.

NEUTRON BEAM RADIATION

Neutrons were discovered in 1932, and research into their potential therapeutic benefits began in 1938. As with protons, gigantic, prohibitively expensive equipment is required to accelerate these particles to the velocities necessary to release their powerful energy.

To treat cancers, high-energy neutron beams are thrown into the target organ, delivering a powerful, damaging blow. The therapy is designed for high-risk, aggressive tumors that would likely prove incurable with other forms of radiation.[13]

On the downside, any contact of the beam with normal tissues causes extreme injury, so neutron treatment carries a high incidence of serious side effects. Like proton beam treatment, the equipment is available in few centers. Given the development of neoadjuvant hormone therapy (hormones given before radiation) that can be used in combination with 3-D conformal therapy with IMRT, it's unlikely that early advantages shown using neutron beams would hold today.

IS EXTERNAL BEAM RADIATION RIGHT FOR YOU?

External radiation can be an excellent choice for men over 70, and for younger men with health problems that make them poor candidates for surgery. Because the prostate is permanently removed with radical prostatectomy, avoiding local recurrences decades later, most experts agree that surgery is the better choice for men in their 40s and early 50s. Between those ages, the decision about whether to opt for surgery or radiation may hinge on your general health, sexual and urinary function, the nature of your cancer, personal preference, and lifestyle issues. (See Chapter 12, Deciding How to Treat Localized Prostate Cancer.)

Radiation may not be for you if you've had prior radiation to the pelvic area. Be sure your doctor knows about any such treatments you've had for whatever reason, no matter how long ago. The damaging effects of radiation last a lifetime, and irradiating an area again can be dangerous.

THE ADVANTAGES OF EXTERNAL BEAM THERAPY

The clear benefit of radiation is that you avoid the immediate side effects of surgery (though radiation does cause short- and long-term side effects of its own). In most cases there is only minimal disruption to normal activities. For men who are not good surgical candidates because of health or age, radiation offers an excellent chance to control the cancer.

For a small, aggressive tumor that may have extended outside the prostate in a way that can be included in the treatment field, radiation may offer a better chance for local cure than surgery. Cancers that have metastasized to distant sites are not suitable for local treatment with surgery or radiation, except in combination with systemic therapy involving hormones and/or chemotherapy.

THE DISADVANTAGES OF EXTERNAL BEAM THERAPY

In surgery, we remove the cancer and the organ that developed the tumor in the first place, preventing late recurrence or the development of a new cancer in the prostate at some later time. With radiation, the prostate is not removed, and no matter how effective the treatment, some normal prostate tissue will remain. Whatever caused the first cancer could give rise to another tumor in the gland. If that happens, further radiation would not be possible. Irradiated organs are given the maximum allowable lifetime dose and changed permanently. Radiation effects are cumulative, and exposing a treated area to more damaging rays can cause serious, irreversible damage to normal tissues.

If radiation fails to control the cancer, your only remaining chance for a cure would be salvage radical prostatectomy, a difficult procedure that should only be attempted by highly skilled, experienced surgeons. Even in the best of hands, the incidence of complications and side effects is considerably higher in salvage surgery than for radical prostatectomy on a gland that has not been irradiated. (See Chapter 14, Surgery, for more details.)

In some cases, logistics can be troublesome. Radiation therapy using 3D-CRT is not available everywhere, and fewer hospitals offer state-of-the-art 3-D conformal radiation with IMRT. Conventional treatment at a lower dose would increase your risk of side effects and limit your chance for a cure. If you don't live near a center that offers good modern technology, a long commute or even a temporary move might prove necessary.

Once you start a course of radiation, you're committed to completing it. You can't take time off in the middle or defer your remaining treatments if something comes up.

HOW TO CHOOSE
A RADIATION PROGRAM

The likelihood that you'll be cured and your risk of serious side effects will hinge heavily on where you get radiation. Be sure to have your treatment with highly trained doctors who use approved modern equipment. This is especially critical with the very high-dose radiation required to destroy prostate cancer.

Effective external beam treatment depends on scrupulous treatment planning, followed by precise, consistent administration of the daily prescribed dose. You'll be best off at a center that uses modern 3-D conformal equipment, preferably with IMRT. Meticulous maintenance of the machines is essential. If you are scheduled to receive 2 Gy (equivalent to 200 centigray or cGy) per day, you don't want to get 2.1 Gy one day and 1.9 the next, and you certainly don't want to receive less than the optimal dose overall. The hospital's radiation team should include a computer planner and a radiation physicist who calibrates the machines frequently to ensure that they're emitting the proper amount of energy.

Radiation disasters happen very rarely, but you don't want them happening to you. Just as you wouldn't expect to see an airline's maintenance record before boarding a plane, you aren't likely to be privy to the center's equipment history or its incidence of serious burns or fistulas (open

---

NOTE: While 70 to 80 percent of centers in the United States now use 3-D conformal radiation and many have purchased the technology required to administer IMRT, using these approaches correctly to administer the high doses needed to kill prostate cancers requires experience and expertise. It's a good idea to question a radiation oncologist's record of long-term cure and to ask about both short- and long-term side effects.

holes). Your best defense is a busy, state-of-the-art facility with an excellent reputation.

THE TREATMENT

One to several weeks before you start treatments, you'll be scheduled for studies to map the size, shape, and location of your prostate. The best centers use a CT scan or MRI to picture your prostate in three dimensions in relation to surrounding tissues. More conventional studies using

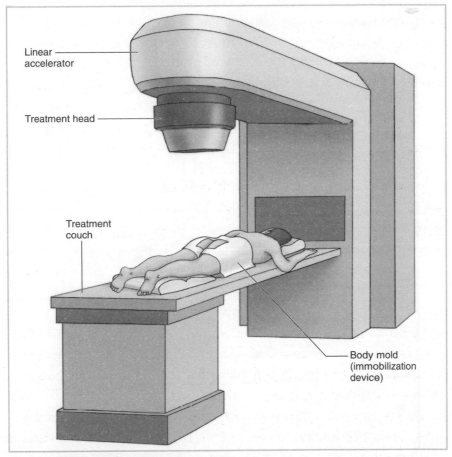

Linear accelerator

Treatment head

Treatment couch

Body mold (immobilization device)

To receive radiation therapy, a patient lies on a table, held in place by a plastic immobilization device, while the radiation is beamed from a linear accelerator.

plain X-ray films and contrast dies to outline the bladder do not offer nearly as precise information about prostate anatomy. In modern centers, a high-tech simulator is used to chart exactly where and how the therapy will be delivered in the three-dimensional field.

A mold of your pelvic area will be made to ensure that you're placed in exactly the same position every day and held in that posture as the radiation is delivered from varying angles. To further ensure consistency, a few tiny dots will be tattooed on your abdomen and back as landmarks.

You'll be scheduled for treatment every weekday for about two months. Treatments last only a few minutes, and the entire process, including check-in and trading your street clothes for a hospital gown, should not take more than about a half hour. Aside from this and some basic suggestions that your radiation oncologist will make regarding skin care, no changes in your normal routine should be necessary. You will not be radioactive during the course of treatment, and close contact, including sexual intercourse, is not a problem.

PSA AND EXTERNAL RADIATION

Because the prostate remains in place after radiation, the PSA drops, but not to zero. It's hard to know what level is low enough to indicate that the cancer has been destroyed. If the PSA starts to rise, a biopsy may be necessary to determine whether cancer cells are present (see Chapter 20, Rising PSA after Surgery or Radiation Therapy). If we find a tumor, it's tough to treat. If we do not, it's difficult to tell whether the biopsy missed cancer cells within the prostate, whether the cancer cells had already spread elsewhere, or whether the PSA is rising from benign growth of the remaining normal prostate tissue. In some men, the PSA level rises after a time and then falls again without treatment. This PSA bounce is difficult to interpret and can cause extreme anxiety.[14] While we wait the necessary interval to determine whether a rising PSA represents a meaningless artifact or a real recurrence, we may miss the window of opportunity for a cure.[15] Interpreting PSA levels becomes especially confusing in a man treated with hormones in addition to radiation. Hormone therapy drives the PSA down to a very low level. When hormones are stopped, the PSA typically rises again until the full effects of radiation kick in and lower it again. For two and a half to three years after radiation, it's virtually impossible to tell for sure whether the cancer has been controlled.

THE SIDE EFFECTS OF EXTERNAL BEAM RADIATION

During the course of external beam radiation, about 15 percent of men complain of decreased energy, altered appetite, weight loss, and fatigue, but the vast majority have no such problems. Skin irritation or burns should never occur with modern radiation techniques. Ten percent of men will have some troublesome (grade II) gastrointestinal problems, such as the urge to defecate with no stool in the rectum (**tenesmus**), dietary intolerance, or rectal bleeding during or soon after treatment. In addition, 40 to 50 percent experience urgency, frequency, and other urinary symptoms. Medication can provide symptomatic relief. Most of these problems clear up about two months after treatment.

Over the long term, the biggest concern with radiation therapy is bowel injury, which may range in severity depending on the type of radiation and the intensity of the dose. **Radiation proctitis** (inflammation of the rectum) can cause diarrhea, tenesmus, bleeding, or ulceration of the rectal wall over the prostate. These problems develop gradually, as treatment effects accumulate. The incidence of bowel injuries, especially serious ones, has been greatly reduced to 17 percent by modern 3D-CRT,[16] and the incidence with IMRT is 2 to 3 percent.[17]

Radiation proctitis tends to be chronic and difficult to treat. Steroid foam or rectal suppositories may offer some relief, as can dietary changes and medications that soften bowel movements. With modern therapy, the need for a colostomy is very rare. (See Chapter 19, Bowel Side Effects, for a further discussion.)

Six to seven percent of patients treated with conventional therapy develop radiation cystitis, an inflammation of the bladder that can cause urinary frequency, burning, and blood in the urine. Very rarely the bleeding is severe enough to require transfusions. Modern 3-D conformal therapy with IMRT greatly reduces the risk of serious urinary side effects by reducing exposure of the bladder to radiation.

After radiation therapy, 40 to 50 percent of patients experience erectile dysfunction. The risk is higher for older men, those who receive hormone therapy along with radiation, and for those whose erections were somewhat impaired before treatment. Seventy-five percent of patients with postradiation erectile loss find medications such as sildenafil helpful.[18]

Over time, radiation causes a reduction in prostate secretions and reduced ejaculatory volume. Sperm production and the passage of sperm to the prostate are also curtailed by scarring and fibrosis. Even though you may continue to ejaculate, it would be rare to be able to father a child after radiation (though this *does not* mean that it's perfectly safe to cease using birth control). If fertility is an issue, you may want to bank sperm before treatment.

BRACHYTHERAPY

The term **brachytherapy,** also known as interstitial therapy or seed implants, derives from the Greek for "short treatment," meaning the dose is delivered at close range. A radiation source—the seed or pellet—is placed directly into the target area, as opposed to external beam therapy, where the dose is delivered from outside the body. The idea is to hit the cancer cells with the bulk of the damaging rays while reducing the effects to surrounding structures. Radiation effects fall off with startling rapidity. When you move a 1/4 inch from the source, there's a sixteenfold reduction in radiation energy.

Almost all brachytherapy today involves the permanent implantation of radioactive iodine or palladium seeds. Each seed is contained in a tiny titanium capsule, shaped like a piece of pencil lead. Five of the implants laid end to end would measure about 1 inch. Each seed emits very low radiation energy, and the therapeutic effect depends on the interaction of multiple seeds positioned in a three-dimensional grid. The required radiation dose depends on the type of seed. With iodine, the minimum radiation dose delivered to the periphery of the prostate must be at least 145 Gy; with palladium it's 125 Gy. This measure, called the **minimal peripheral dose (MPD)**, ensures an adequate dose throughout the gland. Because the energy is time-released over many months, 145 Gy of brachytherapy with iodine seeds is the equivalent of 70 Gy delivered externally, though this could approach 75 or even 81 Gy when therapy is administered expertly. The typical implant involves 50 to 150 tiny seeds, with the highest concentration in the peripheral zone of the prostate, where most cancers arise.[19]

IS BRACHYTHERAPY FOR YOU?

Brachytherapy is *not* for everyone. With the exception of the temporary high-dose iridium implant mentioned above, most experts agree that seed implants are only appropriate for men whose cancers are low-risk, with all favorable features (a low clinical stage of T1 or T2a, a low Gleason score between 2 and 6, with no aggressive Gleason pattern 4 or 5 components, and with a PSA under 10). Patients with *any* high-risk features should opt for surgery or external radiation, both of which offer a greater chance of long-term cancer control.

NOTE: Occasionally, high dose rate (HDR) brachytherapy, using a temporary, very powerful radiation source, is used to treat very large, advanced, or recurring tumors. For this intense treatment, patients are kept in the hospital for thirty hours, during which time high-energy radiation is delivered through a number of slim tubes inserted into the prostate. The procedure—sometimes called the "Andy Grove method" because the Intel cofounder elected to have his prostate cancer treated by HDR in conjunction with external beam therapy—is repeated three times for a few minutes each time under local anesthetic.[20]

Your prostate anatomy is a major consideration. The larger the gland, the harder it is to saturate with seeds. The ultrasound report from your biopsy will include a measure of your prostate size that is far more accurate than the estimate we can make from a digital rectal exam. A small prostate weighing less than 40 grams is ideal. Anything over 50 or 60 grams, even in the most skilled hands, may be too large to treat safely with seeds, increasing the risk of acute urinary retention after the implant and adding to the risk that the prostate will not be saturated with enough seeds to affect a cure. To treat a large prostate with seeds, hormone therapy would be required to shrink the gland before treatment, and that can cause troublesome side effects of its own (see Hormones and Radiation on page 324).

If you're considering brachytherapy, have a thorough examination to establish the precise configuration of your prostate. In some men, the gland has a large median or lateral lobe that extends into the bladder. In other cases, the prostate sits too high under the arch of the pubic bone, making it hard to access. Either of these situations would add to the risks and technical difficulty of an implant. External therapy or surgery may be the better choice.

Whether or not your prostate is enlarged, if you are having difficulty urinating, you would be at high risk of developing acute urinary retention after seed implants, which occurs in 4 to 10 percent of brachytherapy patients nationwide and in 2 percent at Memorial Sloan-Kettering. Bleeding from the multiple needles used to insert the seeds and swelling from the radiation could block the flow of urine completely. Many patients are treated with alpha blockers, such as tamsulosin (Flomax), to relax the prostate and ease voiding.[21]

If you do have difficulty urinating, **urodynamic testing** before the procedure can gauge whether you have urinary obstruction. The test involves passing a catheter into the bladder through the penis, so it's mildly invasive. Also, the test is not available in every community. Another reasonable measure of obstructive symptoms is the speed of your urinary stream (flow rate). A flow-rate test, in which a patient urinates into a special funnel, can be done in the doctor's office. Another good indicator of urinary blockage is the amount of urine that remains in your bladder after you urinate (post-void residual urine). Ultrasound—a noninvasive, widely available, inexpensive imaging technique—can measure this. Finally, a score over eight on a simple questionnaire like the **International Prostate Symptom Score (IPSS)** (see pages 76–77) indicates that you may have urinary obstruction, and the higher the score, the greater the risk of acute urinary retention after seed implants (see Chapter 5, BPH, [Prostate Enlargement]).

Seed implantation is generally not advised for men who have had a previous TURP, commonly dubbed a "Roto-Rooter" procedure, to relieve symptoms of benign prostate enlargement. The operation leaves a shell of the gland rather than a solid sphere. The remaining real estate is typically insufficient to allow effective seed placement.

THE TREATMENT

Before the implant, you'll have routine preoperative exams, including blood tests, a chest X-ray, and an electrocardiogram. Because the radiation dose depends on the interaction of multiple seeds, precise placement of each one is critical. Before brachytherapy, the radiation oncologist will make a detailed, three-dimensional map of your prostate using a CT scan or MRI and transrectal ultrasound. These tests will determine the volume of the gland, which areas of the prostate and how much surrounding tissue should be targeted (target volume), the dose of radiation you'll receive, how many seeds you'll need, and exactly where each one should be placed.

In many centers, these tests are performed one to three weeks before the seeds are implanted. In the operating room, it can be a challenge to match the precise conditions of the planning session. Proper implants require an active collaboration between the radiation therapist who implants the seeds and either a urologist or a radiologist who is expert in using ultrasound. At Memorial Sloan-Kettering, more sophisticated dynamic treatment planning is performed during the implant in real time, allowing the radiation oncologist to make subtle adjustments to ensure an optimal result. A complex software program considers more than 6 million possibilities in determining the optimal placement of each seed.

During the Implant

Seed implants can be done under general or regional (epidural or spinal) anesthetic. As a rule, it's wise to go along with the method your doctor prefers and knows best.

You'll be on your back with your feet raised in stirrups. A metal template is placed on the perineum (between the scrotum and the rectum), and sixteen to twenty hollow needles are inserted through holes in the template at prescribed intervals. Guided by ultrasound through a rectal probe, the radioactive seeds are then loaded through the needles and dropped in place.

After the implant is completed, an imaging study is done in the operating room or within the next day to calculate the actual dose of radiation you've received. If the dosage is inadequate, some radiation oncologists will implant more seeds, but this increases the risk of side effects. Experienced practitioners would rarely have to do this.

Typically, patients go home the day of the implant and return to work and normal activities soon afterward. Before your discharge, you'll be given information about the radiation safety precautions you'll need to take. You may be asked to urinate through a strainer for several days in case any seeds are discharged. If you do pass a seed, use a spoon or tweezers to place it in a small closed container and deliver it to the doctor at your earliest convenience.

A seed can also pass in the ejaculate. For this reason, and because you may experience some pain on orgasm shortly after the implant, doctors sometimes advise that you have five or so ejaculations in private before resuming sexual relations. Some doctors suggest using a condom during intercourse for anywhere from two weeks to a year after brachytherapy. If you are instructed to do this, it's reasonable to question why and whether it's really necessary.

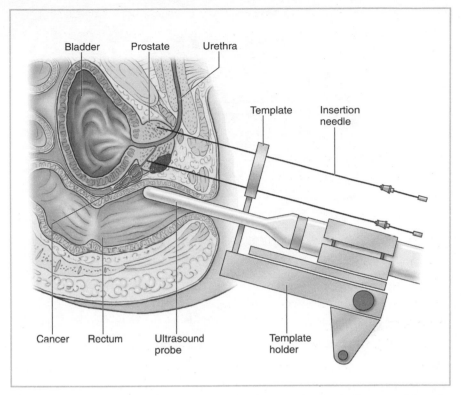

Bladder Prostate Urethra

Template Insertion needle

Cancer Rectum Ultrasound probe Template holder

The setup in the operating room to use ultrasound guidance to place brachytherapy seeds into the prostate.

PSA AFTER BRACHYTHERAPY

With successful eradication of the cancer, the PSA should drop to an al–most undetectable level (preferably less than 0.5) and remain there indef–initely. Sometimes, because the prostate is still in place or the tumor has not been fully destroyed, your PSA may never sink to that ideal low. And it may take as long as three years for PSA to reach its lowest level, which is called the **PSA nadir**. The higher the nadir, the greater the risk that the cancer will eventually recur.

A major source of confusion and anxiety is the PSA bounce,[22] a meaningless rise in the PSA level, which falls again without treatment. Seen in up to 30 percent of patients at about a year and a half to two years after brachytherapy, the bounce phenomenon makes it very diffi-

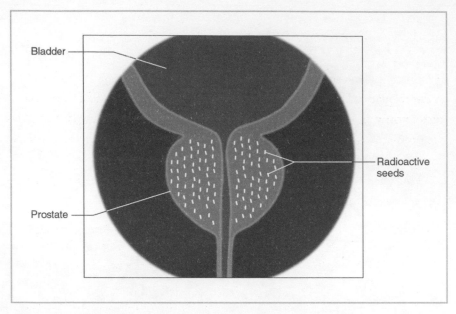

The location of seeds in the prostate on a fluoroscopic image after brachytherapy implantation.

cult to identify a cancer recurrence, and a delay in important treatment may result.

In radiation, treatment is not officially deemed a failure until there are three consecutive rises in the PSA.[23] Our studies suggest that a better measure would be three increasing rises or peaks above the lowest level (nadir), whether or not they are consecutive. If you see three new peaks in your PSA, I'd recommend having a serious discussion with your radiation oncologist and urologist about whether you need a biopsy of the prostate to find out if the cancer is present and growing. Using the current definition of recurrence after radiation, we rarely recognize a failure with brachytherapy or external beam radiation until three to four years after treatment, when the window of opportunity for a cure has passed in most patients.

THE ADVANTAGES OF SEED IMPLANTS

The major attraction of brachytherapy is convenience. You can have the seeds implanted and be home the same day or the next. After the procedure, you will not need a catheter. Typically, you'll have no pain beyond some soreness in the perineal area that can be managed with a simple over-the-counter analgesic such as acetaminophen.

The treatment has few immediate complications and minimal short-term impact on quality of life.

THE DISADVANTAGES OF SEED IMPLANTS

Though side effects are far from inevitable, problems with urinary control and bowel and erectile function develop slowly over months or even years as radiation damage accumulates. While serious side effects are rare, especially in the hands of top experts, 40 to 50 percent of patients have urinary frequency and urgency that can often be alleviated with the use of alpha-blocking drugs.

While the radiation from seeds generally is not harmful to others, you will be told to avoid close contact with small children, young animals, and pregnant women for a few months after the implant, until the radiation dissipates. Being in the same room is not a problem. To expose someone else to radiation from your seeds, you would need to hold the person on your lap or sit right beside them for a prolonged period. Some doctors suggest placing a pillow between yourself and your partner if you like to sleep in the "spoon" position, though others feel that the pelvic bones provide enough natural protection.

Given heightened security in airports and at border crossings, you may want to carry a card that identifies you as an implant patient. Despite the low level of radiation brachytherapy implants emit, you might set off a Geiger counter or other detection device.

Until the radiation is no longer active, it's wise to avoid elective medical procedures, such as a colonoscopy, and elective surgical procedures, such as a hip replacement or dental work, that might put the doctor or dentist at risk of radiation exposure. If you require such procedures, medical personnel should take appropriate precautions.

Treatment results are highly variable and operator-dependent. It takes a very experienced, very meticulous radiation oncologist to do a good job of implanting the seeds. Since side effects and cancer recurrences can take many years to develop or detect, getting reliable information about a particular doctor's track record can be tricky.

Some seeds can migrate out of the prostate, invading adjacent tissues or even distant organs, such as the lungs. Because the energy of individual seeds is very low, stray seeds don't pose a significant health risk.

If treatment fails to control the tumor, you should not receive further radiation. Radiation damage has lifelong effects and is cumulative. Doctors have reported giving external radiation after seeds fail or implanting seeds after an external radiation or brachytherapy failure. I'd warn patients against these approaches, which carry a serious risk of damage to the bowel and urinary tract. We have no good evidence that a second radiation dose is effective against a recurrent cancer.

Salvage surgery can be done after seed implants, but the procedure is far more difficult and riskier than radical prostatectomy on a gland that has not been irradiated. Only a highly experienced surgeon should attempt salvage radical prostatectomy. (See Chapter 14, Surgery.)

THE SIDE EFFECTS OF BRACHYTHERAPY

Immediate side effects are similar to those for a prostate biopsy. There may be some blood in the urine for a few days and some blood in the ejaculate for as long as six to eight weeks. The needles used to implant the seeds can cause mild pain or soreness in the perineum, which usually responds to over-the-counter pain medications such as acetaminophen or an anti-inflammatory drug such as ibuprofen.

The seeds emit their radiation gradually. **Half-life** refers to the number of days required for the radiation source to lose 50 percent of its original strength. Palladium has a shorter half-life (thirty-five days), so it delivers radiation more quickly than iodine, for which the half-life is sixty days. It takes about four to six months for seeds to give off virtually their entire dose of radiation, but it can take years for the damaging effects to accumulate.

It was hoped that modern brachytherapy would yield the same low rates of side effects as early seed implants, but as the dose was increased in an attempt to improve cure rates, complications increased as well. Even in men who have no previous urinary problems, swelling from the implant can cause frequent urination, urgency, or the need to strain to urinate. The symptoms often respond to alpha-blocking drugs such as alfuzosin, tamsulosin, or doxazosin, and most men receive one of these drugs before and after implantation to relax the prostate and bladder neck.

In about 4 to 10 percent of cases (less in the hands of a top expert), irritation and swelling from the implants trigger acute urinary retention, especially in men who have obstructive voiding symptoms before brachytherapy. This sudden inability to urinate could require long-term use of a catheter, the insertion of a suprapubic tube (above the pubic bone at the base of the abdomen), or a transurethral resection of the prostate (TURP). Thirty percent of men who need a TURP (the so-called "Roto-Rooter" procedure) after seed implants develop severe incontinence, requiring placement of an artificial urinary sphincter to regain urinary control.[24]

A month to three months after seed placement, when radiation effects start to accumulate, 20 to 40 percent of patients experience symptoms of radiation urethritis (painful urination, frequency, urgency, and bleeding) or radiation prostatism (a prostate inflammation that causes burning at the tip of the penis), and perineal or lower abdominal pain. As with similar side effects from external beam radiation, these problems are difficult to treat and can persist for years. Anticholinergic drugs and topical anesthetics may provide some relief.

As radiation shrinks the prostate, the amount of fluid produced by the gland diminishes, reducing the volume of ejaculate. Some patients experience painful ejaculations, and virtually all men lose the ability to father children (though this does not mean it's safe to give up birth control unless you've been tested to be sure no viable sperm are present). If fertility is a concern, you may want to bank sperm before the implant.

Over time, there is a gradual loss of erections because of damage to small blood vessels and the erectile nerves. Few good long-term studies have looked at potency after brachytherapy, but a large trial at North Shore Hospital found that 39 percent of patients lost erections by a year after treatment, and a five-year study at Memorial Sloan-Kettering put the impotence rate at 53 percent, though top experts using state-of-the-art methods are beginning to report better results. Some doctors still cite antiquated data from the era of low-dose seeds, when only 10 percent of previously potent men lost erections after brachytherapy, but those numbers do not apply to the higher radiation doses delivered by seeds today. The nerves are so close to the edge of the prostate, and cancer so often grows right at the edge of the gland that it is impossible to dose the entire prostate adequately without exposing the nerves to the same high dose of radiation (see Chapter 2, Normal Male Function).[25]

THE BOTTOM LINE

At Memorial Sloan-Kettering, Dr. Michael Zelefsky has pioneered a far more accurate approach to brachytherapy that uses a sophisticated real-time computer program in the operating room for dose distribution.[26] The program guides seed placement, ensuring an optimal radiation dose to the entire prostate while minimizing damage to the urethra and rectum. By increasing accuracy, Dr. Zelefsky has reduced urinary and bowel side effects substantially while obtaining cancer control rates comparable to those offered by high-dose external beam therapy. But these results are early. Long-term effects on erectile, urinary, and bowel function remain to be seen.

Brachytherapy is a reasonable option for men with prostates smaller than 50 grams and a favorable cancer, especially when convenience is a central issue. Even with the improved techniques at Memorial Sloan-

Kettering, we do not recommend brachytherapy for any patients with a PSA over 10, a Gleason score of 7 or greater, a palpable or visible cancer larger than a centimeter or so, or for patients with more than two biopsy course positive for cancer.

COMBINATION EXTERNAL BEAM AND BRACHYTHERAPY

With conventional therapy (70 Gy radiation delivered externally by a standard linear accelerator), 15 to 20 percent of men have serious bowel and urinary complications. In an attempt to reduce side effects and improve the cure rate, some radiation therapists decided to deliver 40 percent of the recommended dose with seed implants and the other 60 percent by external beam. The first such program was developed by Drs. Phil Hutchins and Eugene Carlton at Baylor College of Medicine in 1965. Following their lead, many major centers started using the combination treatment in the late 1970s and early '80s.

Current advocates of this belt-and-suspenders approach claim that it can deliver higher radiation doses, and, indeed, cure rates with combination therapy are good.[27] Unfortunately, this carries a high price tag of serious complications. Erectile dysfunction is common, as is radiation proctitis (irritation of the bowel), sometimes followed by rectal ulcers. Mild ulcers may respond to anti-inflammatory drugs or steroids, but surgery may be necessary in severe cases.

The problem is prostate anatomy. The gland lies perilously close to the erectile nerves and the rectal wall. At a sufficiently high dose to kill cancers, the combination approach exposes these delicate structures to excessive and highly damaging radiation.

Radiation therapy involves complex decision making by the oncologist and subtle variations in technique. A certain percentage of error, in which normal structures are exposed to damaging X-rays, is inevitable. When both seed implants and external beam therapy are administered, the error rate and resultant side effects may be multiplied. There is no evidence that cancers are cured more effectively with combined approaches. Generally, combination therapy is a low-tech, riskier substitute for modern, high-dose, 3-D conformal radiotherapy.

Given the wide availability of effective, high-dose, modern 3-D conformal radiation and IMRT, I see little justification for the risks involved in the combination approach.

HORMONES AND RADIATION

Radiation works best against a small, manageable adversary. It's easier to wipe out two hundred mosquitoes than two thousand, and the same holds true for cancer cells. Killing off a few insects with a shot of insect repellent has less effect on the environment than saturation crop dusting from a plane. By the same token, a small, highly targeted radiation dose risks less damage to normal surrounding tissues.

Frustrated with the poor cure rates with conventional (70 Gy) external radiation, oncologists designed studies to test whether shrinking the cancer with hormones before radiation would improve the results. Indeed it did, especially for cancers with any aggressive features. In fact, studies clearly showed better survival rates for large (T2b or greater) or high-grade (Gleason 7 or higher) cancers when hormones were combined with conventional doses of radiation.[28] In most studies, hormones were started several months before radiation and continued until the last day of treatment. For particularly aggressive cancers, the best effects were achieved when hormones were continued for two to three years. What we do not know is whether similar cure rates can be achieved with hormones alone, especially if men are willing to stay on hormone therapy permanently. Whether or not radiation therapy works for a high-risk cancer remains to be seen.

In these studies, hormone treatment involves shutting down the production of male hormones with drugs called **LHRH agonists**, administering **antiandrogens** to prevent the cells from absorbing these hormones, or prescribing a combination of the two, known as a **total** or **complete androgen blockade**.

We still don't know whether hormones work by shrinking the primary tumor and increasing the probability that the radiation will kill every cell or by eliminating tiny, undetectable areas of spread, called micrometastases. The latter seems unlikely, since hormones add nothing to cure rates with surgery.

Several studies have shown that hormones plus radiation improve cancer control, but it's unclear why.[29] By shrinking the cancer, hormones may increase the likelihood that a given dose of radiation will completely eradicate the cancer. If so, the same result could be achieved with modern high-dose IMRT. Dr. Steven Leibel at Memorial Sloan-Kettering estimates that combining hormones with radiation is comparable to adding 5 Gy to the dose. At Memorial Sloan-Kettering, about 40 percent of patients are asked to take three to six months of hormone therapy, typically to shrink a large prostate and reduce the size of the field that must be irradiated. Minimizing the area that must be hit with destructive X-rays lowers the risk of damage to the urinary tract, erectile nerves, and rectal wall.

Unfortunately, hormone therapy carries risks of its own. Cutting off the androgen supply can cause troublesome side effects, including hot flashes, loss of libido and erections, loss of muscle mass, changes in the distribution of body hair, breast swelling, and depression.[30] When radiation is combined with hormone therapy, the incidence of permanent erectile dysfunction is greater, though how much greater has not been well studied.

Most men regain normal testosterone production following a short course of three months to a year on hormone therapy, but some don't. Older men and those who started out with low testosterone levels may not regain hormone levels sufficient to restore erectile function or relieve the other side effects.

THE FUTURE

DOSE PAINTING.   This concept shows promise as a way to refine radiation treatments. Researchers are working to develop highly sensitive imaging and staging techniques that would allow us the ability to precisely pinpoint tumors within the prostate. This would allow radiation oncologists to target highly specific areas of the gland while selectively protecting vulnerable adjacent structures, including the erectile nerves, urethra, and rectal wall.[31]

HIGHER RADIATION DOSES.   Doses of 86 and even 91 Gy have been delivered safely using the best modern 3-D conformal therapy with IMRT. Such high doses can eliminate the need for hormone therapy.[32] Dr. Zvi Fuks at Memorial Sloan-Kettering is testing whether a single dose of 22 to 24 Gy, given in a single day, can permanently eradicate cancers even better than the eight-to-ten-week fractioned course of radiation therapy.

SENSITIZING AND PROTECTIVE AGENTS.   A number of substances currently under investigation are designed to increase the effect of radiation on target tissues and reduce the damage to normal adjacent tissues.

SYSTEMIC RADIATION.   This procedure may be used to eliminate undetectable metastases in high-risk patients.

IN SUMMARY

Depending on a man's age and the nature of his disease, good modern radiation can be a highly effective treatment for localized prostate cancer. The dose and precise method of delivery are crucial to maximize your chance for a cure and minimize the risk of side effects. When adjacent organs are exposed to radiation damage, urinary incontinence, sexual dysfunction, and bowel problems can develop over time. If you opt for radiation therapy, be sure to choose an expert radiation oncologist and an excellent, state-of-the-art facility.

16

■

Other Local Therapies

READ THIS CHAPTER TO LEARN:

- What other treatments are available for localized prostate cancer?
- Which are approved by the FDA?
- What is an "investigational" treatment? An "experimental" treatment?
- How can you evaluate these treatments?

Researchers are constantly seeking better ways to search out and destroy prostate cancers. Because the gland is so devilishly difficult to access and the risk of damage to nearby vital structures accompanies all currently accepted treatments, the quest to discover a kindler, gentler, but still effective response continues.

Until a new treatment has been thoroughly tested, proven safe and effective, and practiced for enough time to yield convincing, durable results, we refer to it as investigational. Several investigational treatments are currently available for localized prostate cancer. **Cryotherapy** (freezing the prostate) has been used off and on for over thirty years and is now approved by the FDA, but long-term results are uncertain. Other treatments, such as destroying the tumor with heat (**thermal therapy**) or light (**photodynamic therapy**), or injecting altered genes into the prostate (**gene therapy**), are under intense study as experimental treatments, meaning they are not yet approved by the FDA for routine use. They are being studied in clinical trials, which means their effectiveness has yet to be proven.

In considering any of these approaches, keep in mind that they lack an established track record. While some might eventually earn a place in standard practice, at this point we don't know how safe they are or how successful they will ultimately be in arresting cancers and preventing recurrences. Prostate cancer is typically slow to progress, and it can take many years, or even decades, to demonstrate effects of a therapy on cancer spread and survival. Also, just because a treatment seems "less invasive" or otherwise easier than standard surgery or radiation therapy does not ensure that it will cause fewer side effects or yield better cure rates.

Establishing a new program or center to administer an investigational approach involves considerable expense, time, and energy. Doctors who embrace a novel treatment may stake their financial and professional future on its success. It's wise to be mindful of this as you evaluate these methods and weigh reported outcomes. Physicians studying experimental treatments in clinical trials are ethically bound to disclose whether they or their institution have a financial stake in the outcome of the study. You're well within your rights to ask if a doctor you're considering has such an interest in the treatment he recommends.

FREEZING THE GLAND (CRYOTHERAPY)

Guided by ultrasound, probes are placed in the prostate through the **perineum** (behind the scrotum). Argon gas or liquid nitrogen is delivered through the probes to freeze the gland and surrounding tissues, creating an ice ball. As it forms, the ice ball can be observed by ultrasound, so the surgeon has some control over the extent of tissue damage. At least two cycles of freezing and thawing are required to destroy prostate-cancer cells, and even several cycles provide no guarantee. Normal and malignant prostate cells are remarkably resilient. From biopsy results and elevations in PSA, we know that often some cancer cells persist after freezing. Also, in many cases normal prostate cells remain undamaged, and new cancers may develop years later.

While cryotherapy can effectively destroy cancers in the liver or kidneys, the anatomy of the prostate has restricted its success in treating cancer there. The rectum, the nerves responsible for penile erections, and the urinary sphincter are all situated within millimeters of the capsule of the gland. To destroy cancer, the ice ball must reach the capsule or beyond without destroying these essential surrounding structures. Unfortunately, cryotherapy is not nearly so precise, and the price paid for modestly effective treatment is a high rate of complications and reduced quality of life.

Proponents tout cryosurgery as a minimally invasive, highly effective procedure with minimal side effects. But, in fact, freezing the gland causes virtually all men to lose erections, and few ever recover.[1] Cryoablation can also result in urinary incontinence, scrotal swelling, penile pain or numbness, pelvic pain, urinary obstruction, and, in 1 in 200 cases, a hole (fistula) between the rectum and prostate. Results are highly operator-dependent, varying with the skill and experience of the doctor performing the procedure, and the long-term effectiveness of cryotherapy itself has not been proven. The incidence of serious side effects is higher when cryotherapy is performed for recurrent disease after radiation.[2] Still, using this approach to treat a recurrence may be reasonable considering how few effective alternatives we have. (See Chapter 20, Rising PSA after Surgery or Radiation Therapy.)

FOCAL THERAPIES

THERMAL (HEAT) THERAPY

Thermal therapies, which use various energy sources and delivery methods to effectively cook target tissues, are experimental and not yet approved for use in medical practice outside of a formal clinical trial.

High-intensity focused ultrasound, known as **HIFU**, destroys tissue with the extreme heat generated by high-energy ultrasound waves. The procedure requires regional (spinal or epidural) anesthesia. A probe inserted in the rectum contains two ultrasound transducers, one to image the prostate and identify the target and another to send out the destructive thermal energy.

HIFU has been used successfully to eliminate excess tissue from the central or transition zone of the gland, clearing the urinary blockage caused by benign prostate enlargement (BPH). Preliminary studies in Europe suggest that this approach may eventually have a role in treating relatively small, favorable prostate cancers in elderly men who do not want radiation or surgery.[3] HIFU focuses intense, destructive energy in a tiny cylinder of tissue, measuring about 2×10 millimeters. By lining up these cylinders in the ultrasound image, the urologist can target areas thought to harbor cancers. HIFU and other forms of thermal therapy target small areas of prostate cancer (focal treatment) rather than targeting the whole gland, as is the case with traditional surgery or radiotherapy. Unfortunately, most prostate cancers are multifocal, springing up in several parts of the gland at once. Current imaging techniques are unable to pinpoint all the cancer clusters so they can be destroyed. Generally, larger cancers are more dangerous, but sometimes small, elusive malignancies are aggressive and pose a high risk of spread if not destroyed.

Because of its extreme precision, HIFU appears to be safer than cryotherapy, with few serious side effects reported. Targeting small, suspect areas within the prostate avoids damage to the erectile nerves and urinary sphincter. If a physician tries to treat large cancers using this method, more troubling side effects may occur. Since the dead tissue swells and then sloughs into the urethra, there is a risk of urinary blockage after HIFU. In one study, 33 percent of patients required a TURP to relieve acute urinary retention. Today, TURP is done together with HIFU under the same anesthesia, with better results.

Radiofrequency ablation, known as **RFA**, similarly attempts to eradicate tumor cells by delivering destructive energy through special needles, which are guided into place in the prostate by ultrasound. The procedure, which uses the RITA (radiofrequency interstitial tissue ablation) system, can be done under spinal anesthesia or local anesthesia combined with sedation. RFA has been used to destroy tumors in the kidney and other organs, but since it targets focal areas of the prostate instead of destroying the whole gland, it has the same limitations as HIFU. Also, like HIFU, RFA is relatively new, and long-term results are not available.

PHOTODYNAMIC (LIGHT) THERAPY

An interesting and novel approach to the treatment of localized cancers is photodynamic therapy. Let me disclose at the outset that I have been paid to advise a company that is studying this method.

Photodynamic therapy has been around for decades, stirring little serious interest in the medical community. Recently, however, scientists have developed a new, more powerful chemical derived from plant chlorophyll, nature's premier agent for converting light into energy. The photodynamic agent is administered intravenously. Then, a laser light source is inserted into the prostate, activating the chemical to destroy the cancer along with its blood supply.[4]

Whether the area of tissue destroyed can be controlled precisely, avoiding damage to the surrounding nerves, sphincters, and rectal wall, remains to be proven by carefully performed clinical trials.

The Bottom Line

As yet, no studies have proven that treating specific suspected areas of cancer within the prostate can alter the long-term course of the disease. Other untreated clusters of cancer cells may continue to grow and spread. Still, I find this approach intriguing and well worth investigating. Today, we discover many small cancers that pose little risk but cause so much anxiety that many men insist on treatment nonetheless. If HIFU, RFA, or photodynamic therapy can destroy these tiny tumors with ease and safety and the treatments can be repeated as new cancer clusters are detected, many men may be able to avoid the risks of radical surgery or radiation therapy.

GENE THERAPY
AND ONCOLYTIC VIRUSES

In the 1990s, the research team I led at Baylor College of Medicine in Houston conducted the first successful clinical trial of so-called "suicide" gene therapy for prostate cancer. The idea is to inject a Trojan horse in the form of a virus that infiltrates the cancer cells and leaves behind a gene called thymidine kinase, or tk. Later, we administer an antiviral drug called ganciclovir. The genetically altered cells render the drug far more lethal, and the cancer is destroyed. In several subsequent studies, viruses have been used successfully to introduce suicide genes or to attack cancer cells directly.

Gene therapy by local injection appears to be safe. None of the feared consequences—viruses migrating to other parts of the body and wreaking harm, permanently infecting and destroying the normal gland, or getting into sperm and being transmitted to offspring—has occurred.[5] Unfortunately, the approach has shown limited effectiveness because of the difficulty involved in injecting all of the cancer cells. Development of viral gene therapy has been hindered by its prohibitive cost, the worry about unforeseen consequences of using viruses, and the limited promise of financial reward, which makes the research unattractive to pharmaceutical companies. The pursuit of this treatment has been relegated to the few university laboratories able to afford the research and development costs but appears to be poised for a commercial rebirth.

Most studies to date have tested gene therapy in patients with local recurrences of prostate cancer after radiation therapy. The treatment may yet play a major role when radiation or surgery fails to control a localized prostate cancer, or for very small cancers. Another exciting possibility is that local gene therapy may stimulate generalized immunity to prostate cancer, ridding the body of microscopic metastases that otherwise cannot be controlled.

IN SUMMARY

New treatments for localized prostate cancer are constantly being developed and tested. While some of these novel approaches may become standard practice in the future, they do not have a demonstrated track record of cancer cure, and their long-term risks may be unknown. Be wary of extravagant, unproven claims.

17

■

Urinary Side Effects

READ THIS CHAPTER TO LEARN:

- Why do prostate diseases and their treatments affect urinary function?
- What urinary problems can radiation and radical prostatectomy cause?
- What can be done about urinary side effects?

Urination should be a routine bodily function, but for many men the prostate throws up a major roadblock to that routine. The upper portion of the urethra, the conduit that channels urine from the bladder to the outside, runs directly through the gland. Benign or malignant prostate overgrowth can narrow the passageway, triggering a variety of urinary problems. Symptoms can range in severity from a minor slowing of the urinary stream to a sudden, complete inability to urinate. Acute urinary retention is a medical emergency that requires immediate relief to avoid serious bladder or kidney damage.

Because of the hand-in-glove relationship between the urinary channel and the prostate, treatments for prostate diseases, including surgery and radiation, all carry a risk of urinary side effects. Imagine trying to repair the Lincoln Tunnel without affecting the traffic running through it. Urinary problems can take the form of **obstructive voiding symptoms** (slow stream, hesitancy, intermittency, waking at night to urinate, etc.), **irritative voiding symptoms** (frequency, urgency, blood in the urine, burning, etc.), or urinary **incontinence** (leaking, loss of urinary control).

URINATION AFTER RADICAL PROSTATECTOMY

To cure prostate cancer surgically, we remove the entire gland, the seminal vesicles, and the bladder neck, which runs into and is virtually indistinguishable from the adjacent prostate. Sparing the bladder neck increases the risk of leaving cancer behind. Nevertheless, some surgeons do so in the misguided belief that this is necessary to preserve urinary continence.

The bladder neck contains the **internal urinary sphincter**, a sturdy muscular trapdoor that keeps urine from escaping until you're ready to void. After radical prostatectomy, the **external** (or **outer**) **urinary sphincter**, which normally acts as a second line of defense against accidental leakage, must assume the entire responsibility for keeping you dry.

Typically, the body makes this adjustment uneventfully on its own, though the time it takes to regain full urinary control varies widely. Any leakage that occurs until the transfer of function is completed can usually be managed with the use of small pads that might require changing anywhere from one to several times a day.

NOTE: These pads are specifically designed for this purpose in men and come in a variety of styles. They can be purchased by mail order, online, or in drugstores. (See the Resources section at the back of this book.)

INCONTINENCE

Though prostate cancer commonly evokes an image of severe incontinence and patients often worry that they'll have to use adult diapers or wear a catheter and leg bag, such serious leakage is rare following competent surgery to remove the gland. In the hands of average surgeons nationwide, about 8 percent of radical prostatectomy patients report troublesome incontinence.[1] For those operated on by expert surgeons, any long-term urinary control problem—including minor leakage—is uncommon.[2] Some of my patients are dry as soon as the catheter is removed, and more than half stop needing pads within a few days. By six weeks after surgery, 90 percent achieve social continence, meaning that urinary leakage has ceased altogether or lessened to the point that it has little or no impact on normal activities. Seventy-five percent of these men are sufficiently dry to stop wearing pads altogether, and the rest simply use a small pad to contain minimal leakage. One year after radical prostatectomy, only 1 percent of men I see continue to have leakage troublesome enough to warrant treatment. In general, this holds true for patients of highly experienced surgeons nationwide.

Studies show that recovery after surgery depends to a great extent on the skill of the surgeon.[3] On average in the United States, the return to full urinary control after radical prostatectomy takes six weeks to three months, and about 8 percent of patients continue to be bothered by leakage two years later. When compared with the results of top surgeons, this represents double the time to regaining full control and a four- to eightfold greater risk of lasting incontinence. When choosing a doctor, keep in mind that the quality of your care can have a major impact on your quality of life.

How Much Leakage Constitutes Incontinence?

Though it's common for people to equate the term "urinary incontinence" with the complete lack of bladder control seen in infants, in fact, the generally accepted definition of *severe* incontinence after prostate-cancer treatment is leaking 2 or more tablespoons of urine per day *and* being moderately to severely bothered by it as measured by a question-naire. The response to leaking urine is highly subjective. Some men find it intolerable to lose a single drop, while others are not particularly trou-bled by the need to use a few small, unobtrusive pads per day to keep their clothing dry.

> NOTE: The number of pads used is not a good way to measure the severity of urinary control problems. Some men elect to change a pad every time it gets the least bit damp, while others are content to wait for total saturation.

When weighing the risk of side effects, keep in mind that doctors may differ enormously in what they mean when they report their results. If you see one surgeon who sets his incontinence rate at 30 percent and another who claims only a 1 percent incidence, they could be describing entirely different outcomes. The former doctor might be telling you about every patient who leaks even a small amount of urine for a short time after surgery, while the latter only counts patients as incontinent if they have severe, intractable leakage that persists for years. Be sure to ask physicians you consult to define their terms.

Who Is at Risk for Incontinence?

Age plays a significant role. Men over 65 have more difficulty regaining urinary control, and after age 70, the problems tend to be even greater. Older men may be more susceptible to incontinence because of benign enlargement of the prostate, preexisting bladder outlet obstruction, or the reduced muscle mass that typically accompanies advancing age.[4]

Men who need to have erectile nerves removed to cure their cancer experience greater problems with urinary control. Having these nerves intact appears to play a role in normal voiding—an important reason to have nerve-sparing surgery where possible, even if sexual function is not a concern.

Urinary incontinence is much more likely in men who develop a stricture (see page 340). But your risk of incontinence is not affected by an enlarged prostate, a previous TURP, symptoms of prostatitis, your weight, or the size of your cancer.

Leaking Urine During Sex

Some men recover erections while they are still experiencing lapses in urinary control. Worries about losing urine while with a partner during intercourse or orgasm can inhibit sexual activity and hamper recovery of erectile function. In most cases, the problem clears up on its own. If it doesn't, exercises, medications, or, though rarely, further surgery may be indicated. Definitely discuss this and any other postoperative concerns with your doctor. Open communication with your sexual partner is also a good idea. Something you view as a major issue may not concern your partner. Also, rest assured that urine is sterile, and a little leakage is harmless.

> NOTE: When it comes to sensitive, private concerns about urinary and sexual function, many men are tempted to "grin and bear it," but this won't get the problems solved. Today, treatments exist for most side effects.

What Can You Do about Early Problems with Urinary Incontinence?

In patients who continue to experience some leakage more than six weeks after surgery, the problem is typically minor, requiring the use of no more than one to two pads per day, and it usually resolves over time on its own. Some men have **stress urinary incontinence (SUI)** after surgery and only lose urine when they stand up, sneeze, cough, or bend, or when then engage in strenuous physical activity, such as swinging a golf club, jogging, or lifting weights. Paradoxically, some highly conditioned athletes only have a problem when they're relaxed. Early on, it's not uncommon for men to lose urine when they are tired or have been drinking alcohol, both of which relax the sphincter muscle. Some men urinate at night, during deep sleep, without realizing it, so even if you experience no leakage during the day, a protective pad on the mattress may be a good idea for the first month or two.

NOTE: Radical prostatectomy alters your anatomy. By making some minor adjustments, you may be able to reduce or even avoid urinary leakage. Simple actions like emptying your bladder more frequently might improve your urinary control. Be aware of factors, such as fatigue, that increase your probability of losing urine. In situations where you are likely to drink alcohol or engage in strenuous physical activities that test your ability to stay dry, you may want to wear a pad as a precaution.

For the first six weeks or so after surgery, extra vigilance can help you avoid any embarrassment. If you're scheduled to be in busy social situations or in the spotlight, such as an actor onstage, a lawyer presenting to a jury, or a public speaker delivering a speech, it's wise to empty your bladder beforehand and wear a pad.

Thankfully, most of these issues clear up without intervention. By a year after surgery, only 4 to 5 percent of men I see continue to need a pad. If you experience persistent, severe incontinence (most often this occurs in men who had urinary problems prior to surgery), it's a good idea to have a detailed evaluation by an urologist who specializes in lower urinary tract function, a field known as urodynamics. Thorough **urodynamic testing** can rule out possible contributory causes such as an unstable bladder or urethral stricture and ensure that you'll get the most appropriate treatment. (See Treating Persistent Incontinence, on page 347).

STRICTURES

Since the urethra runs through the prostate, it must be severed and then reconnected when the prostate is removed. The cut ends are sewn back together in an end-to-end connection called an anastomosis. If excessive scar tissue forms at this juncture, the urethra narrows and urinary flow slows severely. We call this scarring a **urethral stricture**. Patients with strictures may appear to recover continence early because the scarring acts as a natural dam, but since strictures get in the way of normal voiding, these men have a higher incidence of incontinence in the long run.

A **stricture** generally develops at four to six weeks after surgery. The urinary stream gradually slows, becoming weaker, and some men have to strain to urinate. Voiding may be incomplete, with urine left in the blad-

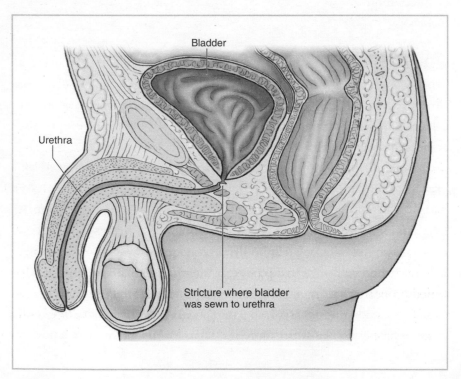

Scarring at the site where the bladder is sewn to the urethra can form a urethral stricture, blocking the urinary channel and causing symptoms.

der, which can lead to overflow incontinence. The urinary reservoir is always at or near capacity, so the slightest increase in abdominal pressure causes spillover.

Treatment of simple, early strictures involves passing a flexible or metal catheter called a "sound" through the urethra to stretch the constricted area. If the scarring is too thick or too firm, a doctor can visualize the urethra through a scope and incise the stricture in a procedure called an internal urethrotomy to relieve the blockage. In certain cases, scarring is in a location that impedes the sphincter mechanism. If treating the stricture requires cutting, the sphincter could be damaged.

> NOTE: The national average incidence of strictures after radical prostatectomy is 10 to 20 percent. For experienced surgeons, no more than 1 percent of patients develop the problem. Strictures appear to be rare after radical laparoscopic prostatectomy. This may be because only the best laparoscopic surgeons are reporting their results.

OTHER URINARY SIDE EFFECTS OF SURGERY

In rare instances (2 in 1,000) surgery causes a ureteral obstruction. One of the slender tubes (ureters) that lead from the kidneys to the bladder gets damaged or caught in a suture. This might cause flank pain, but it can also be symptom-free, where the only warning is an increased blood creatinine level that signals a possible reduction in kidney function. To avoid kidney damage, surgery must be done to relieve the obstruction. Also rare is a urinary fistula, where the bladder and urethra are not rejoined properly and urine leaks out. This can cause scarring and increase the risk of incontinence. Experienced surgeons know how to avoid both of these problems.

Importance of Surgical Skill and Technique

Outcomes vary widely, depending on precisely how a radical prostatectomy is performed. Surgeons differ in fine details of the procedure, and that can make a major difference in the incidence and severity of side effects.

But even among the busiest surgeons, results can be all over the lot. Our study of men 65 and over found that incontinence rates a year or more after radical prostatectomy ranged from 1 percent to a whopping 50 percent, depending on surgical know-how and technique.[5] For example, it's important to avoid shortening the external urinary sphincter, which is called upon to take over the job of holding back urine after the internal sphincter is removed during radical prostatectomy. Highly experienced surgeons are more likely to know this and incorporate it in their standard procedure. Doctors who perform radical prostatectomy rarely may fail to consider important nuances that can make a major difference in results. Make sure you know your surgeon's track record and put yourself in the care of someone with a demonstrated capacity to avoid serious side effects such as urinary incontinence.

NOTE: Incontinence is far more common when the prostate is removed in a so-called **salvage radical prostatectomy**, when a man's prostate cancer recurs after external beam therapy or brachytherapy. These treatments often inflict incidental damage on the external urinary sphincter, which must take charge of urinary control after the prostate and the inner sphincter are removed. Salvage surgery leaves two men in four incontinent, one in four severely enough to require surgical correction (see Treating Persistent Incontinence, on page 347).

URINARY SIDE EFFECTS
OF RADIATION

In treating prostate cancer, radiation therapists face a delicate balancing act. The challenge is to deliver enough radiation to kill the cancer without inflicting unacceptable damage on healthy innocent bystanders like the erectile nerves, the bowel, and the urinary tract. Lower radiation doses cause less injury to neighboring structures, but they also increase the chances that the cancer will recur. Higher doses raise the probability of cancer cure, but that comes with a greater risk of collateral damage.

The problem is compounded by the fact that some organs are far more susceptible to the effects of radiation than others. Destroying prostate tissue requires a hefty dose that would severely harm more vulnerable surrounding structures, including the bladder and urethra.

Although external beam radiation and seed implants leave some men with urinary control problems, the incidence is greater immediately after surgery. Fortunately, incontinence after radical prostatectomy tends to be short-lived and generally resolves on its own. With radiation, symptoms begin later, after the damaging effects set in. The problems persist longer and may worsen over time.

EXTERNAL BEAM THERAPY

Radiation of any kind causes inflammation and irritation. During the typical nine-week course of external beam therapy, the lining of the urethra may sustain damage and cease to provide an effective barrier to urine. This can cause bleeding, irritation, and pain. Depending on the target area or "field" of radiation, a patient may develop an inflammation of the urethra (radiation urethritis) or, if the bladder is exposed, **radiation cystitis**. Both of these conditions cause urinary frequency, urgency, burning, pain, and the need to get up during the night to urinate. During external beam therapy, 10 to 20 percent of men develop these symptoms of irritation. Typically, the problems appear after four to six weeks of treatment, continue to worsen for one to three months after therapy is completed, and then spontaneously resolve.

Until symptoms clear up, an analgesic, such as Pyridium taken orally, may soothe the pain, though it will also turn your urine bright orange. Anticholinergics, such as tolterodine (Detrol) and oxybutynin (Ditropan), reset the bladder's trigger point, quieting the signals that prompt the frantic urge to urinate. Some men undergoing radiation find it difficult to void because of inflammation and swelling, and alpha blockers, such as tamsulosin, terazosin, and alfuzosin, which relax smooth muscles in the bladder neck and prostate, help to alleviate the problem.

In the long term, radiation can cause ulceration in the sensitive lining of the urethra and consequent bleeding and pain. Blood vessels in the field may become abnormal and more prone to bleed spontaneously. Conventional radiotherapy targets a box-shaped area, and the bladder receives a great deal of incidental injury. Problems with serious bleeding, requiring transfusion or, in the worst cases, removal of the bladder, are far less common with modern radiation therapy involving 3-D conformal technology or, better yet, 3-D conformal radiation with IMRT. Still, 1 to 3 percent of patients experience serious bleeding from radiation.

BRACHYTHERAPY

This involves the placement of dozens or even a hundred or more radioactive seeds through multiple needles inserted in the prostate. The implant causes swelling in the gland that can obstruct urinary flow. In severe cases, a patient is suddenly unable to urinate. Treating acute urinary retention may necessitate prolonged use of a Foley catheter through the penis, a suprapubic tube inserted into the bladder through the lower abdomen or an emergency TURP to remove obstructing tissue in the prostate. In a third of cases after brachytherapy, TURP results in severe incontinence. For this reason, it's ill-advised for men who have prostates over 60 grams or prior bladder outlet obstruction to have seed implants, since they run a greater risk of developing acute retention.[6]

Sometimes symptoms of urinary obstruction are apparent from the patient's responses on a questionnaire such as the International Prostate Symptom Score (IPSS) (see pages 76–77). Still, since it's possible to have obstruction without symptoms, the best way to determine whether seed implants are appropriate is to have a urinary flow test, a measure of the amount of urine left in the bladder after urinating (post-void residual urine), and urodynamic studies. To avoid the risk of acute retention, all brachytherapy patients typically take alpha-blocking drugs before the implant and continue to take them for several months afterward.

As damage from the implanted seeds accumulates, other urinary problems can develop. Radiation can damage the sensitive lining of the urethra, leaving the area raw and highly sensitive like a scraped knee. Without this protective lining, urine passing through the urethra causes inflammation, burning, and pain.

Brachytherapy is associated with symptoms of lower urinary tract irritation, including frequency, urgency, painful urination, and waking at night to urinate, sometimes as often as every hour. Such problems affect 30 percent of brachytherapy patients and persist for an average of two years, but they can take as long as six to seven years to clear up. Medications may offer some, though often not total, symptomatic relief. Dr. Michael Zelefsky, a brachytherapy expert at Memorial Sloan-Kettering, has shortened the time course of irritative symptoms to a mean of six to eight months by using three-dimensional, real-time treatment planning during seed implantation.

> NOTE: Despite a commonly held belief to the contrary, drinking cranberry juice or taking vitamin C do nothing to alleviate these symptoms. Such home remedies cannot change the pH of urine.

In less than 1 percent of cases, bleeding around the needle sites after the implant is serious enough to require catheterization to wash out the blood clots in the bladder. Long-term urinary bleeding (**hematuria**) after radiation is more common with external beam therapy, though 1 to

3 percent of men receiving modern brachytherapy develop blood in the urine from radiation urethritis or radiation damage to blood vessels in the area.

URINARY SIDE EFFECTS OF OTHER LOCAL TREATMENTS

When seed implants are combined with external beam therapy to boost the radiation dose, the risk of urinary side effects increases. All the problems described above for external beam radiation and for brachytherapy are far more common with the overlapping doses of combined radiotherapy.

Adding hormone therapy to radiation does not increase urinary side effects. On the contrary, by shrinking the prostate, hormone therapy relieves obstruction and reduces the risk of sudden urinary blockage.

Cryotherapy causes more urinary problems than radiation and about the same long-term risk of incontinence as radical prostatectomy. Freezing is designed to kill both normal and malignant prostate tissue. As the dead tissue sloughs off, it can block the urinary channel. Some patients require drainage with a catheter or suprapubic tube (through the base of the abdomen) for three to six weeks after cryotherapy. Urinary frequency, urgency, pain, and a weak stream may persist for months.[7] Some patients need a TURP to remove the dead, obstructing tissue. In the long run, about 3 to 7 percent of patients complain of persistent incontinence. The most devastating complication of cryotherapy is a rectourethral fistula—a hole between the rectum and urinary tract that requires a colostomy to divert feces away from the damaged site. Fortunately, this occurs rarely and only in the hands of inexperienced cryosurgeons.

High-intensity focused ultrasound (HIFU), radiofrequency ablation (RFA), and photodynamic therapy are not yet approved for treatment of prostate cancer in this country. These investigational approaches may cause urinary obstruction but rarely cause incontinence.

WILL AVOIDING TREATMENT PREVENT URINARY PROBLEMS?

In the short term, avoiding treatment does mean you avoid the risk of urinary complications. But over time, all but the most favorable prostate cancers enlarge, eventually blocking the urinary channel and invading the urinary sphincter. In a Swedish study comparing radical prostatectomy and watchful waiting, the untreated patients experienced more urinary problems. Surgery patients had a greater incidence of urine leakage, but watchful waiting patients had far more urinary obstruction requiring invasive treatments, and their urinary quality of life was substantially worse. An unchecked cancer can also grow into the bladder, obstructing the ureters that drain the kidneys.

TREATING PERSISTENT INCONTINENCE

The best-case scenario is to avoid the problem. A major cause of incontinence after radical prostatectomy is a shortened external sphincter. Highly skilled, experienced surgeons know how to leave this critical mechanism with sufficient length to function properly and prevent leakage. A doctor's record of results should reflect this know-how. If you're going to have surgery, seek someone whose patients rarely have serious trouble with long-term urinary control.

Because they run an increased risk of incontinence, older men, especially those over 70, are often better served by radiation therapy than by radical prostatectomy. Nevertheless, some older men who are anxious to have the cancer removed opt to have surgery anyway. If this applies to you, make sure you fully understand the nature and extent of potential problems.

Incontinence after radiation can best be avoided by making sure you receive good modern 3-D conformal radiation, preferably with IMRT. A highly skilled radiation oncologist knows how to target the appropriate field, while minimizing injury to the urethra and bladder. Seed implants are not a good idea if you have a large prostate or symptoms of bladder outlet obstruction.

EXERCISES

In 1932, a New York obstetrician named Joshua W. Davies theorized that women troubled by incontinence after childbirth could regain control by strengthening the muscles used to interrupt the urinary stream. Davies recommended that his patients contract these pelvic floor muscles voluntarily several times a day, but many women found it difficult or impossible to isolate them. They did the exercises incorrectly, squeezing abdominal, thigh, or buttocks muscles instead. The effort proved useless and, in some cases, actually made the incontinence worse.

A breakthrough occurred in the mid-1940s, when Arnold Kegel, a Los Angeles gynecologist, invented the world's first biofeedback device: the Kegel Perineometer. A probe placed in the vagina was connected to a gauge that registered successful contractions of the target muscles. Though this invention and the pioneering discovery of biofeedback won Kegel little recognition, his name continues to be widely associated with simple isometric exercises that may help to restore urinary control in men and women.[8] After radical prostatectomy, Kegel exercises can be used to strengthen the muscles that act like scaffolding to support the urethra.[9]

To isolate the correct muscles, try stopping and starting the urinary stream several times. Be sure to keep your thigh, abdominal, and gluteus muscles relaxed. If you have difficulty doing this on your own or are unsure that you're doing it correctly, your doctor can refer you for biofeed-

NOTE: One in four to five men do these exercises improperly, so biofeedback training is a good idea.

back training. A probe is placed in the anal canal, and a gauge indicates when you're stimulating the right muscles.

Kegel exercises should not be performed while the catheter is in place. After it's removed, wait a day or two to see if you actually leak. Many men never need Kegel exercises. If you do have leakage, try forcefully contracting the pelvic floor muscles and holding the contraction for ten to fifteen seconds, and then relax for five seconds before squeezing again. By doing ten repetitions three times a day, you may strengthen the supporting muscles sufficiently to reduce urinary leakage. As with any physical conditioning, the process could take weeks or even months.

NOTE: While doing Kegel exercises may help and should not cause any harm, overdoing them is inadvisable. You could fatigue the muscles and exacerbate the problem.

IDENTIFYING AND TREATING SECONDARY CAUSES

If incontinence persists, you should discuss it with your doctor. A secondary cause might be the culprit. **Urinary tract** infections can compromise urinary control. They are easy to diagnose and treat with antibiotics.

Another possible secondary cause for incontinence is a urethral stricture. Scar tissue narrows the urinary channel and can make it difficult to empty the bladder completely (see page 340). Urine left in the bladder after voiding, also known as post-void residual urine (PVR), sets you up to leak with any increase in intra-abdominal pressure, as occurs when you bend, lift, sneeze, or cough. Your doctor can check for strictures by examining the urethra through a cystoscope inserted in the penis. The presence of post-void residual urine can be determined by an abdominal sonogram. A urinary flow test can point to the existence of a stricture or other obstructions that impede normal voiding and increase problems with urinary control.

MEDICATIONS

Though no drugs have been FDA-approved as yet for the treatment of stress incontinence, tricyclic antidepressants are sometimes prescribed to treat incontinence, because they can relax the bladder muscle and stimulate the muscular urinary sphincter. Another antidepressant, duloxetine, is awaiting FDA approval for the treatment of stress incontinence.

Drugs for radiation cystitis and urethritis are targeted to the symptoms. If radiation causes urinary frequency, anticholinergics such as tolterodine (Detrol) or oxybutynin (Ditropan) are prescribed. When pain is the primary symptom, the preferred medications are anti-inflammatories or urinary anesthetics such as phenazopyridine (Pyridium).

BULKING AGENTS

Beefing up the urinary sphincter can increase its resistance to urinary flow. Originally, Teflon suspended in an aqueous solution was used for this purpose, but the substance tended to migrate to other areas of the body. Currently, two bulking agents, Durasphere and Contigen, are FDA-approved to treat incontinence.

Contigen, derived from bovine collagen, causes allergic reactions in about 3 percent of patients, so an allergy test must be conducted four weeks prior to treatment. Durasphere, made of tiny carbon-coated beads, does not provoke allergic responses, but, like Contigen, it has limited effectiveness, and with both substances, calibrating the correct amount to implant can be tricky. Too little material will fail to stop the leak; too much may result in a total inability to urinate. Finding the "just right" amount can be hit or miss. Fifty percent of patients improve with bulking agents, but it often takes four to five expensive injections to achieve a satisfactory outcome. Also, results are not permanent or even durable, lasting only a few years.[10]

Both agents carry a risk of infection, bleeding, and urinary retention. In rare instances, the leakage gets much worse after the injections. Other

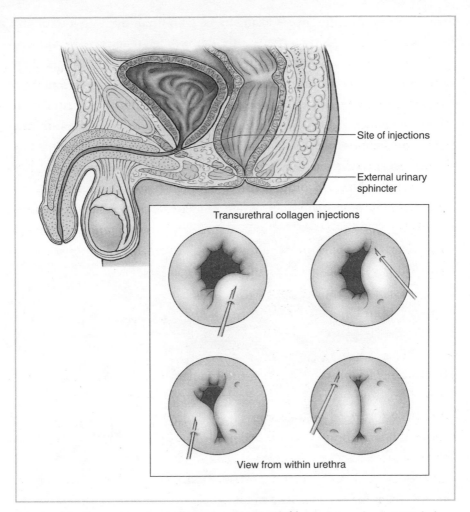

Injection of collagen or another bulking agent into the bladder neck to reduce urinary leakage after radical prostatectomy.

bulking materials are in current development with an eye toward offering improved durability, safety, and effectiveness.

SLING PROCEDURES

Though they are a relatively new way to treat incontinence after radical prostatectomy, **sling procedures** have been used in thousands of women.

Stress urinary incontinence—losing urine with strenuous activity, coughing, sneezing, etc.—is far more common in women than men. In women, when the problem does not respond to medication or exercises, a sling operation is the corrective procedure of choice. The simplest sling used in men after radical prostatectomy is a silicone model made by American Medical Systems. Held in place by metal screws that are fixed to the pelvic bone, the sling compresses the urethra below the sphincter just enough to keep the patient dry. The operation is a fairly simple, one-day surgery procedure, and so far, the results appear promising.[11] It's too soon to know how many men will develop infection, erosion, or break

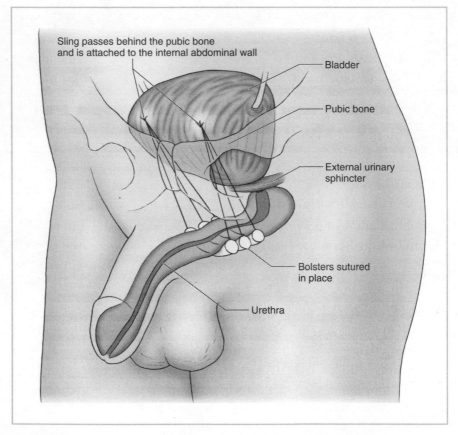

Sling passes behind the pubic bone
and is attached to the internal abdominal wall

Bladder

Pubic bone

External urinary
sphincter

Bolsters sutured
in place

Urethra

One type of sling or suspension operation to treat stress urinary incontinence after radical prostatectomy.

down over time. At least the sling burns no bridges. If it fails, patients can have an artificial sphincter implanted.

ARTIFICIAL SPHINCTER

For patients with severe incontinence that doesn't respond to exercises or medications, an artificial sphincter can provide excellent relief. Ninety-five percent of people who have the device implanted see considerable improvement, though they still may have to wear one or two small pads per day.[12]

Surgery to implant an artificial sphincter is not trivial. The procedure is sometimes done on an outpatient basis, but an overnight hospital stay

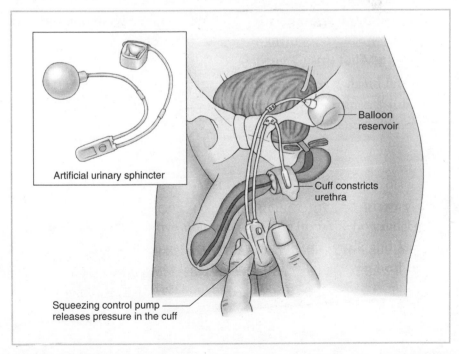

Artificial urinary sphincter

Balloon reservoir

Cuff constricts urethra

Squeezing control pump releases pressure in the cuff

Surgical implantation of an artificial urinary sphincter is the most effective procedure for treating severe, persistent stress urinary incontinence.

may be required. Patients continue to leak for six weeks afterward, since the implant cannot be activated until the area heals.

Complications include infection that could necessitate long-term antibiotics or require that the device be removed or replaced. An artificial sphincter can erode the urethra, causing infection and necessitating removal. Every year 3 to 5 percent of men experience mechanical failure or erosion and need to have further surgery to replace or remove the device. Still, 95 percent of patients are very satisfied with this treatment. All in all, the artificial sphincter sets the gold standard for effective treatment of severe urinary incontinence.

IN SUMMARY

Prostate cancer and all treatments for the disease carry a risk of urinary complications. Many men do not suffer urinary side effects or do so only for a short time. For those with persistent, troubling symptoms, we have several highly satisfactory means to solve the problem.

18

Sexual Side Effects

READ THIS CHAPTER TO LEARN:

- How do erections work, and what causes erectile dysfunction?
- What are the sexual side effects of radical prostatectomy, radiation therapy, and hormone treatment?
- What can be done about erectile dysfunction?

In 1941, Charles Huggins made the groundbreaking discovery that prostate cancer required male hormones to grow and spread.[1] By removing the testicles or administering the female hormone estrogen to counteract the effects of testosterone, Huggins achieved dramatic—though sadly temporary—regression of advanced prostate cancers. In a matter of days, men who had been bedridden with debilitating pain from bone metastases were able to resume their former active lives.

This spectacular improvement came at a cost. In addition to other troubling symptoms (see Chapter 21, Treating Metastatic Prostate Cancer), patients on hormone therapy suffered a loss of libido and erections. This led to the common and persistent assumption that treating prostate cancer always meant the end of sexual function.

Not long ago, that view was fairly accurate. Until the development of nerve-sparing surgery in the early 1980s, a loss of erections was seen as the price men had to pay to get their prostates out (though some patients, inexplicably, confounded their doctors' expectations and regained sexual function after radical prostatectomy).

In the 1960s, radiation became the preferred treatment choice for prostate cancer because it was thought to have no sexual side effects. That assessment proved to be unrealistically optimistic. During treatment and soon after radiation, sexual function appeared to be unchanged, but as damaging effects accumulated, patients often found that their erections steadily diminished. Because many of these men were not followed regularly after treatment, researchers were slow to recognize the negative sexual effects of radiation. When patients did report erectile loss over time, doctors often chalked it up to a normal consequence of aging.

WHY THINGS CHANGED

In the pre-PSA era, many prostate cancers went undetected until they were advanced and incurable. Sexual concerns took a distant backseat to keeping men alive. Before PSA testing, the disease was typically diagnosed in older men, whose sexual function had already declined, making it more difficult to restore satisfactory erections after treatment. Given the patient's age, sexual function often was not seen as a major issue (though that supposition is often incorrect). Until the FDA approved sildenafil (Viagra) in 1996, we had no simple, reliable means to promote the early recovery of erections after cancer treatment and preserve sexual health.

Thankfully, things have changed. We detect most prostate cancers while they are small, contained, and curable. The median age at diagnosis has declined steadily down from 71 in 1995 to 69 in 1999, and the average age at radical prostatectomy is 58. An ever-increasing number of prostate cancers are now diagnosed before age 60, so we see the disease much more commonly in healthy, vital men for whom sexual function is of major importance. Advances in radiation and surgery have reduced the incidence of sexual side effects, and a variety of highly effective therapies can alleviate, or even reverse, the problems that occur. After treatment, most prostate-cancer patients can look forward to resuming an active, satisfying sex life.

ERECTILE DYSFUNCTION (ED)

Erectile dysfunction (ED) refers to the inability to produce and maintain erections satisfactory for sexual relations. In professional parlance, the term is now generally preferred over **impotence**, though the meaning of both terms is largely synonymous.

Note that the definition of ED uses the term "satisfactory," highlighting the fact that only *you* can be the judge of whether your sexual abilities are adequate to suit your needs. For some men, sex is not an issue. To others, sexual performance is so crucial that they rank it above survival on a questionnaire to assess their priorities.

NORMAL ERECTIONS

The penis has two large erection chambers—the **corpora cavernosa**—and one small chamber surrounding the urethra—the corpus spongiosum—filled with spongy erectile tissue (corporal sinusoids). Triggered by direct genital stimulation, psychological arousal, or REM (dream) sleep, a number of nerves and hormones relax the smooth muscle in the walls of these three chambers, allowing a rapid inflow of blood. Under sufficient pressure, the penile veins are compressed, causing a valve-like effect, which traps blood in the penis and keeps it rigid until orgasm occurs or the stimulus that caused the erection stops. The same hydraulic principle applies when you inflate a bicycle tire. To make the tire rigid, you have to force in sufficient air and then keep it contained under pressure. A leaky valve would make it impossible to maintain rigidity, and the tire would quickly go flat.

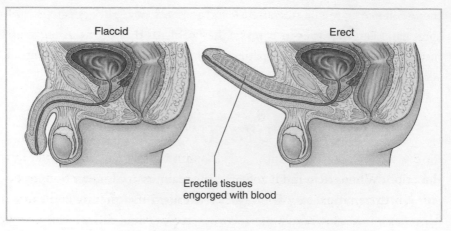

A view of the flaccid and erect penis from the side.

Men who cannot achieve erections can still experience the pleasure and release of orgasm. After radical prostatectomy, erection and orgasm can occur even though patients no longer ejaculate. (See Chapter 2, Normal Male Function.)

NOTE: *Orgasm, erection, and ejaculation are separate, independent functions.* Erections require good blood flow and intact nervous impulses to the penis. Ejaculation relies on fluid production by an intact prostate and seminal vesicles followed by nerve and muscle action to force the fluid out. Orgasm is a psychological event, requiring nothing beyond a healthy, well-functioning brain.

WHAT CAUSES ED?

An erection is a marvel of engineering that hinges on a series of intricate, interdependent events. As in a factory, damage to any aspect of the complex mechanism can cause the entire system to break down. Erectile problems can result from a single factor or have multiple causes. The problem may be psychological, physical, or, most commonly, both.[2]

PSYCHOLOGICAL CAUSES OF ED

Stress, anxiety, and depression are all common triggers for erectile dysfunction. While excitement and arousal are necessary for erections to occur, an extreme excess of either can overload the circuits and cause a shutdown.[3] Under psychological siege, your body shifts into combat mode, pumping extra adrenaline that directs blood flow away from peripheral structures like the penis into core organs. This reaction serves people well in emergencies—if you were fleeing a foe or a fire, you'd need maximum heart and lung capacity and a fully alert brain, not a firm, reliable erection.

Unfortunately, this crucial survival mechanism can kick in and cause problems when no real or imminent danger exists. It's common for men to experience a loss of erections when they're worried about finances, relationships, or troubles on the job. Erectile failure can trigger a vicious

NOTE: Men normally have an average of five erections per night, each lasting about thirty minutes and associated with REM (dream) sleep. Tests of **nocturnal penile tumescence (NPT)**, in which an elastic gauge linked to a monitor is placed around the penis, determine whether or not you're having these erections.

Until recently, if a man had normal erections during sleep, the problems he had while awake were thought to be psychological. We now know that this is not necessarily the case. Only 10 to 15 percent of ED is currently thought to have primarily emotional roots, though in as many as 85 percent of cases, a loss of erections will have a secondary psychological impact that makes matters worse.

cycle, causing performance anxiety, which leads to further erectile dysfunction, which intensifies the performance anxiety, and so on.

Losing a partner can also result in self-perpetuating erectile dysfunction. Widower's syndrome refers to erectile problems caused by depression, performance anxiety, or guilt following the death of a spouse. The condition may lead men to retreat from social and sexual situations, which, naturally, exacerbates the problem.

PHYSICAL CAUSES OF ED

Vascular (blood vessel) disorders are the most common physical culprit, responsible for 10 to 20 percent of erectile dysfunction. Heart disease, hypertension and the drugs used to treat it, and high cholesterol with resultant hardening of the arteries all can impair circulation to the penis, making it impossible to fill the organ with enough blood to induce rigidity.[4]

If blood flow is insufficient, the erection chambers may not exert sufficient pressure to compress the veins. The condition is tantamount to a loose drain plug in the bathtub. The blood runs out, and the erection cannot be sustained.

Nervous System (Neurogenic) Causes
Damage to the autonomic (involuntary) nervous system, which regulates dilation and contraction of the blood vessels that lead to the penis, can interrupt the electrical impulses required to trigger erections, causing the equivalent of a power outage. Multiple sclerosis, Parkinson's disease, and spinal-cord injury are common causes of neurogenic erectile loss, as is damage to the erectile nerves by surgical trauma, radiation, or freezing during cryotherapy.

Hormones
A deficiency or excess of thyroid hormone or an abnormal increase in the pituitary hormone prolactin can lead to a loss of erections. So can anabolic steroid abuse.[5]

> NOTE: Be aware that "neutraceuticals" such as **DHEA**, which are often touted as having "miracle" sexual performance-boosting and anti-aging properties, are unregulated. Their safety and effectiveness have not been rigorously tested or proven. In addition, there is concern that these substances may cause serious side effects, including an increased risk of prostate cancer.

Hypogonadism (low testosterone), which can be congenital, caused by damaged testicles or from central nervous system diseases that affect the pituitary or hypothalamus glands, may retard sexual development, causing infertility and erectile dysfunction. While erections can sometimes occur despite a low testosterone level, a paucity of the hormone does cause a lack of libido and a general weakening of erections.

Diabetes
Diabetes causes both nerve and vascular damage, putting patients at high risk for erectile dysfunction.[6]

Smoking
Though it has not been proven to be a direct cause of impotence, smoking increases the risk of cardiovascular diseases such as atherosclerosis, which impair erectile function. The risk of erectile dysfunction increases with the number of cigarettes smoked per day.

Alcohol and Drugs
In moderate doses, alcohol may help you relax and heighten your sex drive. But because alcohol acts as a powerful nerve inhibitor, heavy drinking markedly depresses erections. The same is true of recreational drugs, such as marijuana and heroine. Cocaine users also risk **priapism**, a persistent erection lasting four hours or more that can cause severe, permanent damage to the penis.[7] Chronic drug abuse can lead to permanent vascular and neurological damage and a consequent loss of erectile function.

A wide variety of medications, including anti-anxiety drugs, antide-pressants, chemotherapeutic agents, drugs for heart disease and hyper-tension, and glaucoma treatments put men at risk for erectile dysfunction.

PROSTATE CANCER AND ED

Because the prostate lies in such close proximity to the male sexual ap-paratus, all treatments for cancer in the gland carry some risk of sexual side effects. Your particular outcome will depend on the nature of your cancer and the quality of care you receive. Larger, more aggressive tu-mors typically require more extensive treatments, increasing the proba-bility that potency will be impaired. Highly skilled surgeons and radiation oncologists know how to minimize damage to erectile nerves and reduce the incidence of ED. Keep in mind that how well you are treated may have a greater impact on your outcome than which treatment you decide to have.

NOTE: Fear of erectile dysfunction is *not* a sound reason to avoid treat-ment, especially for a young, healthy man. Left alone, prostate cancer can penetrate the capsule of the gland and grow into the erectile nerves, causing a loss of erections. Should the cancer spread and metas-tasize, hormone therapy, which destroys libido and erectile function, would be necessary to slow progression of the disease and ease symp-toms. You would lose the chance for a cure while still risking erectile failure.

SEXUAL SIDE EFFECTS OF RADICAL PROSTATECTOMY

Erectile Function

Erections depend on triggering signals from the **cavernous (erectile) nerves,** which run along the prostate like string on a package. During radical prostatectomy, surgeons using accepted modern techniques attempt to spare these nerves unless doing so would compromise cancer cure. Still, erectile nerves are exquisitely delicate. Even with a top-notch nerve-sparing procedure, it's difficult to remove the gland without causing some temporary trauma to these fragile fibers. The nerves suffer the equivalent of a bad concussion, leaving them temporarily dazed and unresponsive. As a result, most men experience some loss of erectile function for the first few months following radical prostatectomy (though some are able to function right away!).

During the healing process, inflammation and scarring around the nerves can deliver what amounts to a further blow that can interrupt or delay sexual recovery. Some men who regain erections early lose them again after a month or two, putting them back at square one in the recuperative process.

In some cases, one or both erectile nerve bundles must be removed to cure the cancer. Surgeons skilled in nerve grafting can insert a nerve from the ankle (sural nerve) or groin (genitofemoral nerve) between the cut ends of the lost erectile nerve. The sheath of the graft provides a conduit through which the cut nerves can regenerate. At Memorial Sloan-Kettering, in our patients with grafts, 33 percent of men who lost both nerves were able to recover erections, versus none without the graft. Replacing one lost nerve with a graft substantially improved recovery compared to those with no graft.[8] (See Chapter 14, Surgery.)

While the main artery that supplies blood to the penis (the pudendal artery) lies well away from the prostate, other important collateral arteries can be injured during radical prostatectomy. Insufficient blood flow means the erectile chambers will not fill completely and the penis will not achieve full rigidity.

Some men have functional erections a few weeks after surgery, but typically recovery is a long, gradual process. The average patient takes four months to achieve an erection sufficient for intercourse. Older men, patients with diminished erections before the operation, and those with damage to or removal of a nerve will be slower to recover. Healing can continue for several years. One patient came to see me three and a half years after surgery, having long since given up hope of ever having sexual intercourse without drugs. "You can have all those medicines back," he said. "I'm *finally* back to normal."

LOSS OF EJACULATION

After radical prostatectomy, you can continue to enjoy normal sensation in the penis, experience normal desire, and have orgasms. Removing the gland means you will no longer ejaculate when you climax (dry orgasm). The effect of this change is unpredictable. After surgery, some men experience heightened orgasms and some judge their climax to be less intense, but most men report no significant difference.

PAIN DURING ORGASM

For a time after surgery, 20 percent of men report pain in the penis, scrotum, or perineum during orgasm (**dysorgasmia**). Typically, this clears up without treatment.

PENIS SIZE AND SHAPE

Removing the prostate does not pull the penis into your body and make it shorter. The penis and urethra are fixed to the bones of the pelvis and

How Great Is the Risk of ED after Surgery?

In the care of average surgeons nationwide, about 40 to 45 percent of men who were fully functional before the operation recover workable erections by two years after radical prostatectomy. Surgeons with special expertise in nerve sparing report a 75 to 90 percent potency rate. Here again, the skill of the surgeon can make an enormous difference in how well you're likely to fare.

cannot be dislodged. When the prostate is removed, the bladder is brought down and sewn to the urethra. The urethra *is not* pulled up with an effect like a retracted hose!

Still, some men observe that their penis seems smaller or shorter after surgery. I'm aware of three reasons for this—two misleading and one real. If there is intense scarring between the lower part of the abdominal incision and the penis, as the scar retracts, the penis may be pulled toward the pubic bone and appear shorter. Alternatively, after the operation, some men gain weight for a variety of reasons, including sexual frustration. Fatty deposits over the pubic area can cover part of the penis, making it appear smaller. In both instances, there is no actual shortening, though the penis looks shorter to the patient. When erection occurs, the penis fills out and functions normally.

Genuine penile shortening can result from the long-term effects of damaged nerves and the absence of erections, not directly from the removal of the gland. While the mechanism remains a mystery, in some men the delicate vascular channels of the penis atrophy and become hard and inelastic (fibrotic). Fibrous tissue does not expand when the penis fills with blood, so the organ remains shorter and erections may not be as firm. Some men report curvature of the penis with erections, or a penis that is rigid near the body but softer near the tip.

Rarely, large blocks of fibrous tissue form along the walls of the erectile bodies, mimicking the hard plaques of **Peyronie's disease**. This condition ranges in severity from small, inconsequential areas of thickening to a serious, painful bend in the shaft that can make intercourse impossible.

These changes are uncommon but are certainly troublesome when they occur. Fibrosis after radical prostatectomy is an area of intense research. We do not know how fibrotic changes occur after surgery or which men are at greatest risk. Men in the prostate-cancer age group can develop Peyronie's disease spontaneously. There have been no studies of penile fibrosis after external radiation or seed implants, even though these treatments can cause impotence in 40 to 56 percent of patients over five years after treatment. We don't know whether hormone therapy, either alone or in combination with surgery or radiation, makes fibrosis worse or prevents it.

Penile Rehabilitation

Many doctors urge prostate-cancer patients to use any effective means to have regular, frequent erections after surgery. This may promote full recovery of erectile function and possibly prevent fibrosis. In two published studies, a program of penile rehabilitation, including the early, regular use of injections two to three times a week for six months or a nightly 50 or 100 milligram dose of sildenafil (Viagra) for nine months to induce regular erections, resulted in better spontaneous erections a year after surgery.[9] While these studies are suggestive, more intensive research is needed to confirm whether penile rehabilitation really promotes recovery of erections.

Infertility

After radical prostatectomy, you will no longer ejaculate. If fathering children is a current or potential future issue, you should bank sperm before the operation. Plan on making at least six to ten deposits, spaced several days apart.

If you haven't banked sperm and later wish you had, they can sometimes be harvested directly from the testicles in a simple procedure involving a small biopsy-like needle under local anesthetic. Using a method called ICSI (intracytoplasmic sperm injection) a single sperm is then injected into an ovum in the lab. Pregnancy results in about 65 percent of cases.

WHAT PUTS MEN AT RISK FOR SEXUAL PROBLEMS AFTER SURGERY?

Recovery of erections after radical prostatectomy depends on your age, the quality of your erections before the operation, the degree of preservation of the nerves during the procedure, and how skillfully the surgery is performed. Men with diabetes, high cholesterol, hypertension, or coronary artery disease as well as cigarette smokers all have some intrinsic lowering of blood flow to the penis that will make recovering erections less likely after radical prostatectomy.

Men under 60 years old and those with good erectile function before surgery are more likely to recover full potency afterward. If you have weak or unreliable erections prior to the operation, they *will not* be better afterward.

If both nerves are spared, your chances for sexual recovery will be greater than if one nerve is removed or severely damaged. All things

NOTE: Dr. John Mulhall, an erectile dysfunction specialist, encourages patients not to give up if the surgeon reports that he had to remove both nerves. In Mulhall's experience, 15 percent of such men are able to achieve good erections with the help of sildenafil or similar drugs. Erectile nerves are a large group (plexus), not a single fiber. Sometimes, less experienced surgeons leave a portion of the nerve behind inadvertently, so a trial with an erection-inducing drug is a good idea.

considered, removing one nerve reduces the chance of erectile recovery by half. When I deliberately excise both erectile nerves to control cancer, none of my patients has recovered erections unless a nerve graft procedure was performed.

SEXUAL SIDE EFFECTS OF RADIATION

Unlike radical prostatectomy, the effect of radiation on erections may not become evident until years after treatment. Radiation causes a gradual loss of erections by injuring the erectile nerves and blood vessels that provide crucial circulation to the penis. Direct damage to the erectile tissue can compound the problem. Forty to 50 percent of a conventional radiation dose is absorbed by the part of the penis nearest the body. This exposure is reduced with modern 3-D conformal radiation, especially with IMRT.

The impact of radiation on erections depends on the seriousness of the cancer, the specific nature of the therapy, and the skill of the specialist delivering it. More aggressive disease requires higher-dose radiation to a wider field with more resultant damage.

The type of radiation you get is crucial as well. Conventional therapy with a linear accelerator bombards a broader, box-shaped area with damaging rays. 3-D conformal therapy narrows the field, but the penis is still exposed to part of the dose. With IMRT, that exposure is reduced by 40 percent.[10] In brachytherapy (seed implants), the precision of the implant will affect how much incidental damage is inflicted on crucial blood vessels, erection chambers, and erectile nerves. Since the erectile nerves lie within a few millimeters (about 1/10 of an inch) of the prostate, it is impossible to irradiate the gland sufficiently and still completely avoid injuring those nerves.

INFERTILITY

Radiation causes damaging mutations in sperm cells. It would be rare for a man to be able to father a child after treatment. While radiation to the prostate should not be considered a guaranteed method of birth control, if fathering children in the future is important to you, it would be wise to bank sperm before treatment begins (see page 366).

SEXUAL SIDE EFFECTS OF HORMONE THERAPY

Prostate cancer relies on male hormones to grow and spread. Blocking these hormones can slow progression of the disease or shrink the cancer to facilitate treatment.

Removing the testicles will stop testosterone production, and some patients with advanced prostate cancer still opt for this approach. Drugs called **LHRH agonists** shut down testicular function and reduce testosterone to the same level achieved by surgical castration. **Antiandrogens** block the effects of testosterone on hormone-responsive cells. **Estrogens** (female hormones) lower testosterone levels by blocking the natural secretion of hormone-stimulating substances by the brain. In treating advanced prostate cancer, a combination of these drugs is sometimes given to produce a complete androgen blockade.

Some experts believe that the resultant low hormonal levels cause permanent scarring of the erectile tissues (though children born with low levels do not suffer such damaging effects, so this seems unlikely). Administering hormone therapy intermittently might avert any possible damage. Once the drugs succeed in driving down the PSA, a patient may be taken off therapy for a while, during which time testosterone levels rebound and sexual function is regained. If your treatment involves hormone therapy, you may want to discuss the possibility of cycled therapy with your doctor. The negative effect on sexual function is one reason to delay hormone therapy as long as possible.[11] Monitoring PSA is such an effective way to gauge the course of the cancer that at Memorial Sloan-Kettering we generally recommend delaying hormone treatment until the PSA is rising so fast that problems from the cancer are imminent. (See Chapter 20, Rising PSA after Surgery or Radiation Therapy.) Hormone therapy should definitely be started before metastases appear.

PREVENTING AND TREATING ED

The primary goal of treatment for ED is to restore spontaneous, functional erections as soon as possible after radical prostatectomy and to maintain functional erections in the long run after radiation treatment.

ORAL MEDICATIONS

The first-line treatment for erectile dysfunction is the family of erection-inducing medications that include sildenafil (Viagra), vardenafil (Levitra), and tadalafil (Cialis), all of which act to relax smooth muscles in the penis. This encourages blood flow, allowing the penis to become firmer and remain so longer. These drugs work by blocking the enzyme phosphodiesterase-5 and are therefore also known as PDE-5 inhibitors.[12] Sildenafil boasts an 80 percent response rate, longer-lasting tadalafil is said to work in 88 percent of men, and 90 percent report improved erections with vardenafil, which is faster acting than sildenafil. For most men, these drugs can be used daily with no ill effects, but two to three times per week is considered sufficient to help restore normal erections after surgery, and most prescription drug programs that cover these medications limit payment to that.

Remember, these pills are a catalyst, not a catapult, and they do not act as aphrodisiacs. Physical stimulation or psychological arousal is neces-

NOTE: If you are on any form of nitrates or nitroglycerin, including recreational drugs containing nitrates such as "poppers," you *must not* take PDE-5 inhibitors. These medications can interact dangerously, causing a profound drop in blood pressure that could lead to sudden death.

Makers of vardenafil and tadalafil also caution against using those medications if you are taking alpha blockers for hypertension or benign prostate enlargement, if you've had a recent stroke or heart attack and have low or uncontrolled high blood pressure, or if you have a rare irregularity in your heart rhythm, known as a Q-T prolongation.

sary to induce an erection once the medication takes effect. In the absence of stimulation, the penis remains flaccid. An erection is maintained only as long as the sexual stimulus persists.

Because food reduces absorption of sildenafil by 30 percent, it's important to take the drug on an empty stomach. (Vardenafil absorption can be slowed by a high-fat meal, and tadalafil is not affected by food intake.) For most men, that means waiting two hours after a meal or thirty minutes before eating to take sildenafil. Normally, this drug takes sixty to ninety minutes to work. If you take it on an empty stomach, a glass of ice water may speed the effect. Men with diabetes, whose digestion may take longer, should wait three hours after eating. Given that heavy drinking can interfere with erections, you should minimize alcohol consumption when trying these drugs.

Sildenafil and vardenafil provide about a six-hour window of opportunity for erectile function, though in some men, effects last up to twelve hours. Tadalafil acts for twenty-four to thirty-six hours, so three weekly doses allow men to be ready for sexual encounters whenever the mood strikes.

Some men fail to respond to these drugs. Others experience unacceptable side effects, which may include headache, nasal stuffiness, stomach upset, sensitivity to light, and in the case of sildenafil, distortions in the perception of the color blue.

INJECTIONS

Ninety percent of men with erectile dysfunction who do not respond to or can't tolerate oral medications have good results with direct injection of an erection-inducing drug into the penis. The drug takes five minutes to work, and results last for twenty to ninety minutes. Though some men are squeamish about injecting themselves, the therapy uses a tiny 29-gauge needle (29 would fit in 1 inch), only ⅜- to ½-inch long and causes no more discomfort than a mosquito bite. With training, most patients get past their aversion to the needle and find this therapy highly satisfactory. If it seems preferable, your partner can be trained to administer the medication for you.

Caverject, which works for 65 percent of men, is the only FDA-approved injectable medication for erectile dysfunction. It comes prepackaged in a syringe with a drug called alprostadil that causes blood vessels in the penis to dilate, permitting blood to rush in and fill the erection chambers, causing rigidity.[13] On the downside, the drug can cause burning penile pain when used in the first few months after radical prostatectomy. For 90 percent of men, Trimix, a mixture of papaverine, phentolamine, and alprostadil, provides good workable erections with far less risk of the burning sensation because it only contains a small amount of alprostadil. The combination is not commercially available and must be compounded by your pharmacy or hospital. A four-month supply costs about $200 to $250, and it's rarely covered by insurance.

Side Effects of Injections

Alternating the injection site minimizes the risk of fibrosis or scarring from the needles, which only occurs in about 1 in 3,500 cases. The most serious potential problem is **priapism**, a persistent erection lasting more than four hours that can damage the penis, but with adequate instruction and training this is very rare.

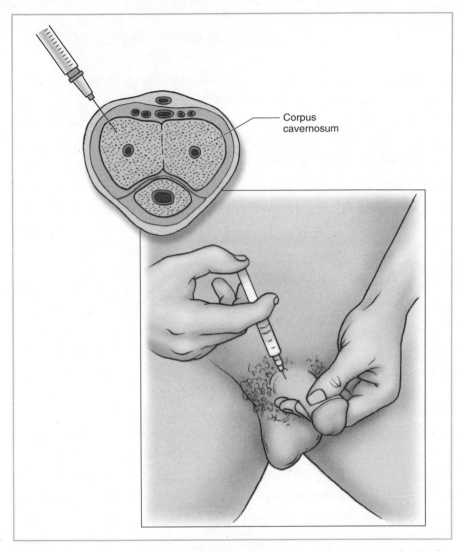

Corpus
cavernosum

Erections can be achieved by injecting drugs that dilate blood vessels into an erectile chamber (corpus cavernosum). Note that the site of injection should be near the body, on the side of the penis.

NOTE: If your erection lasts for more than three hours, call your doctor or go to the nearest emergency room right away! The erection can usually be reversed with injection of a vasoconstrictor like phenylephrine.

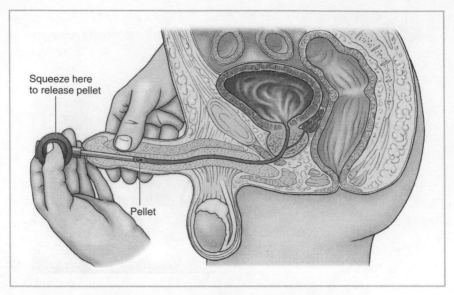

Squeeze here
to release pellet

Pellet

Insertion of a pellet of alprostadil (MUSE) to aid erections.

SUPPOSITORIES

For some men who do not do well with oral medications and cannot deal with injections, the MUSE (medicated urethral system for erection) provides a satisfactory alternative. The treatment involves insertion of a small pellet containing alprostadil into the urethra, through an applicator introduced into the tip of the penis.

The procedure can be awkward. Men must urinate first, insert the drug, and then massage the penis for ten to twenty minutes while standing, until an erection occurs. Results are inconsistent, and some men lose their erection when they lie down. The medication causes burning and penile pain in about 50 percent of cases, especially in the first few months after radical prostatectomy. Two percent of men get dizzy when they first use MUSE and some faint, so initial trials should be done under medical supervision.[14] Nevertheless, MUSE, like oral medications and injections, dilates blood vessels. This increases blood supply to the penis and may help to promote healthy penile tissue. While not especially powerful alone, some men have been successful using MUSE in combination with oral medications.

CONSTRICTING RINGS

Erections that are not quite stiff or durable enough for intercourse can be bolstered by using a **constricting ring** or band like the one that comes with the VED (see below). The adjustable or elastic band is lubricated and then placed around the base of the penis before arousal. This helps to retain blood in the penis after an erection is achieved, while not interfering with the overall circulation or arterial inflow. These bands are inexpensive and readily available, but they have been underutilized in men who have some difficulty maintaining full erections after surgery or radiation.

VACUUM ERECTION DEVICES (VEDs)

A tube is placed over the penis and an erection is induced by pumping out the air in the tube to create a vacuum. A rubber ring placed at the base of the penis maintains rigidity. **Vacuum erection devices (VEDs)** do not produce an actual physiological erection and therefore don't promote the circulation of fresh, oxygenated blood. Consequently, they may not help avoid fibrosis after radical prostatectomy.

VEDs are simple to use, and they come with an instructional videotape, but the apparatus is cumbersome. The resulting erections are rigid and lasting, but they neither look nor feel normal. The penis remains 1° F below body temperature, so it registers as cold and looks rather blue. Nevertheless, some men prefer these relatively simple devices to oral medications or injections.

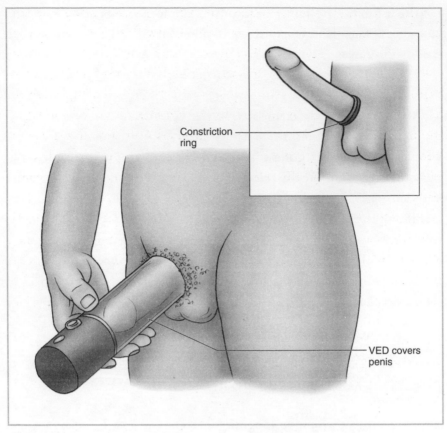

Constriction ring

VED covers penis

A vacuum erection device (VED) with a constriction ring is a simple way to achieve a firm, workable erection.

PENILE IMPLANTS (PROSTHESES)

For men who can't use oral medications, suppositiories, or injections, and are not satisfied with bands or VEDs, penile implants can be an excellent means to restore functional erections.[15]

The prostheses can be semirigid or inflatable. Semirigid devices are simpler to implant and have a lower risk of mechanical failure, but they do not provide normal-looking erections and, since they remain semirigid all the time, can be difficult to conceal under clothing and could make showering in a locker room awkward.

With inflatable implants, erectile chambers are surgically implanted in the penis. There are two different types—a two-piece device and a three-piece device. The two-piece device has a pump in the scrotum which forces the fluid in these chambers to move forward, causing rigidity. To reverse the process, a man bends the penis at mid-shaft to release the fluid, and the erection subsides. In the three-piece device, the scrotal pump forces fluid into the erectile chambers from a reservoir in the abdomen to which it returns after sexual activity is completed. It is deflated by pressure on the release valve. The non-erect penis appears nearly normal.

Implants do involve surgery and anesthesia. Two to 3 percent of men will have postoperative infections, and 15 percent experience mechanical or other failure requiring a second surgery to repair or replace the de-

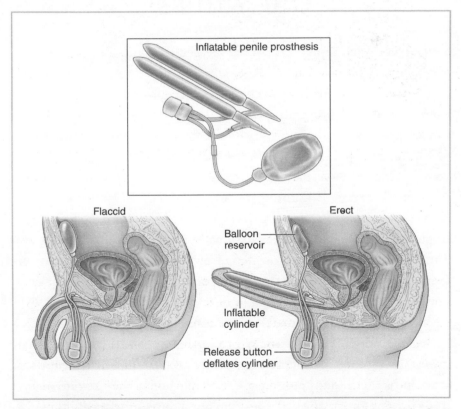

The three-part inflatable penile prosthesis (top panel) shown in the flaccid and erect states after it is implanted.

vice. The procedure is permanent and irreversible. It does not result in increased penile girth or length.

> NOTE: Since it can take two to three years to recover erections completely after radical prostatectomy, men should postpone permanent interventions like penile implants until their level of recovery is clear. Partial erections may continue to improve gradually. If a man has no hint of erections eighteen to twenty-four months after surgery, he will not recover workable erections. At that point, an implant is reasonable.

THE FUTURE

Several promising tools are being developed to improve sexual function for men with prostate cancer. Recently, drugs used to prevent rejection of transplanted organs have been found to be powerful neuroprotective agents, capable of preventing damage to erectile nerves from prostate-cancer treatment. These investigational drugs have proven effective in animal models, and studies are under way to evaluate their ability to prevent or reverse nerve damage in a wide variety of diseases, including Alzheimer's disease, Parkinson's disease, and diabetes.

We are conducting clinical trials to see how effective these drugs might be in reducing erectile dysfunction after radical prostatectomy. Similar studies are planned for men receiving radiation therapy and certain types of chemotherapy that cause peripheral neuropathy (damage to nerves in the hands and feet that leads to chronic pain).

In addition, we're testing the "use it or lose it" hypothesis by comparing recovery of erections in men given regular injections of alprostadil with those of men who use only pills like sildenafil for the first six months after radical prostatectomy. While preliminary studies suggest some benefit to regular injections or nightly doses of sildenafil for six to nine months after the operation, proof awaits further studies. Until we have more data, I encourage my patients to be sexually active as early as possible after radical prostatectomy, which may promote penile health, decrease the chances of scarring and fibrosis, and optimize the recovery of good erections.

IN SUMMARY

Prostate cancer and treatments for the disease can cause erectile dysfunction. Many men recover good sexual function after radical prostatectomy, though this can be gradual and in some cases takes years. Following radiation, problems with erectile function may appear slowly as damage from the treatment accumulates. Hormone therapy causes a loss of erections and libido. Fortunately, we have excellent means to deal with these problems. Most men are able to resume a satisfactory sex life after treatment for prostate cancer.

19

Bowel Side Effects

> READ THIS CHAPTER TO LEARN:
>
> • How can prostate cancer and treatments for the disease affect bowel function?
> • What can be done about bowel problems?

Mention prostate cancer, and other than the prospect of dying of the disease, the thing patients worry most about is a loss of erections or urinary control. Though problems with bowel function can have a greater impact on quality of life than urinary incontinence or impotence, men with this disease are typically unconcerned about these side effects. In fact, most patients (and many physicians) have no idea that the risk of such problems exists.

This general lack of awareness is unfortunate though certainly understandable. The effects of prostate cancer treatments on gastrointestinal function have been sparsely investigated and scarcely mentioned in literature in the field. For the most part, the problem has been simply, inexplicably ignored. Bowel side effects have been treated like the metaphorical elephant in the room that no one talks about, as if that magically might make it cease to exist. Unfortunately, for the men affected by them, this particular elephant looms undeniably real and very large indeed.

The rear of the prostate sits mere millimeters from the anterior (front) rectal wall (see illustration on page 18). Given this anatomical coincidence and the fact that the prostate is buried deep in the pelvis and otherwise extremely hard to reach, doctors who specialize in diagnosing and treating prostate diseases have come to rely on the lower end of the bowel, also known as the rectum, as the equivalent of an access road or service entrance to the gland. To conduct a DRE, a doctor places a gloved finger in the rectum and examines the rear of the prostate for abnormalities. The needles used for prostate biopsies, along with the ultrasound that guides them, are inserted through the rectum. Transrectal ultrasound can also be used to gauge the size and shape of the prostate and may show the shadow of a large cancer in the gland—both pieces of information significant for diagnosis and treatment planning. Endorectal MRI, another sophisticated imaging technique, allows us to visualize the prostate and may help to gauge the location and seriousness of cancers in the prostate, seminal vesicles, and pelvic lymph nodes.

Being so close to the prostate renders the rectum both useful in cancer treatments and vulnerable to their effects. When we conduct a search-and-destroy mission to eradicate cancer in the prostate, bowel function can be an accidental casualty.

DOES RADICAL PROSTATECTOMY AFFECT BOWEL FUNCTION?

To remove the prostate, the rear of the gland must be peeled away from the rectum. In doing so, there's always a risk that the surgeon will nick or even perforate the rectal wall. Fortunately, these small tears occur rarely (about 1 in 150 cases), and when they do, they can be irrigated with antibiotic solution and immediately and uneventfully repaired. A course of intravenous antibiotics will prevent infection from fecal contamination. In extremely rare cases, less than 1 in 1,000, a serious rectal injury could necessitate a temporary colostomy, meaning the colon is diverted to the outside through the abdomen until the wound heals, at which point normal function is restored. This almost never happens in the hands of a skilled surgeon.

Removing the prostate leaves a space into which the rectum can expand. This can lead to a temporary decrease in rectal tone and an increased vulnerability to constipation. For about six weeks after surgery, until things return to normal, it's important to avoid constipation by drinking plenty of water, eating food rich in fiber, and getting adequate exercise. Simple stool softeners such as docusate (Colace) or Metamucil, taken by mouth twice a day for six weeks after surgery, will help to keep you from having to strain to move your bowels. Doing so could damage your incision and increase the risk of a blood clot moving to your lungs.

> NOTE: During this time, you *should not* use enemas, which could risk perforating the rectal wall. Suppositories should not be a problem.

While it usually takes four to five days after a radical prostatectomy before your first bowel movement and a week or two to resume normal regularity, most men notice no other changes in their bowel habits after surgery. In fact, one advantage of surgery is that it is the least likely to cause bowel problems of all the standard treatments for localized prostate cancer.

BOWEL SIDE EFFECTS OF RADIATION

To effectively treat prostate cancer, radiation oncologists must bombard the entire gland with damaging rays. In doing so, it's impossible to spare the rectum completely from radiation exposure and injury. To make matters worse, the rectal wall is far more susceptible to radiation damage than the prostate gland.[1]

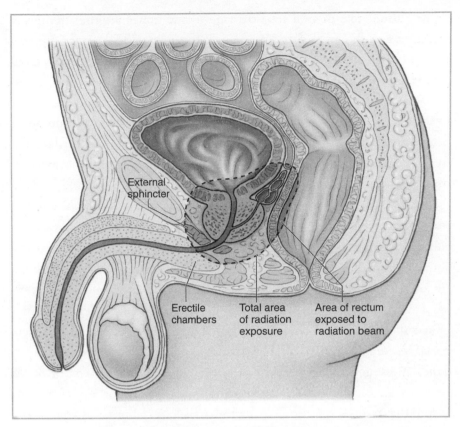

External
sphincter

Erectile
chambers

Total area
of radiation
exposure

Area of rectum
exposed to
radiation beam

Area exposed to the full dose of radiation during external beam radiation therapy for prostate cancer. Note that some part of the rectal wall receives a full dose of radiation.

All normal cells in the human body are programmed to grow for a time, die off, and then replace themselves. Radiation works by damaging the genetic blueprint (DNA) cells rely on to reproduce, and a sufficient dose shuts the replication process down completely. As a result, the faster cells turn over, the more quickly and dramatically they register radiation's destructive effects. Radiation sensitivity varies from organ to organ, depending on the speed of that turnover and the number of delicate blood vessels in the organ. Prostate cells are analogous to the brick house in the tale of the three little pigs—very difficult to destroy. Cells lining the rectal wall are the straw house equivalent, highly vulnerable to external assaults.

Key predictors of radiation damage to the bowel are the strength of the dose and the area of the rectal wall hit by that dose. Anything over 50 Gy risks damage to the rectum, and treatment for prostate cancer involves a dose of 70 Gy or higher. Still, bowel symptoms rarely occur unless a significant portion of the rectal wall receives that much radiation.[2] Early on, 6 to 8 percent of all radiation patients develop symptoms of acute **proctitis** (inflammation of the rectum), which can cause diarrhea, frequent passage of mucus (tenesmus), and rectal bleeding that requires men to use tampons or pads.

As radiation injury accumulates after treatment, other troubling and more intractable bowel side effects can appear. Radiation damage and resultant exposure to bacteria can lead to erosion or ulceration of the anal canal, causing painful bowel movements and bleeding. One study found that a year after radiation, 26 percent of patients were troubled by intestinal cramps, 38 percent reported moderate to severe flatulence, 17 percent suffered with chronic diarrhea, 12 percent experienced persistent rectal bleeding or mucus discharge, and 30 percent had rectal pain. In another investigation, 35 percent of men reported problems with bowel urgency a year after external beam radiation. Yet another large study found that two years after treatment, diarrhea, rectal urgency, and bleeding continued to plague men who had opted for external beam radiation or seed implants.[3]

Dietary changes, such as increasing bulk and fluids, can relieve constipation, as can stool softeners, while medications may alleviate diarrhea. Bleeding used to be common, but thankfully it's rare now and typically clears up on its own. With modern 3-D conformal radiation, less than 1 in 1,000 men have bleeding severe enough to require transfusion. The risk of rectal bleeding is higher in frequent aspirin users.

Radiation damage can reduce the effectiveness of the anal sphincter, decrease rectal capacity, or increase sensitivity in the lining of the rectal wall. Some patients develop **fecal incontinence** as a result, and some men are unable to control the expulsion of gas. Radiation damage can also exacerbate hemorrhoids, which can bleed and cause pain. Overall, about 10 to 15 percent of radiation patients have problems with liquid or solid soiling, though one study found the incidence to be as high as one man in four. These problems can lead to major alterations in lifestyle, seriously hindering social interactions and triggering depression. Fecal incontinence and persistent rectal bleeding after radiation have also been associated with chronic, debilitating fatigue.

REDUCING THE RISK

The incidence and severity of gastrointestinal problems is highly related to the type of treatment you get. With conventional external beam therapy that irradiates a box-shaped area around the prostate, about 30 percent of men develop serious proctitis (rectal inflammation). 3-D conformal therapy reduces the incidence to 14 percent, and only 2 percent of those who receive 3-D conformal therapy with IMRT develop bowel frequency, urgency, tenesmus, or bleeding. For men who opt for modern seed implants, 3 percent experience severe rectal inflammation early on, and 10 to 15 percent develop moderate irritative bowel symptoms, such as flatulence, urgency, bleeding, and cramps. Severe bleeding, requiring multiple cauterizations, occurs in 2 to 3 percent of men who receive conventional radiation, occasionally leading to a colostomy. With seed implants or 3-D conformal radiation with IMRT, serious bleeding requiring such drastic measures is very rare.

With all types of radiation, side effects increase in direct proportion to the size of the dose and—more important—the area of the rectum that's included in the field.[4] If more than 14 square centimeters of the rectal wall are exposed to radiation, the risk of side effects goes up markedly. For this reason, computer-assisted treatment planning is essential to limit the side effects of radiation therapy. In some cases, the particular relationship of the rectal wall to the prostate makes it impossible to deliver an adequate dose of radiation to the cancer without risking damage to the rectum. Prudent radiotherapists refer such patients to a surgeon.

To avoid bowel problems, 40 percent of men receive a short course of reversible hormone therapy with LHRH agonists and/or antiandrogens to shrink the prostate before radiation, reducing the size of the field and the area of the rectum that will be bombarded by damaging rays.

Certain medical conditions place you at greater risk for serious bowel problems after radiation. Men with anticoagulation or bleeding problems are not good candidates for external beam therapy or seed implants. The same may be true for patients with Crohn's disease or ulcerative colitis, depending on the severity of the disease, whether they've needed surgical procedures, and how well the illness is controlled by medication.

Combination therapies, including brachytherapy with external beam radiation, increase the risk of bowel problems. So does treatment with outmoded technology, such as a conventional linear accelerator. If you decide to have brachytherapy or external beam radiation, make sure you're treated by a highly experienced radiation oncologist at a facility that offers state-of-the-art equipment.

CAN YOU PREVENT BOWEL PROBLEMS BY AVOIDING TREATMENT?

Prostate cancer rarely grows around the rectum or blocks the intestinal tract. But if your cancer is serious enough or you are young enough to require treatment and you are concerned about the gastrointestinal effects of radiation, you should consider having surgery instead. Even men with previous rectal surgery, such as total removal of the colon (colectomy) with the small bowel connected to the rectum (ileorectal anastomosis), can have a radical prostatectomy safely. If your age, health, or the extent of your cancer excludes surgery as an option, and radiation is the right treatment choice, consider taking hormone therapy to reduce the area of rectal wall that will be exposed. In the final analysis, the risk of bowel problems can best be minimized by seeking optimal treatment from highly skilled and experienced experts.

THE FUTURE

Studies are under way to determine whether novel radioprotective agents can prevent damage to rectal tissues from external beam therapy or seed implants. In one such trial in Greece, an experimental drug called amifostine significantly reduced acute symptoms of bowel inflammation after radiation.[5] As we learn more about the way radiation therapy works to destroy cancers, we will discover other drugs that promote cancer eradication or protect normal tissue.

IMRT was a major advancement in radiation therapy that substantially reduced side effects and increased cure rates for prostate cancer. Gastroenterologists at Memorial Sloan-Kettering report far fewer serious bowel complications of prostate cancer radiation today than they saw ten years ago, before IMRT was developed. This technique continues to be refined as we explore the optimal dose for each type of prostate cancer and study ways to combine high-dose radiotherapy with hormone therapy more effectively.

IN SUMMARY

Though it is rarely discussed and little known, treatment for prostate cancer can alter or impair bowel function. For several weeks after surgery, men must avoid constipation. After radiation, some men suffer bowel inflammation, urgency, and fecal incontinence. These problems can be troubling and difficult to manage.

20

■

Rising PSA after Surgery
or Radiation Therapy

READ THIS CHAPTER TO LEARN:

- Why do some prostate cancers recur?
- Does a rising PSA always mean cancer?
- What can be done about a rising PSA after surgery or radiation?

While modern surgery and radiation are highly effective against prostate cancer, 25 to 40 percent of patients will eventually have a recurrence of the disease that is first evidenced by a rising PSA.

Local treatments cannot cure cancers that have already spread, and even the best modern tests are incapable of detecting tiny clusters of cancer cells that may exist elsewhere in the body before surgery or radiation. Sometimes, even when the tumor is locally contained, the surgeon may fail to remove all the cancer (positive surgical margins) or mistakenly leave some normal prostate tissue behind (benign surgical margins). In the first case, the tumor would eventually grow again. In the second instance, the remaining prostate tissue or a new cancer that develops within it might grow. Either of these situations could cause the PSA to rise.

Radiation leaves the gland in place. The prostate tissue that remains continues to produce PSA, which is why most men have a detectable PSA after radiation therapy. If all the cancer cells are not killed, the tumor will recur and the PSA level will rise. Even if the original cancer is eradicated completely, a new cancer could develop within the gland at some future time.

DOES A RISING PSA ALWAYS MEAN CANCER?

PSA tests can be a source of intense, or even debilitating, anxiety. After surgery or radiation, many men anticipate the test with dread and await the outcome like the verdict in a capital case. Occasionally, an elevation in the PSA represents nothing more than a laboratory error, a benign condition, or meaningless background noise. One study showed that less than half of men who at some point had a PSA that registered 0.2 or higher after surgery ever experienced a genuine rising PSA over time. After radiation, PSA levels tend to fluctuate for the first few years, sometimes for no apparent reason. (See PSA Bounce, on page 400.)

Even when the PSA is genuinely rising because of cancer, it suggests trouble on the distant horizon, *not* an imminent threat. A cancer recurrence may be contained in the prostate area and curable with further (**salvage**) treatment. Sometimes the PSA rises so slowly (suggesting that the cancer is growing very slowly as well) that no treatment is needed for many years. In an older man with a limited life expectancy, further treatment may never be required. The disease may not cause any problems in his lifetime.

PSA AFTER RADICAL PROSTATECTOMY

After the prostate is surgically removed, your PSA should become unde-tectable. By taking out the gland, we destroy the PSA factory, and no more of the enzyme is produced. Residual PSA is flushed from the bloodstream in a few weeks, eliminating the final inventory.

This creates a peculiar conundrum. It's impossible to measure some-thing that does not exist. Proving there is no PSA is like trying to demon-strate as a certainty that there is no arsenic in the drinking water. How do we know we looked everywhere? Couldn't there have been a few PSA molecules that we failed to detect among the trillions in the tube? The best a laboratory can do is report that, in the sample they studied, the PSA was found to be less than some very low, arbitrary number they predeter-mine in an attempt to avoid reporting insignificant background noise. In our lab at Memorial Sloan-Kettering, the threshold for an undetectable PSA is 0.05, but other facilities set that number considerably higher. The quality of these tests and the laboratories running them can differ widely.

In two to three of every hundred tests, a reported elevation turns out to be false. The problem could be laboratory error or some other inno-cent artifact. If, after treatment, you have fifty or more PSA tests over the years, chances are one or more of them will show a spurious elevation.

PSA AFTER RADIATION

After brachytherapy or external beam radiation, it's difficult to deter-mine the cause of a rising PSA. The prostate is not removed as it is with surgery. Any PSA we detect may be coming from benign overgrowth or inflammation of normal prostate tissue, not necessarily from cancer.

As radiation kills cancer cells, the PSA slowly declines until it reaches its lowest level, which we refer to as the **PSA nadir**. During the course of radiation, the PSA may actually rise at first and not begin to fall until six months after the treatment course is finished. The average time it takes to reach PSA nadir is eighteen months, but it can take as long as three years. Ideally, we want that lowest number to be 0.5 or less. The PSA rarely becomes undetectable as it does after radical prostatectomy. The nadir is predictive of how you're likely to fare. The lower the PSA goes, the smaller the chance that your cancer will recur.

The American Society for Therapeutic Radiology and Oncology (ASTRO) defines radiation failure as three consecutive rises from the PSA nadir, measured at six-month intervals. If your PSA goes up twice and the next test shows a lower level, you are not viewed as having a recurrence, and the count begins again.[1]

Using this definition, it's possible to ignore a tumor recurrence for a very long time and miss a second chance for a cure. Ideally, the PSA should fall to a low and stay there. If it begins to rise from the lowest point, is higher than 1, and reaches three new peaks or highs, even if they're not consecutive, I'd advise you to meet with your radiation oncologist and urologist to consider the next steps.

The purpose of the three-peak rule is to make sure the PSA increase is genuine. But if your level begins to rise above the nadir, I believe it's prudent to wait three months—not six—to repeat the test with an eye to further assessment and possible treatment if you see three new peaks.

WHAT IF THE PSA LEVEL BEGINS TO RISE?

There is no need to panic. Even if cancer is the cause of the PSA elevation, you could enjoy many, many years with no symptoms of recurrence, often without any further treatment. Your doctor can help you evaluate how long a horizon remains until the next level of trouble, and what course of action makes sense. Try not to let worries about what may happen down the road stand in the way of enjoying the present.

The first order of business is to repeat the test. You'll want to make sure the elevation is not a fluke. To be significant, your PSA must be both reliably measurable and unequivocally rising. Typically, we look for a steady rise on three subsequent tests, though these need not be consecutive.

NOTE: PSA can fluctuate for no reason from day to day by as much as 36 percent for men who still have the gland in place after radiation therapy, so you're bound to see some meaningless ups and downs. After surgery, the PSA should become undetectable and remain so.

After radical prostatectomy, if your PSA reaches a level of 0.2 or more and continues to rise steadily, it's reasonable to assume that there has been a regrowth of prostate tissue, which could be benign or malignant. Properly done, radical prostatectomy should remove the entire gland. There should be no benign prostatic tissue left in the patient. Unfortunately, that does not always happen. Residual prostatic tissue, if it is benign, may cause no health risk at all. But if it begins to grow or becomes inflamed, the PSA can become detectable and continue to rise, causing considerable consternation for the patient and his doctor, since the apparently benign tissue might harbor a focus of cancer that can be difficult to diagnose.[2]

THE CAUSE OF A RISING PSA: BENIGN PROSTATE TISSUE OR CANCER?

If your PSA level increases after radical prostatectomy, the usual cause is cancer. But it's also possible that normal prostate tissue was left behind by an inexperienced surgeon or one who mistakenly focused on something other than the primary goal, which is removing the entire prostate and the seminal vesicles to cure the cancer. Some surgeons erroneously believe that it's necessary to spare the bladder neck or the apex (bottom tip) of the prostate to preserve urinary continence. The prostate and bladder neck intersect like woven fingers, so it's virtually impossible to remove the entire gland and leave the bladder neck intact. Some surgeons excise too little tissue in an attempt to save erectile nerves, inadvertently leaving some normal prostate tissue behind.

If a rising PSA comes from remaining bits of benign tissue, the PSA usually rises slowly and peaks at a low level, about 1. How soon the elevation occurs depends on how much prostate tissue is left in place and the sensitivity of the PSA assay. If the lab examining the blood sample has a very low threshold, less than 0.05, BPH can usually account for an increase within the first year or two, though in rare cases a rising PSA can take six years or more to show up.

Where the rise is more rapid or goes above 1, the cause is more likely a return of the tumor. With cancer, the PSA will continue to rise until you have treatment. To decide what to do, we have to determine whether the cancer has recurred locally or spread beyond the prostate area. Diagnostic tests like bone scans are rarely able to detect where the cancer is until the PSA is greater than 10 to 20.[3] Sometimes local regrowth of cancer can be seen with an MRI or transrectal ultrasound. Typically, we must make an educated guess about where the cancer is likely to be. We base that judgment on how quickly the PSA is rising, the amount of time that passed between surgery and the first detectable PSA, and the characteristics of your cancer at the time of surgery.[4]

HOW DANGEROUS IS A RISING PSA?

PSA DOUBLING TIME

The rate at which your PSA rises is a critical indicator. The longer it takes for the PSA to double, the longer the time before metastases appear. Ten months is the typical cutoff. If the PSA doubles in less than ten months, the cancer is more serious, with a greater chance of metastases, while a doubling time longer than ten months suggests local recurrence. Doubling times less than three months are ominous indicators of early metastases.[5]

Doubling time is a complex and dynamic measure. You cannot plot the slope correctly by simply looking at your first and most recent test

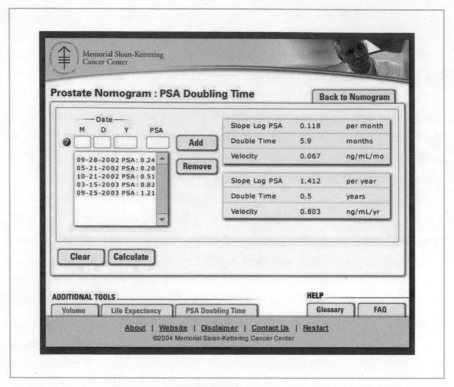

PSA doubling time calculator available online on the Memorial Sloan-Kettering Web site or at www.nomogram.org.

results. To get an accurate picture of how rapidly your PSA is rising, you should accumulate all of your available scores and use a doubling calculator such as the one you can find online at: http://www.mskcc.org/mskcc/html/10088.cfm.

Remember that PSA doubling time does not necessarily remain constant. It should be recalculated from time to time to gauge the effects of treatment or any change in the rate of tumor growth.

NOTE: Combining the PSA doubling time, the time to first rise, and the information from your pathology report improves our ability to assess whether a recurrence is local or distant.

TIME TO FIRST RISE

The longer your PSA remained undetectable after surgery before it began to rise, the greater the chances that the recurrence is local rather than metastatic. A PSA that starts to rise within the first two years suggests distant metastases, while an increase that begins two years or more after radical prostatectomy points to local recurrence.

OTHER PROGNOSTIC INDICATORS

Another important consideration is the nature of your original tumor. If your cancer was confined to the gland with a Gleason grade of 7 or less but you had positive surgical margins, meaning the cancer was not completely removed, any recurrence is likely to be localized to the prostate area. If you had positive lymph nodes or seminal vesicle invasion and a high Gleason sum of 8 to 10, chances are far greater that the cancer had already spread before treatment and has metastasized beyond the prostate area.[6]

WHAT FURTHER TESTS ARE NEEDED IF THE PSA BEGINS TO RISE?

An annual digital rectal exam (DRE) should be part of the standard monitoring after radical prostatectomy. If the doctor feels a suspicious area on DRE, a biopsy of the suspect tissue is indicated. Cancer regrows in the prostate bed (the area left behind after surgery) with disturbing frequency. In several studies, cancer was detected on biopsy in a whopping 40 percent of patients who had a rising PSA after radical prostatectomy. I have sometimes been surprised and dismayed to find an obvious residual segment of the prostate or the entire seminal vesicles left behind by surgeons after a so-called "radical" prostatectomy (which should remove the entire gland and the seminal vesicles).

The location of a cancer recurrence is hard to pin down. Biopsies of the prostate area after the gland is removed only detect about half of existing cancers, so a negative result does not rule out the possibility that the tumor has recurred. In this situation, an endorectal MRI may be illuminating. Using MRI after surgery, Drs. Hedvig Hricak and Howard Scher at Memorial Sloan-Kettering found signs of tumor recurrence in or around the urethra or bladder neck with surprising frequency, areas difficult to examine with DRE alone. As an added benefit, the MRI allowed a good look at pelvic lymph nodes and pelvic bones, frequent sites of cancer spread. These endorectal MRIs even found areas of cancer in men with PSA levels less than 2.

It's extremely rare for bone scans, CT scans, or plain X-rays to find anything if the PSA is less than 10. In fact, such tests are unlikely to detect any sign of metastases until a man's PSA rises over 20. At lower levels, these imaging tests are generally useless. To predict the likelihood of a positive bone scan, we've developed a nomogram that combines the PSA level, PSA doubling time, the time since surgery, and other relevant factors. (See Memorial Sloan-Kettering prostate nomograms on pages 394 to 397.)

A number of cutting-edge investigational tools show promise in allowing us to identify areas of metastatic spread. A PET scan may be able to pick up a cancer anywhere in the body. Studies are under way at our institution and at other cancer centers to determine whether this technology used in conjunction with various tumor markers might be able to identify the site of a prostate-cancer recurrence.

Monoclonal antibodies are substances produced in the laboratory that can track down and bind with cancer cells. Essentially, these are detective molecules that locate and attach to the suspect tumor cells with the equivalent of chemical handcuffs. While the first generation of these scans (**ProstaScint**) has not produced consistently reliable results, a new form of monoclonal antibody, developed by Neil Bander of Weill-Cornell College of Medicine, appears to be safer and better able to detect tiny amounts of prostate cancer.[7]

TREATING A RISING PSA AFTER SURGERY

WATCHFUL WAITING

One possibility is to simply wait and continue to monitor the situation regularly. Every treatment carries some risk of side effects. If your PSA is low and doubling very slowly, and your cancer was favorable at the time of surgery, it may be ten or even twenty years before you face the

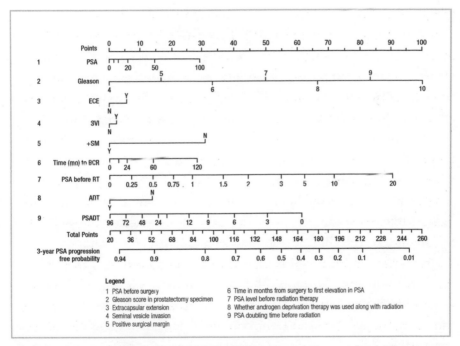

Nomogram to predict chances of a favorable response to radiation for men with a rising PSA after surgery. To use the nomogram, drop a line straight down from the "points" line to the value of each factor (PSA, tumor stage, etc.) to determine the points for each factor. Add the sum of points for each, then drop a line from the "Total Points" line to determine the "predictive value" or probability that the cancer is indolent.*

---

* Source: Modified from Stephenson, A. J., and K. M. Slawin. "The Value of Radiotherapy for the Treatment of Recurrent Prostate Cancer after Radical Prostatectomy." *Nature Clinical Practice Urology* 1, no. 2 (2004): 90–96.

likelihood of symptoms from local growth or metastases. Depending on your age, general health, lifestyle, and personal preferences, periodic checkups may be all you need. The key tests to monitor the cancer are the PSA doubling time and the absolute level of PSA. The Memorial Sloan-Kettering nomograms, available at http://www.mskcc.org/mskcc/html/10088.cfm, can help you and your doctor to assess how imminent and serious a risk your recurrence poses and help you decide when additional therapy might be indicated.

Of course, the main goal is to keep the cancer under control, hopefully for the rest of your life. The best thing to do is watch closely to make sure to be ready to institute treatment if and when it becomes necessary.

SALVAGE RADIATION

If the recurrent tumor is restricted to the prostate area, radiation offers a second chance for a cure. In fact, radiation is the only available therapy that has the potential to cure a patient with a rising PSA after radical prostatectomy. Keep in mind that the window of opportunity is limited. After the PSA rises above 2, the odds for a cure decline significantly.[8] There is a high likelihood that you'll respond to radiation if your PSA is less than 2 with a doubling time greater than ten months, especially if your surgical margin was positive (meaning some cancer was likely left behind) and the Gleason score was less than 8 (see Memorial Sloan-Kettering nomograms for salvage radiation at www.nomogram.org).

Radiation after radical prostatectomy does have a downside. Lacking a clear map of where the tumor lies, the radiation therapist cannot take advantage of precise, modern, conformal techniques and instead must target the general area. Consequently, the side effects are higher for any given dose. There is a significant probability that **salvage radiation** to treat a recurrence will impair erections, and 3 percent of patients treated with this approach will develop incontinence. That number is even higher in men who are still having stress incontinence after radical prostatectomy. If possible, it's best to wait until urinary continence has been regained and stabilized after surgery before beginning salvage radiation. This is feasible as long as the PSA remains low.

Because more of the bladder and more of the rectum are included in the targeted field, the incidence of **radiation proctitis** (bowel irritation) and **cystitis** (bladder irritation) is as great as if you were getting full-fledged radiotherapy to treat a primary cancer.[9] This is true even though the dose is lower for salvage radiation. If you have a low, slowly rising PSA and no nodule that the doctor can feel on DRE, along with a negative ultrasound or negative MRI, the salvage dose can be kept to about 64 to 68 Gy. If a definite area of cancer can be located by biopsy or MRI, we recommend increasing the dose to 70 to 75 Gy and adding hormone therapy in the form of LHRH or antiandrogens to the treatment program. The increased possibility of long-term cure justifies the added risk of erectile dysfunction from higher radiation doses or hormone therapy.

DETECTING CANCER RECURRENCE AFTER RADIATION

Because the prostate is still in place, it can be a real challenge to prove that a rising PSA indicates that the cancer has recurred. Given that radiation kills cancer gradually, a biopsy would not yield any meaningful information for about two years after treatment. Cancer cells found in a biopsy done earlier could be lethally irradiated, though not yet dead. Radiologists often recommend waiting two and a half years for the full effects of treatment to kick in, but generally an expert pathologist can tell at two years whether there's a radiation effect. If undamaged cancer cells remain at this point, they're not going to disappear.

After radiation, a bone scan or CT scan rarely shows any sign of cancer before the PSA reaches 20. We have found that performing an endorectal MRI of the prostate with spectroscopy can be helpful in detecting local recurrence of cancer within the prostate, especially if a comparable MRI was done before radiotherapy and we can compare the results.[10] I always prescribe this sophisticated imaging study before doing a biopsy of the prostate in this situation. The results help guide where I will place the biopsy needles and how I should treat the cancer if it has recurred.

> NOTE: If the PSA dips only slightly after radiation and then begins to rise, it may be wise to do a biopsy earlier. Some men receive grossly inadequate radiation. If the cancer has not spread, a salvage radical prostatectomy might still offer the chance for a cure (see page 402).

PSA BOUNCE

Though the reason remains unclear, in 30 to 40 percent of brachytherapy patients and 5 to 15 percent of men who have received external beam therapy (without hormones), the PSA level goes up for a while and then falls again without any additional treatment. This PSA bounce tends to occur within the first three years. The level can rise long and steadily enough to meet the ASTRO definition of a radiation failure (see page 391). If this happens within the first two years, we have to consider that the PSA elevations we see might represent an innocent bounce that will spontaneously return to low levels. Of course, an early rise may continue, indicating recurrent cancer. The uncertainty of PSA levels after radiation can lead to a crucial delay in starting further, curative treatment. Normally, a bounce doesn't go very high and the slope is gradual, but the phenomenon confounds our ability to diagnose a recurrence soon after radiation.[11]

If the PSA begins to rise two to two and a half years after radiation therapy, a biopsy may be in order. If the results are negative, indicating no cancer, we would continue to follow the PSA and plot its doubling time. Since with radiation the prostate and surrounding tissues were not removed and examined (as they are after surgery), we have no way of knowing whether the cancer had already spread to the seminal vesicles or lymph nodes when you were first diagnosed. All we have to go on after radiation are your original PSA, the clinical stage and grade of your cancer at the time of biopsy, how low your PSA went after radiation (PSA nadir), the amount of time that elapsed after radiation before your PSA began to rise, and your PSA doubling time. A high-risk cancer with an initial Gleason grade of 8 to 10, a PSA over 10, and an extensive tumor points to a higher risk of distant spread, as would a nadir higher than 1, a rise that begins less than two years after treatment, and a doubling time of less than six months.[12]

RISING PSA AFTER RADIATION WITH HORMONES

Hormone therapy shrinks the prostate and the tumor, providing a better chance of cure at low radiation doses. Once the treatment is stopped, almost everyone has a PSA bounce. Hormone therapy acts by curtailing testosterone production or blocking its effects. When medication is withdrawn, testosterone returns and the PSA goes up. This can make it difficult to diagnose a recurrence, and critical treatment could be delayed.

TREATING A RISING PSA
AFTER RADIATION

WATCHFUL WAITING

Doing nothing beyond continuing to monitor the PSA is a reasonable alternative, especially for older men, those with significant health problems aside from prostate cancer, and patients unwilling to risk the side effects of available treatment options. This approach is especially attractive if a biopsy of the prostate turns up no local cancer, the PSA is low, and the PSA doubling time is longer than six months.

SALVAGE RADICAL PROSTATECTOMY

Removing the prostate after primary radiation treatment may cure the cancer if it is still locally contained. In our series of radical prostatectomies at Memorial Sloan-Kettering, 50 percent of patients remained cancer-free ten years after salvage surgery, and 35 percent still show no sign of recurrence at fifteen years.[13] Because this is a risky, technically challenging procedure, it should *only* be attempted by highly skilled, experienced surgeons.

Before considering salvage surgery, it's important to be certain that your PSA rise really signifies a cancer recurrence and not an innocent artifact or the PSA bounce. In men who have had hormone therapy in conjunction with radiation, an increase in PSA is especially difficult to assess. Careful interpretation of the biopsy is critical as well. Radiation can cause cells to look abnormal, and an inexperienced pathologist might have trouble distinguishing these innocent changes from cancer.

If the cancer has spread beyond the local area, removing the prostate will not cure it. In evaluating whether a patient is a good candidate for salvage surgery, I take a look at the original Gleason grade, stage, and PSA to judge whether the cancer was initially curable. If the original PSA was over 20 or the Gleason sum was over 7, and the cancer extended through the capsule, it was not curable then and it is not curable now. If after radiation therapy the PSA has risen above 4, there is invasion of the seminal vesicles, or the biopsy shows extensive, high-grade cancer in most of the cores, the cancer is probably not curable and an operation to remove the gland would not be appropriate.

If the cancer is more favorable and potentially curable with salvage surgery, the next question is whether you are otherwise healthy and have a long enough life expectancy to justify the operation. Salvage radical prostatectomy may make sense if you have a life expectancy greater than ten years. For older men or men in poor health, hormone therapy will likely keep the cancer in check for many years. Finally, you must be willing to accept the increased risks that salvage surgery entails.

Even in the best of hands, the incidence of side effects—especially incontinence and erectile dysfunction—is considerably higher with a salvage operation than it is for radical prostatectomy on a gland that has not been irradiated. Still, given the best modern techniques, this procedure has become increasingly successful and less hazardous. Rectal injuries are rare (no more than 1 to 2 percent), and dramatic bowel damage no longer occurs. Half of men regain normal urinary continence, though about 20 percent require an artificial sphincter to restore satisfactory urinary control. The risk of urinary stricture is 10 percent higher than it is for surgery on a gland that has not been irradiated. After salvage radical prostatectomy, most men (84 percent) do not recover spontaneous sexual function, even with medication like sildenafil. To cure the cancer, we generally have to remove the erectile nerves, though nerve sparing is possible if the recurrent cancer is found early. Because of radiation damage, the results of nerve grafts with salvage prostatectomy have not been as promising as they have in men who have not had radiation treatment.

CRYOTHERAPY

For cancer that recurs in the prostate area after radiation, freezing the gland is a reasonable option. Cryotherapy is less invasive than salvage radical prostatectomy and carries a lower risk of incontinence. Ten to 15 percent of cryotherapy patients develop serious urinary control problems, as opposed to 25 to 30 percent of men after salvage surgery. Impotence, however, is more common, and nearly all men lose erections after cryotherapy.[14] Also, though the incontinence rate is lower, the procedure does cause other bothersome urinary complications. Freezing kills the gland, and the dead tissue sloughs off into the urethra, where it can cause a blockage. This may require the use of a suprapubic catheter (a tube placed through the lower abdomen into the bladder) or a Foley catheter (a tube through the penis into the bladder) for up to six weeks.

With cryotherapy, you can be out of the hospital the same day, and catastrophic complications are rare. Unfortunately, the cure rate is not impressive. Most men convert to a negative biopsy after the gland is frozen, but many will later develop a rising PSA, indicating a recurrence of the tumor.

Other recently developed local therapies include **HIFU (high-**

intensity focused ultrasound) and **RFA (radiofrequency ablation)** using the "RITA" system, both of which effectively cook tumor cells with heat generated by soundwaves. Though it's too early to determine long-term results, both approaches seem to inhibit the local growth of cancer with reasonable safety. Since they are designed to treat focal areas of cancer rather than the entire prostate, these therapies are best for local tumor control, where cancer cure is not the goal.

INVESTIGATIONAL TREATMENTS

These include **gene therapy**, injections of cytotoxins (cell destroyers), and oncolytic viruses (viruses capable of infiltrating and killing cancer cells) as alternative possibilities for patients opposed to salvage prostatectomy. A promising new approach just being studied is photodynamic therapy, where laser light is beamed into the prostate to activate an intravenously delivered chemical agent derived from chlorophyll that destroys tumor cells and the blood vessels that feed them. Care for people involved in clinical trials to test the effectiveness of new methods is often better than standard care, and entering such a trial gives you access to treatments that would otherwise be unavailable. (See page 416 for more on clinical trials.)

THE FUTURE

Investigational treatments include chemotherapy, new biological agents, and immunotherapy. For most other malignancies, recurrences are not detected until the disease has progressed enough to become visible on imaging studies or has caused debilitating symptoms. With prostate cancer, you have a unique opportunity. You're likely to remain symptom-free for many years after your PSA begins to rise. In fact, one study found an average of 11.3 years from the first rising PSA to the development of metastases. Another investigation reported a median of 8 years until metastases appeared, and 5 more years before the average man with a rising PSA succumbed to prostate cancer. This gives you ample time to look into newer forms of treatment, many of which do not have the side effects of hormone therapy. Medicine is changing rapidly. Clinical trials are in progress to test the effectiveness of prostate cancer vaccines that may be able to arm your own body to seek out and destroy tumor cells. Monoclonal antibodies may be able to defeat the cancer after tracking it down. We are testing ways to alter immune cells or genes so that they turn against the cancer while leaving normal cells alone.

Vitamin D shows promise as a means to slow the growth of prostate cancer, though it may not lower your PSA. In fact, vitamin D treatment and certain other drugs may cause a wild cancer to become more like normal prostate cells. As a result, the PSA may actually rise, which makes it tricky to judge whether these strategies are beneficial.

Modern chemotherapy appears to be as effective in prostate-cancer treatment as it is in treating breast cancer, and recent clinical trials have shown a clear survival advantage for chemotherapy in men with advanced prostate cancer (see Chapter 21).[15] About 60 percent of men show regression of their tumors with combination chemotherapy, using agents such as docetaxel, carboplatin, and estramustine (which combines estrogen with a cytotoxin that kills cells).

IN SUMMARY

PSA is an important and often useful diagnostic tool, but it is far from magical or infallible. Like many tests, it has limitations and inherent variability, especially at the low levels we see after radical prostatectomy or radiation treatment.

Still, the test offers a significant advantage. A rising PSA gives us six to eight years, on average, before any scan or X-ray would show a cancer recurrence, and the time before symptoms of metastases can be as long as twenty years. If your tumor recurs in the local prostate area, radiation or salvage surgery can be curative, and hormones and investigational treatments can control the cancer, often for a man's remaining lifetime, or at least for many, many years.

21

■

Treating Metastatic
Prostate Cancer

READ THIS CHAPTER TO LEARN:

- What can be done about prostate cancer that has metastasized?
- How can you judge clinical trials and experimental treatments?
- What about alternative and complementary therapies?
- What strategies are available to effectively manage discomfort and pain?

Each year in the United States, 50,000 men with prostate cancer develop a steadily rising PSA after treatment. If the cause is a recurrence in the local prostate area, salvage radiation or salvage radical prostatectomy offers a second chance to cure the disease. But sometimes we find evidence that the cancer has spread to lymph nodes, bones, or other organs—a far more serious situation. At this stage, the cancer is metastatic, and the treatment focus shifts from cure to control. Our goal is to delay progression of the cancer for as long as possible, prolong survival, and maintain the best possible quality of life. Medicine in this setting is closer to art than science, as we work carefully to optimize the benefits of available treatments and minimize their risks. The good news is that we now have effective treatments for metastatic prostate cancer. Traditional hormone therapy works dramatically well, at least for a time. Many new molecular and immunological therapies are being studied, and we finally have clear proof that the right chemotherapy prolongs life.

TREATMENT OPTIONS

If your PSA is rising and the tumor cannot be shown to have recurred in the prostate area, we must presume that the cancer has spread to distant sites. Even so, there are several treatment choices, including watchful waiting, hormone therapy, chemotherapy, and clinical trials of investigational agents.

WATCHFUL WAITING

This is a reasonable option, since there is no proven way to cure prostate cancer in this situation, and though a few trials have suggested that early hormone treatment may prolong survival, we lack definitive evidence that this is the case. The goal is to keep you feeling well and symptom-free for as long as possible, hopefully for the rest of your natural life. Many physicians recommend careful monitoring with regular checks of the PSA level and postpone hormone treatment and its side effects for as long as possible. Annual bone scans and periodic MRIs of the pelvis are reasonable studies that may alert us to actual sites of spread. The PSA level and its doubling time are the best indicators of when it may be necessary to intervene. Treatment can reasonably be postponed as long as you have no symptoms, imaging scans show no cancer, and your PSA doubling time is greater than six months.

Hormone Therapy

The second option for cancer that has spread beyond the local prostate area is hormone therapy or **androgen deprivation**, as it is often called. Prostate cancer requires male hormones (androgens) to grow and thrive. Deprive the cancer cells of these vital chemicals, and they rapidly die in a process called apoptosis.

Testosterone, the principle androgen, is produced in the testicles. Historically, the preferred means to withdraw male hormones was surgical castration. The testicles were removed in an operation known as **orchiectomy**. By the mid-1980s, medications called LHRH agonists were developed that could block hormone production without surgical excision of the testicles. Today, few men opt for orchiectomy, which is irreversible and can exact a psychological toll. Proponents of surgical castration emphasize that the procedure is simple, less expensive than prolonged medication, and may avoid some side effects of drugs (though the side effects of androgen withdrawal are identical whether castration is accomplished medically or surgically). Those patients who choose to have their testicles removed can have the doctor implant silicone prostheses shaped like testicles at the time of surgery. Limited operations, such as subtotal orchiectomy, in which the pulp but not the capsule of the testicles is removed, have been discredited because they leave too much androgen-producing tissue behind.

In sufficient doses, LHRH agonists such as leuprolide (Lupron or Eligard) or goserelin (Zoladex), given as an injection monthly, every three months, or every four months, shut down the testosterone-generating Leydig cells in the testes, bringing androgen output from these glands to a halt. At first, these drugs ironically boost testosterone production, but within two weeks the level falls below 20 ng/ml compared to normal testosterone levels of 300 to 1,000 ng/ml. Since 5 percent of the body's androgen is produced by the adrenal glands, medical or surgical castration will not drive the level to zero.

Another class of drugs was later developed to block the effects of any remaining androgens on the cancer cells. These so-called antiandrogens, such as flutamide (Eulexin), bicalutamide (Casodex), and nilutamide (Nilandron), can be taken in conjunction with LHRH agonists to achieve what is known as a complete or total androgen blockade. Flutamide, which requires a dosing schedule of two pills, three times per day, is more cumbersome than the one-a-day bicalutamide or nilutamide. Antiandrogens have not been shown to offer any significant advantage when used in a man who has had an orchiectomy. Their main benefit seems to be averting the effects of the flare, or sudden rise, in testosterone during the first two weeks after an LHRH agonist injection. After that, their effect is marginal. Years of study have shown that life expectancy is slightly prolonged when a complete androgen blockade is compared to LHRH agonists alone. Still, given their cost and side effects, the benefit of long-term use of antiandrogens in addition to LHRH agonists is debatable.

NOTE: For a time, the female hormone estrogen, in the form of DES, was used in hormone therapy for prostate cancer. DES is an inexpensive pill that reduces testosterone and controls cancer as well as orchiectomy. But at maximally effective doses, DES proved dangerous, causing heart attacks, emboli, and strokes, and it is rarely recommended today. Whether a low dose, 1 to 3 milligrams a day, would be equally effective without these side effects has never been adequately tested.

The major decisions in hormone therapy are whether it is necessary, when to begin treatment, and whether to administer the drugs on a continuous or intermittent basis.[1]

To decide if hormone treatment is indicated, doctors should consider the age and health of the patient (i.e. life expectancy) in light of the seriousness of his disease. For example, Tom J. is 75 years old with heart disease and diabetes. His cancer at the time of diagnosis was a low-risk Gleason 6, stage T1; and his PSA doubling time is more than twelve months. In his case, hormone treatment may never prove necessary, and monitoring the disease is the most sensible approach. On the other hand, Ben B. is a vigorous 61-year-old with no serious health problems apart from his prostate cancer. His PSA started to rise only a few months after radical prostatectomy, which was not surprising, given that his original tumor was a Gleason 8 with seminal vesicle invasion. In Ben's case, hormones will be required.

Experts disagree about the value of early versus late hormone therapy.[2] We even lack consensus about what constitutes "early" or "late," though basically, early treatment means starting hormones soon after the PSA begins to rise, and late means beginning the therapy when symptoms or clinical signs of metastases seem imminent. There is general agreement that it's probably *not* necessary to begin hormone treatment and deal with the unpleasant side effects at the very first sign of a rising PSA. Most experts also concur that waiting until a man has signs or symptoms of metastases is unwise. Unfortunately, we have no crystal ball that can predict with certainty exactly when metastases will appear. In deciding when to begin hormone treatment, we look at the seriousness of the original tumor. If the cancer was high-grade (Gleason 8 to 10, stage T3a or higher) before radiation treatment, or if the pathologist found cancer in the seminal vesicles or pelvic lymph nodes after surgery, metastases are likely to develop sooner than they would in someone whose original tumor was Gleason 7 or below and stage T1 or T2. A short PSA doubling time of less than ten months also predicts more rapid distant spread. Be sure to communicate carefully with your physician to ensure that you understand and agree with his philosophy about hormone treatment and that your personal needs and preferences are taken into account.

If you participate in a clinical trial (see Experimental Therapies on page 415 and the section on Investigational Treatments on page 404), the rules of the study may govern when your treatment will begin. If you don't enter a trial, I certainly recommend beginning hormone therapy before a bone scan or other tests identify a definite site of metastases. If your PSA is followed regularly, your doctor can monitor the PSA level and doubling time and start you on hormone treatment when the pace of cancer growth starts to accelerate. In my view, you're probably best off delaying hormone therapy until it appears necessary. I've seen inadequate evidence to date that starting this treatment earlier prolongs life, and withdrawing hormones does cause troubling side effects. When we studied men given hormone therapy for rising PSA after radical prostatectomy at Memorial Sloan-Kettering, we found that 50 percent responded for ten years, meaning the PSA dropped and stayed low. But ten years is a long time to deal with the side effects of androgen deprivation, which can include loss of libido and erectile function, hot flashes, decreased muscle mass, thinning of bones and increased risk of fracture, breast enlargement and tenderness, anemia, and possibly diminished mental acuity. The benefits of early androgen deprivation would have to be substantial to balance these negative effects. Nevertheless, anxiety drives many men to demand hormone therapy early, and they are understandably reassured by the dramatic fall in PSA.

NOTE: I recommend a cautious approach to hormone therapy for metastatic prostate cancer. While it can be comforting to have your PSA fall dramatically or even become undetectable, the relevant issue is what's really happening to your cancer and how you can enjoy the best quality of life for as long as possible.

Some experts advocate intermittent hormone therapy.[3] Patients are given hormone-suppressing drugs until the PSA drops to undetectable levels. When it does, they are taken off the medication. Testosterone production resumes, and side effects associated with its absence (including sexual dysfunction) can resolve. When the PSA rises, hormone treatment begins again.

Intermittent therapy offers a false promise that men can enjoy more time free of the side effects of hormone therapy. In fact, the major benefit is during the first cycle, when patients can be on the drugs for 60 percent of the time and off for 40 percent. With subsequent cycles, the time to a rising PSA shortens, and treatment must resume sooner. Since it takes a while after the drugs are stopped to regain functional testosterone levels, the actual amount of time that a man can be sexually active and relieved of other side effects such as weight gain, mood swings, anemia, lethargy, and hot flashes may boil down to only 10 to 15 percent of his remaining lifetime. PSA is such a powerful, effective early warning system that overall quality of life may be better if we simply postpone hormone treatment until the PSA reaches 20 or so, or there are other signs of impending trouble.

All hormone treatments for prostate cancer result in infertility. Without adequate testosterone, sperm production stops. (This does not mean that you should cease using birth control as soon as you being hormone therapy. Before doing so, you should be evaluated to ensure that you're no longer fertile.)

> NOTE: Men vary widely in their tolerance of hormone therapy. Side effects range in severity, and, though common, they are not universal or inevitable. Also, while it can cause side effects, *hormone therapy is not dangerous.* Radiation and surgery both carry more serious risks.

WHEN HORMONE THERAPY STOPS WORKING

Depriving a prostate tumor of testosterone only works for a time. Eventually, cancer cells learn how to thrive without male hormones and become hormone refractory. Though the mechanism is not clear, one theory holds that a small fraction of the cells in every cancer are paradoxically programmed to flourish in the absence of male hormones. Another suggests that withdrawing androgens induces some cancer cells to learn to live without them, finding alternative ways to survive and grow. Recent research suggests that increased sensitivity to tiny amounts of androgens or androgen-like drugs and hormones as the trigger for the renewed growth of cells after the withdrawal or blockade of androgens.[4]

Second-line Hormone Therapy

All prostate cancers eventually find a way to grow in the absence of androgens. Typically, the first sign that this has occurred is a steadily rising PSA. At this stage ("disease state") the cancer is referred to as **hormone refractory**, though recent studies have suggested that this may not in fact be the case. Like breast cancer, prostate cancer may continue to respond favorably to changes in hormone levels. If a man has been taking LHRH agonists alone, we would try adding an antiandrogen like bicalutamide. If the patient is already on the combination of drugs, we might stop the antiandrogen.

Other secondary hormonal manipulations that work equally well include switching from a hormone-blocking agent like bicalutamide to adrenal-blocking drugs like ketoconazole (Nizoral) or aminoglutethamide. Sometimes, corticosteroids like hydrocortisone or prednisone are effective, and they are often added to adrenal-blocking drugs to prevent adrenal insufficiency. For years, we have used high-dose estrogens as second- or third-line agents, though they increase the risk of blood clots. The idea is to keep trying to slow the growth of the cancer and allow patients to survive symptom-free for as long as possible.

CHEMOTHERAPY

For many other cancers, chemotherapy has long been a standard weapon in the treatment arsenal. Traditionally this has not been the case with prostate cancer, but recent studies have altered our thinking and practice. Only a decade ago, chemotherapeutic agents used to treat this disease seemed to offer a poor ratio of benefits to risks. Even when the most potent drugs were combined, few cancers responded, and few patients with advanced prostate cancer improved. Doctors specializing in cancer therapy, whether urologists or medical oncologists, became skeptical of the value of chemotherapy and leery of the side effects.

The first study that hinted at any real benefit from chemotherapy was published only a few years ago. Patients treated with the anticancer drug mitoxantrone (Novantrone) plus steroids had substantially better pain relief and slightly longer survival than patients treated with steroids alone.[5] Still, the real breakthrough came in 2004, when two large studies proved that combination chemotherapy clearly prolonged life compared to a regime of mitoxantrone and prednisone (a steroid). The chemotherapy combinations in both studies included the powerful Taxol-related drug, Taxotere. In one study, Taxotere was combined with the estrogenlike estramustine; in the other, with prednisone. In both trials, the combined chemotherapy "cocktails" prolonged life by three to four months compared to the previous standard that used pain-relieving mitoxantrone and prednisone.[6] While a few months do not constitute a huge improvement, it is an encouraging start. These patients were at the end of their rope. All other treatments had failed. Prolonging their lives proved that traditional chemotherapy does work in prostate cancer and strongly suggests that if these drugs were used earlier in the course of the disease, the benefit might be much greater.

Past trials of chemotherapeutic drugs for prostate cancer failed because of flawed study design, using the wrong drug combinations, and not understanding how to minimize side effects. Modern chemotherapy works because newly available drugs are less toxic, better tolerated, and can be administered with far less disruption on an outpatient basis. Serious side effects, such as an overwhelming infection (sepsis) along with a dangerous drop in white blood count (leucopenia), are generally preventable, and in those rare instances when they do occur, they can be managed by administering powerful antibiotics.

Modern chemotherapy "cocktails" involving multiple agents are likely to prolong survival even more than the two-drug combinations. We are entering a new era, when chemotherapy for prostate cancer will be embraced as lifesaving, as it has been for decades in breast cancer.

EXPERIMENTAL THERAPIES

Medical science is in the midst of a historic revolution. Research and practice are changing dramatically, ushering in the age of molecular medicine. In this new approach, medical treatment targets microscopic cells and molecules rather than the traditional—and often overly complex and confounding—organ or systemwide assaults on disease. I have never witnessed a more exciting time in the field, when new technology holds such promise for men with advanced prostate cancer.

Biological profiling is effective in breast-cancer therapy and may enable us to identify and target specific prostate cancer–promoting genes. Antisense refers to synthetic genetic agents that slow or stop the growth of cancer cells. Antisense drugs, such as BCL2, may make prostate-tumor cells more susceptible to medications that induce cell death (apoptosis). Ansamycins might stem the growth of prostate cancers by destroying the receptors that enable cells in the gland to absorb cancer-promoting hormones. Monoclonal antibodies directed against specific targets on prostate-cancer cells can seek out and destroy these cells or deliver a killer payload of toxic medication. Various vaccines under investigation may be able to enhance the body's ability to battle prostate cancer on its own.

Cancers are extraordinarily complex, but the essential features they require to grow and spread are steadily being identified. To survive in the body, cancer cells must be able to divide, to avoid apoptosis, to break through normal tissue barriers, to spread through the bloodstream or lymphatic system, and to induce the growth of the blood vessels (angiogenesis) they require for oxygen and nutrients. Each of these activities is controlled by a number of enzymes, signaling proteins, and growth regulators, all of which are potential targets for therapeutic assault. Major research efforts are currently in progress to develop drugs that will bring the cancer to its knees by arresting these conspirators and putting them out of commission for good.

Because bones are a magnet for prostate-cancer spread, a second major research focus is on agents designed to target, protect, and strengthen bones. Drugs that seek out and destroy cancer cells in bone (radioisotopes such as Strontium 89) may be able to prevent or curtail the growth of bone metastases. Bisphosphonates, such as pamidronate (Aredia), clodronate (Bonefos), and zoledronic acid (Zometa) protect bones from the destructive effects of disease and from the bone loss and bone weakening that can result from hormone therapy and other cancer treatments.[7] Today we believe that these agents are so effective that every patient placed on permanent androgen deprivation should also take a bone-protective drug to prevent osteoporosis and reduce the risk of metastases in the spine.

IS A CLINICAL TRIAL RIGHT FOR YOU?

Though many people initially balk at the idea of entering a clinical trial, experimental or investigational treatments actually offer several distinct advantages. Patients enrolled in a study are typically offered top-notch care and scrupulous monitoring. Experts in various disciplines review planned trials carefully to make sure they are well thought out and that the potential benefits outweigh the risks before investigators get the go-ahead to proceed.

Since we have no approved medications as yet that cure advanced prostate cancer, a new drug or novel combination therapy may be the best way to improve your odds. A clinical trial gives you an early opportunity to try a novel therapy that might eventually prove to be more effective than treatments that are currently available. Remember, every drug treatment we have to battle diseases today was once experimental.

Through these trials, scientists using impeccable methodology may devise groundbreaking treatments. Most trials are rigorously designed and overseen by experts, but do be aware that a small percentage of research efforts is unquestionably misguided. Beware of trials you might find on the Internet that are not in the Physician Data Query (PDQ) database of the National Cancer Institute, conducted under the auspices of the NCI, or overseen by a major cancer center. To decide whether a given approach makes sense in your particular situation, it's important to understand how studies and clinical trials are constructed. (See the Resources section at the back of this book, and the NIH, NCI, PDQ Web sites).

A medical study or clinical trial seeks to answer a question about the cause, treatment, or prevention of a medical condition or disease. The questions vary enormously. A trial may look at imaging techniques or pathology, or it may be designed to demonstrate the effectiveness of a new medication or medical device. To win approval by the Federal Drug Administration (FDA) or similar agencies in other countries, new drugs and devices are put through a series of increasingly challenging, rigorous, and expensive hoops.

Phase 1 clinical drug trials involve twenty to eighty subjects. These preliminary studies are intended to demonstrate that the drug under investigation can be safely administered to humans after their safety has been established in a laboratory setting. During a phase 1 trial, scientists observe the impact of the experimental drug and monitor its side effects at varying dose levels.

Once a treatment appears safe in a phase 1 trial, a *phase 2 clinical drug trial* evaluates the drug's effectiveness on a larger group of patients who have the target condition or disease. Risks and side effects are carefully monitored, but the main goal of the trial is to see whether the drug works.

During *phase 3 clinical trials,* a drug that has been proven safe and effective in smaller studies is administered to many hundreds or even thousands of patients to examine the overall risks and benefits. Usually, phase 3 trials compare new treatments to standard approaches. If an experimental regimen passes phase 2 and phase 3 trials, the sponsor applies for FDA approval to market the drug.

Once a regimen is approved, *phase 4 drug trials* may be conducted in an effort to learn more about an approved drug's optimal dosage level, long-term effectiveness, and negative effects.

The value and validity of clinical trials hinge on how strictly they conform to the long-established principles of scientific investigation. Medical studies can range from the observation of a few people (which can yield highly misleading results) to scientifically rigorous assessments involving large groups that are carefully controlled to prevent extraneous factors from affecting the outcome. Prospective studies, where a question is asked and then the experimental groups are formed and followed over time, are considered more reliable than retrospective ones, though we have derived valuable information from retrospective studies as well, and sometimes retrospective information is all we have to go on.

While participants in clinical trials are fully informed about the nature of the study, to prevent bias that can affect results they may be kept in the dark about which arm of a trial they are in. Experimental subjects get the drug under study, while control subjects get a standard medication or a placebo (see below). In single-blind studies, medical personnel know which therapy subjects are getting, but the patients remain unaware. Double-blind trials withhold this information from both patients and physicians, whose perceptions or practice might be influenced by the knowledge.

A placebo is an inactive substance that looks identical to and is administered in precisely the same way as an experimental drug. In clinical trials, placebos are often used to ensure that the observed effects are actually the result of the therapy being studied and not some extraneous factor such as a patient's expectation that he'll get better or experience fewer symptoms. Large, placebo-controlled, double-blind studies in which experimental subjects are carefully matched ("case-controlled") and randomly assigned to treatment and control groups are far more likely to yield reliable results than a study involving a small number of subjects and a less rigorous experimental design. The gold standard in

> NOTE: In clinical trials for men with metastatic prostate cancer, placebos would not be used. Men in both arms of a study would get potentially beneficially treatment, so valuable time would not be lost.

medical investigation is the large, randomized, prospective, double-blind clinical trial.

The endpoint refers to the predefined event or outcome that completes the study. In medical investigations, total mortality or the overall survival rate is considered the easiest endpoint to define and the least subject to reporting bias (not to mention of crucial importance to patients). Did the experimental subjects live longer, and if so, how much longer? If there was a survival advantage, how long was it, and what percentage of subjects were alive five or ten years later?

Cause-specific survival refers to the numbers of deaths that resulted from the disease being studied. While this may say more about the effectiveness of the drug than overall survival, the measure is more subject to investigator bias. When a subject dies, the cause of death can be a judgment call. Pneumonia or the spread of prostate cancer to the lungs could reasonably be entered on the death certificate and in the researcher's databank.

Even when they do nothing to increase survival, therapies may confer other important benefits, such as symptom control. Treatments that improve quality of life are of critical importance to patients, and many studies focus on endpoints related to well-being in deciding whether a therapy should be included in medical practice. Did the treatment alleviate pain? Did the experimental subjects have fewer bowel problems than those in control groups? Were the experimental subjects able to have better erections and more satisfactory sexual function than those in the control groups?

Other endpoints focus on surrogate or secondary issues such as the amount of time subjects remain free of any signs of the disease (i.e. a measurable PSA after radical prostatectomy), the amount of time that elapses before their disease progresses (e.g. a new abnormality on bone scan), or how much tumors shrink as a result of the treatment. Since prostate cancer can take many years or even decades to become lethal, surrogate endpoints such as freedom from metastases or from a rapidly rising PSA can be highly useful in gauging the effectiveness of a new therapy.

NOTE: Famed British statesman, orator, and novelist Benjamin Disraeli noted that, "there are three kinds of lies: lies, damned lies and statistics." Study outcomes can be affected by subtle alterations in interpretation or experimental design. Clinical trials can cost many millions of dollars, and a company's fortunes, or even its very survival, might hinge on the outcome. It's wise to be aware of who sponsored a study and what, if anything, that sponsor had to gain. Where results are confusing or contradictory, experts should be able to help you sort things out and assess what is most significant and believable.

ALTERNATIVE AND COMPLEMENTARY MEDICINE

Alternative medicine utilizes substances such as vitamins and herbal or homeopathic remedies whose safety and effectiveness have not been established by proven scientific means. These "natural" agents are exempt from government oversight, and no agency guarantees their purity or consistency. In a particularly egregious example, shipments of PC-SPES, which contains eight Chinese herbs and appears to be effective in some men with hormone refractory prostate cancer, were recently found to be contaminated with female hormones and hazardous blood thinners to counteract the blood clots those hormones cause. Obviously, the company that added these dangerous drugs did not believe in the efficacy of PC-SPES alone. Understandably, people are often drawn to such treatments by extravagant (though also unregulated and generally unproven) claims. In fact, if they were appropriately tested and scrupulously manufactured, some of these agents would be found to be harmless, while others might prove useful. The problem is separating the innocent suspects and positive players from those capable of doing serious harm.

If you decide to take alternative substances, be sure to discuss them with your doctor. Investigate any agent you plan to take—whether a supplement, an herb, or any other "natural" remedy—thoroughly before you start. Consider carefully the possible effects of the dose you plan to take. Beware of the foolhardy concept that if a little is good, a lot must be better. Some supplements and herbs can interact dangerously with prescribed medications. Others may drive your PSA down artificially without affecting the cancer, or change your testosterone level with the attendant side effects. If your physician is unaware that you're taking these drugs, the diagnostic significance of a change in these values could be misinterpreted, triggering a risky modification in your treatment.

Complementary medicine refers to therapies designed to improve well-being by reducing symptoms or making them more tolerable. Common approaches include prayer, meditation, acupuncture, guided imagery, and massage. Increasingly, complementary methods are gaining acceptance in conventional medical circles, and medical insurance may cover some of them.

An estimated 70 percent of all cancer patients turn to alternative and complementary methods at some point in their treatment. If you decide to do so, be sure to seek referrals to reputable practitioners and substances that are considered safe. A reasonable doctor should be willing to explore these options with you and help you to take advantage of interventions that might ease the course of treatment and improve your quality of life.

NOTE: For an up-to-date, comprehensive, and scientifically accurate evaluation of current alternative and complementary strategies, see *The Alternative Medicine Handbook* by Dr. Barrie Cassileth.[8]

PAIN MANAGEMENT AND PALLIATION

For patients with metastatic disease, pain is a central concern. Many of us remember losing relatives or friends to cancer, and those memories are often shadowed by the specter of suffering. Historically, pain control took a backseat to issues considered more medically relevant, such as prolonging life or alleviating dangerous symptoms. Today, in recognition of the enormous impact that pain and discomfort can have on quality of life, palliation and pain management receive far greater attention. In fact, pain management has spawned its own medical discipline. Most hospitals have pain-management teams dedicated to keeping patients comfortable throughout all stages of any given disease and reducing the pain and discomfort associated with treatments. Where no such team exists, attending physicians can and should see to the important business of keeping patients comfortable.

Nevertheless, an estimated 50 percent of cancer patients worldwide still receive inadequate analgesia. Sometimes this results from a discrepancy between the level of pain patients experience and how much discomfort doctors judge them to have. In some cases, physicians are reluctant to prescribe adequate pain relief, fearing that the patient may become addicted, develop a tolerance that would render the drugs ineffective, or experience unacceptable side effects. Patients may refuse to request sufficient pain medication for the same misguided reasons. Also, with serious illness, the primary focus still tends to be on medical issues such as prolonging life and relieving dangerous symptoms, rather than pain control. Nevertheless, adequate analgesic relief is critical to a patient's overall sense of well-being, central to how well he tolerates and complies with necessary treatments, and, quite possibly, crucial to how long he lives.

Recognizing this, the World Health Organization (WHO) recommends a sequential "ladder" approach to pain management and palliation for cancer patients. Following this approach, more than 80 percent of people with advanced cancer have their pain relieved.[9]

Under the WHO guidelines, a primary goal is to prevent the onset of pain by administering analgesics at regular intervals, rather than waiting for the pain to become severe and then try to relieve it with drugs. "By the clock" dosage is determined after a careful evaluation of how long an analgesic drug stays in the system (**half-life**) and the duration of its palliative effects. The best pain control is carefully tailored to meet each patient's needs, with constant adjustments as necessary to achieve the best pain control with the fewest possible side effects. Ideally, analgesics should be simple to administer so they can be taken by the patient or given by family members at home. For this reason, oral medications, patches, and nasal sprays are preferable to those that must be injected or administered intravenously.

Mild pain can often be managed with non-opioid drugs such as paracetamol (acetaminophen, Tylenol) or NSAIDs (aspirin, ibuprofen, Motrin, Advil). As a tumor grows, it can trigger the synthesis and release of substances called **prostaglandins**, which cause inflammation in adjacent tissues. NSAIDs work by blocking prostaglandin production, allowing the inflammation and the pain it causes to subside.

All drugs have effects and side effects. Taken persistently in high doses, NSAIDs can cause indigestion, nausea, and vomiting. Regular monitoring is necessary to ensure that serious problems such as ulcers or gastrointestinal bleeding do not develop. Extended use may compromise normal kidney function and lead to swelling in the extremities or cause easy bruising of the skin.

Non-opioids have limited analgesic effects. Above a certain recommended level, increasing the dose would only increase the risk of side effects while failing to alleviate the pain. At that point, it's necessary to add or switch to low-dose opioids, such as codeine or tramadol for mild to moderate pain, or stronger opioids, such as morphine, methadone, hydrocodone, buprenorphine, or fentanyl, if the pain is moderate to severe.

Morphine has long been the mainstay in pain management for advanced cancer. Though it has provided blessed relief for so many, patients (and some health professionals) continue to misunderstand and mistrust it. With this and all opioids, they worry about severe sedation, though, in reality, doses can be carefully regulated to minimize this risk. They believe that morphine will suppress breathing, but with proper dosing this is not the case. Addiction is not a concern in a patient with intractable pain from metastatic cancer.

Oral morphine comes in two forms. The short-release variety works in twenty to ninety minutes and effects last for four to six hours. The twelve-hour, slow-release variety requires only two doses per day. Morphine can also be administered by rectal suppository, by skin patch, or by injection.

Methodone, despite its unfortunate association with illegal narcotics, is a powerful, long-acting pain reliever that avoids some of the side effects of morphine. Hydromorphone is faster-acting (though not as long-lasting), and fentanyl is seventy-five times as potent as morphine. Several other powerful opioids are approved for the treatment of severe pain, and the best relief may require a trial of several of these alone or in combination.

Opioids can cause some sedation, constipation, and nausea, as well as many other unpleasant effects. Additional (adjuvant) drugs might be needed to counteract these problems and keep you comfortable. The treatment arsenal includes antidepressants, laxatives, amphetamines, cor-ticosteroids, and anti-emetics (to counteract vomiting), to name a few. Some patients have severe anxiety or difficulty sleeping, requiring the use of tranquilizers. Anorexia or malnutrition may call for appetite stim-ulants. Anticonvulsants may be necessary if the disease causes damage to the nervous system.

Pain is a subjective sensation, and successful pain management de-pends on a careful assessment of and response to each patient's needs. A person's pain tolerance or pain threshold can be boosted by such simple measures as adequate rest, diverting activities, understanding, and empa-thy. On the other hand, psychological negatives like fear, anger, fatigue, isolation, or depression, all common in patients with advanced disease, can make pain seem worse and harder to tolerate. Cultural, spiritual, physical, and psychological issues also factor into our highly personal perception and tolerance of pain.

Try to think of your doctor as your quarterback, there to run inter-ference, plan strategic moves, and ease your way past the problems and obstacles that arise. Be sure to discuss pain management before it be-comes an issue and to seek help for issues like depression, fatigue, and anxiety that can make symptoms harder to tolerate. If you are not re-ceiving adequate relief, or if the pain medication is causing unacceptable side effects, don't hesitate to request a more effective regime. Your med-ical team should work with you to alleviate symptoms and keep you feel-ing and functioning well for as long as possible.

In addition to pain medications, bone-seeking radiopharmaceuticals like Strontium 89, bisphosphonates, targeted external beam radiation, and chemotherapy are useful tools to alleviate the pain of bone metastases.[10]

IN SUMMARY

Given steady advances in our understanding of prostate cancer and the emergence of novel, increasingly effective therapies, the outlook for men with metastatic disease has improved considerably and continues to brighten all the time. The average survival for men with bone metastases has risen from two to three years in the 1980s to five to six years today. As new drugs under investigation become part of the standard treatment arsenal, we will move ever nearer to the goal of eliminating suffering and death from this disease for all men. As we work toward that goal, we are also developing ever better means to palliate symptoms and prolong survival for men with metastatic disease.

NOTES

CHAPTER 1: THE PROSTATE

1. Carter, H. B., and D. S. Coffey. "The Prostate—An Increasing Medical Problem." *Prostate* 16, no. 1 (1990): 39–48; and Greene, D. R., S. Egawa, D. K. Hellerstein, and P. T. Scardino. "Sonographic Measurements of Transition Zone of Prostate in Men with and without Benign Prostatic Hyperplasia." *Urology* 36, no. 4 (1990): 293–9.

CHAPTER 3: CHANGES WITH AGING

1. Committee on Assessing the Need for Clinical Trials of Testosterone Replacement Therapy. *Testosterone and Aging: Clinical Research Directions*. Edited by C. T. Liverman and D. G. Blazer. Washington, DC: National Academies Press, 2004.

CHAPTER 4: PROSTATITIS

1. Roberts, R. O., M. M. Lieber, T. Rhodes, C. J. Girman, D. G. Bostwick, and S. J. Jacobsen. "Prevalence of a Physician-Assigned Diagnosis of Prostatitis: The Olmsted County Study of Urinary Symptoms and Health Status Among Men." *Urology* 51, no. 4 (1998): 578–84; and Collins, M. M., R. S. Stafford, M. P. O'Leary, and M. J. Barry. "How Common Is Prostatitis? A National Survey of Physician Visits." *J Urol* 159, no. 4 (1998): 1224–8.
2. Stamey, T. A. "Prostatitis." *J R Soc Med* 74, no. 1 (1981): 22–40.
3. Schaeffer, A. J. "NIDDK-Sponsored Chronic Prostatitis Collaborative Research Network (CPCRN) 5-Year Data and Treatment Guidelines for Bacterial Prostatitis." *Int J Antimicrob Agents* 24 Suppl 1 (2004): 49–52.
4. Roberts et al.
5. Bjerklund Johansen, T. E., R. N. Gruneberg, J. Guibert, A. Hofstetter, B. Lobel, K. G. Naber, J. Palou Redorta, and P. J. van Cangh. "The Role of Antibiotics in the Treatment of Chronic Prostatitis: A Consensus Statement." *Eur Urol* 34, no. 6 (1998): 457–66.
6. Schaeffer, A. J. "Etiology and Management of Chronic Pelvic Pain Syndrome in Men." *Urology* 63, no. 3 Suppl 1 (2004): 75–84.
7. Batstone, G. R., A. Doble, and D. Batstone. "Chronic Prostatitis." *Curr Opin Urol* 13, no. 1 (2003): 23–9.
8. Krieger, J. N., R. E. Berger, S. O. Ross, I. Rothman, and C. H. Muller. "Seminal Fluid Findings in Men with Nonbacterial Prostatitis and Prostatodynia." *J Androl* 17, no. 3 (1996): 310–8.
9. Bjerklund et al.
10. Nickel, J. C., B. Johnston, J. Downey, J. Barkin, P. Pommerville, M. Gregoire, and E. Ramsey. "Pentosan Polysulfate Therapy for Chronic Nonbacterial Prostatitis (Chronic Pelvic Pain Syndrome Category IIIA): A Prospective Multicenter Clinical Trial." *Urology* 56, no. 3 (2000): 413–7.

11. Cassileth, B. R. *The Alternative Medicine Handbook.* New York: W. W. Norton & Co., 1998.

12. Liatsikos, E. N., C. Z. Dinlenc, R. Kapoor, and A. D. Smith. "Transurethral Microwave Thermotherapy for the Treatment of Prostatitis." *J Endourol* 14, no. 8 (2000): 689–92.

13. Potts, J. M. "Prospective Identification of National Institutes of Health Category IV Prostatitis in Men with Elevated Prostate Specific Antigen." *J Urol* 164, no. 5 (2000): 1550–3.

14. Hu, J. C., G. S. Palapattu, M. W. Kattan, P. T. Scardino, and T. M. Wheeler. "The Association of Selected Pathological Features with Prostate Cancer in a Single-Needle Biopsy Accession." *Hum Pathol* 29, no. 12 (1998): 1536–8.

15. Eastham, J. A., E. Riedel, P. T. Scardino, M. Shike, M. Fleisher, A. Schatzkin, E. Lanza, L. Latkany, and C. B. Begg. "Variation of Serum Prostate-Specific Antigen Levels: An Evaluation of Year-to-Year Fluctuations." *JAMA* 289, no. 20 (2003): 2695–700.

16. Pontari, M. A., and M. R. Ruggieri. "Mechanisms in Prostatitis/Chronic Pelvic Pain Syndrome." *J Urol* 172, no. 3 (2004): 839–45.

CHAPTER 5: BPH (PROSTATE ENLARGEMENT)

1. Isaacson, Walter. *Benjamin Franklin: An American Life.* New York: Simon & Schuster, 2003.

2. Murphy, L. J. T. *The History of Urology.* Springfield, Ill.: Charles C. Thomas, 1972.

3. Ibid.

4. McNeal, J. E., E. A. Redwine, F. S. Freiha, and T. A. Stamey. "Zonal Distribution of Prostatic Adenocarcinoma. Correlation with Histologic Pattern and Direction of Spread." *Am J Surg Pathol* 12, no. 12 (1988): 897–906.

5. Jacobsen, S. J., C. J. Girman, and M. M. Lieber. "Natural History of Benign Prostatic Hyperplasia." *Urology* 58, no. 6 Suppl 1 (2001): 5–16; discussion 16.

6. Farnsworth, W. E. "Estrogen in the Etiopathogenesis of Bph." *Prostate* 41, no. 4 (1999): 263–74.

7. Imperato-McGinley, J., R. E. Peterson, T. Gautier, and E. Sturla. "Male Pseudohermaphroditism Secondary to 5 Alpha-Reductase Deficiency—A Model for the Role of Androgens in Both the Development of the Male Phenotype and the Evolution of a Male Gender Identity." *J Steroid Biochem* 11, no. 1B (1979): 637–45.

8. Gormley, G. J., E. Stoner, R. C. Bruskewitz, J. Imperato-McGinley, P. C. Walsh, J. D. McConnell, G. L. Andriole, J. Geller, B. R. Bracken, J. S. Tenover, et al. "The Effect of Finasteride in Men with Benign Prostatic Hyperplasia. The Finasteride Study Group [see comments]." *N Engl J Med* 327, no. 17 (1992): 1185–91.

9. Rushton, D. H. "Androgenetic Alopecia in Men: The Scale of the Problem and Prospects for Treatment." *Int J Clin Pract* 53, no. 1 (1999): 50–3.

10. Carter, H. B., and D. S. Coffey. "The Prostate—An Increasing Medical Problem." *Prostate* 16, no. 1 (1990): 39–48.

11. Lanes, S. F., S. Sulsky, A. M. Walker, J. Isen, C. E. Grier, 3rd, B. E. Lewis, and N. A. Dreyer. "A Cost Density Analysis of Benign Prostatic Hyperplasia." *Clin Ther* 18, no. 5 (1996): 993–1004.

12. Pearson, J. D., H. H. Lei, T. H. Beaty, K. E. Wiley, S. D. Isaacs, W. B. Isaacs, E. Stoner, and P. C. Walsh. "Familial Aggregation of Bothersome Benign Prostatic Hyperplasia Symptoms." *Urology* 61, no. 4 (2003): 781–5.

13. Sutaria, P. M., and D. R. Staskin. "Hydronephrosis and Renal Deterioration in the Elderly Due to Abnormalities of the Lower Urinary Tract and Ureterovesical Junction." *Int Urol Nephrol* 32, no. 1 (2000): 119–26.

14. Gretzer, M. B., and A. W. Partin. "PSA Markers in Prostate Cancer Detection." *Urol Clin North Am* 30, no. 4 (2003): 677–86.

15. http://www.nsc.org.

16. Ramsey, E. W. "Benign Prostatic Hyperplasia: A Review." *Can J Urol* 7, no. 6 (2000): 1135–43.

17. Bjork, T., B. Ljungberg, T. Piironen, P. A. Abrahamsson, K. Pettersson, A. T. K. Cockett, and H. Lilja. "Rapid Exponential Elimination of Free Prostate-Specific Antigen Contrasts the Slow, Capacity-Limited Elimination of PSA Complexed to Alpha(1)-Antichymotrypsin from Serum." *Urology* 51, no. 1 (1998): 57–62.

18. McConnell, J. D., R. Bruskewitz, P. Walsh, G. Andriole, M. Lieber, H. L. Holtgrewe, P. Albertsen, C. G. Roehrborn, J. C. Nickel, D. Z. Wang, A. M. Taylor, and J. Waldstreicher. "The Effect of Finasteride on the Risk of Acute Urinary Retention and the Need for Surgical Treatment Among Men with Benign Prostatic Hyperplasia." *N Engl J Med* 338, no. 9 (1998): 557–63.

19. McConnell, J. D., C. G. Roehrborn, O. M. Bautista, et al. "The Long-Term Effect of Doxazosin, Finasteride, and Combination Therapy on the Clinical Progression of Benign Prostatic Hyperplasia; the Effect of Finasteride on the Risk of Acute Urinary Retention and the Need for Surgical Treatment Among Men with Benign Prostatic Hyperplasia. Finasteride Long-Term Efficacy and Safety Study Group; the Effect of Finasteride in Men with Benign Prostatic Hyperplasia. The Finasteride Study Group." *N Engl J Med* 349, no. 25 (2003): 2387–98.

20. Thompson, I. M., P. J. Goodman, C. M. Tangen, et al. "The Influence of Finasteride on the Development of Prostate Cancer." *N Engl J Med* 349, no. 3 (2003): 215–24.

21. McConnell, J. D., C. G. Roehrborn, O. M. Bautista, G. L. Andriole, Jr., C. M. Dixon, J. W. Kusek, et al. "The Long-Term Effect of Doxazosin, Finasteride, and Combination Therapy on the Clinical Progression of Benign Prostatic Hyperplasia." *N Engl J Med* 349, no. 25 (2003): 2387–98.

22. Cassileth, B. R. "Evaluating Complementary and Alternative Therapies for Cancer Patients." *CA Cancer J Clin* 49, no. 6 (1999): 362–75.

23. Cassileth, B. R. *The Alternative Medicine Handbook*. New York: W. W. Norton & Co., 1998.

24. Schatzl, G., S. Madersbacher, B. Djavan, T. Lang, and M. Marberger. "Two-Year Results of Transurethral Resection of the Prostate Versus Four 'Less Invasive' Treatment Options." *Eur Urol* 37, no. 6 (2000): 695–701.

25. Wasson, J. H., D. J. Reda, R. C. Bruskewitz, J. Elinson, A. M. Keller, and W. G. Henderson. "A Comparison of Transurethral Surgery with Watchful Waiting for Moderate Symptoms of Benign Prostatic Hyperplasia. The Veterans Affairs Cooperative Study Group on Transurethral Resection of the Prostate." *N Engl J Med* 332, no. 2 (1995): 75–9.

26. Hammadeh, M. Y., S. Madaan, M. Singh, and T. Philp. "A 3-Year Follow-up of a Prospective Randomized Trial Comparing Transurethral Electrovaporization of the Prostate with Standard Transurethral Prostatectomy." *BJU Int* 86, no. 6 (2000): 648–51.

27. Hoffman, R. M., R. MacDonald, J. W. Slaton, and T. J. Wilt. "Laser Prostatectomy Versus Transurethral Resection for Treating Benign Prostatic Obstruction: A Systematic Review." *J Urol* 169, no. 1 (2003): 210–5; and Te, A. E. "The Development of Laser Prostatectomy." *BJU Int* 93, no. 3 (2004): 262–5.

28. Schatzl, et al.; and van Melick, H. H., G. E. van Venrooij, and T. A. Boon. "Long-Term Follow-up After Transurethral Resection of the Prostate, Contact Laser Prostatectomy, and Electrovaporization." *Urology* 62, no. 6 (2003): 1029–34.

29. Pomer, S., and Z. F. Dobrowolski. "The Therapy of Benign Prostatic Hyperplasia Using Less-Invasive Procedures: The Current Situation." *BJU Int* 89, no. 7 (2002): 773–5.

30. Yang, Q., P. Abrams, J. Donovan, S. Mulligan, and G. Williams. "Transurethral Resection or Incision of the Prostate and Other Therapies: A Survey of Treatments for Benign Prostatic Obstruction in the UK." *BJU Int* 84, no. 6 (1999): 640–5.

31. Tunuguntla, H. S., and C. P. Evans. "Minimally Invasive Therapies for Benign Prostatic Hyperplasia." *World J Urol* 20, no. 4 (2002): 197–206; and de la Rosette, J. J., M. P. Laguna,

S. Gravas, and M. J. de Wildt. "Transurethral Microwave Thermotherapy: The Gold Standard for Minimally Invasive Therapies for Patients with Benign Prostatic Hyperplasia?" *J Endourol* 17, no. 4 (2003): 245–51.

32. Hill, B., W. Belville, R. Bruskewitz, M. Issa, R. Perez-Marrero, C. Roehrborn, M. Terris, and M. Naslund. "Transurethral Needle Ablation Versus Transurethral Resection of the Prostate for the Treatment of Symptomatic Benign Prostatic Hyperplasia: 5-Year Results of a Prospective, Randomized, Multicenter Clinical Trial." *J Urol* 171, no. 6 Pt 1 (2004): 2336–40.

33. Mulligan, E. D., T. H. Lynch, D. Mulvin, D. Greene, J. M. Smith, and J. M. Fitzpatrick. "High-Intensity Focused Ultrasound in the Treatment of Benign Prostatic Hyperplasia." *Br J Urol* 79, no. 2 (1997): 177–80; and Madersbacher, S., G. Schatzl, B. Djavan, T. Stulnig, and M. Marberger. "Long-Term Outcome of Transrectal High-Intensity Focused Ultrasound Therapy for Benign Prostatic Hyperplasia." *Eur Urol* 37, no. 6 (2000): 687–94.

34. Canto, E. I., H. Singh, S. F. Shariat, D. J. Lamb, S. D. Mikolajczyk, H. J. Linton, H. G. Rittenhouse, D. Kadmon, B. J. Miles, and K. M. Slawin. "Serum BPSA Outperforms Both Total PSA and Free PSA as a Predictor of Prostatic Enlargement in Men without Prostate Cancer." *Urology* 63, no. 5 (2004): 905–10; discussion 10–1.

CHAPTER 6: PROSTATE CANCER FACTS

1. American Cancer Society, Cancer Statistics Presentation 2004, available at http://www.cancer.org/docroot/pro/content/pro_1_1_cancer_statistics_2004_presentation.asp; last accessed on 10/07/2004.

2. Prostate Cancer Foundation, Report to the Nation, available at http://www.prostatecancerfoundation.org/atf/cf/{705b3273-F2ef-4ef6-A653-E15c5d8bb6b1}/pcf%20monograph-final1.pdf; last accessed on 10/07/2004.

3. Jemal, A., T. Murray, A. Samuels, A. Ghafoor, E. Ward, and M. J. Thun. "Cancer Statistics, 2003." *CA Cancer J Clin* 53, no. 1 (2003): 5–26.

4. Folkman, J. "What Is the Evidence That Tumors Are Angiogenesis Dependent?" *Journal of the National Cancer Institute* 82, no. 1 (1990): 4–6.

5. Scardino, P. T., R. Weaver, and M. A. Hudson. "Early Detection of Prostate Cancer." *Human Pathology* 23, no. 3 (1992): 211–22.

6. McNeal, J. E. "Origin and Development of Carcinoma in the Prostate." *Cancer* 23, no. 1 (1969): 24–34.

7. Ohori, M., T. M. Wheeler, J. K. Dunn, T. A. Stamey, and P. T. Scardino. "The Pathological Features and Prognosis of Prostate Cancer Detectable with Current Diagnostic Tests." *J Urol* 152, no. 5 Pt 2 (1994): 1714–20.

8. Ibid.

9. McNeal, J. E., E. A. Redwine, F. S. Freiha, and T. A. Stamey. "Zonal Distribution of Prostatic Adenocarcinoma. Correlation with Histologic Pattern and Direction of Spread." *Am J Surg Pathol* 12, no. 12 (1988): 897–906.

10. Greene, D. R., T. M. Wheeler, S. Egawa, J. K. Dunn, and P. T. Scardino. "A Comparison of the Morphological Features of Cancer Arising in the Transition Zone and in the Peripheral Zone of the Prostate." *J Urol* 146, no. 4 (1991): 1069–76.

11. Albertsen, P. C., D. G. Fryback, B. E. Storer, T. F. Kolon, and J. Fine. "Long-Term Survival Among Men with Conservatively Treated Localized Prostate Cancer." *JAMA* 274, no. 8 (1995): 626–31; and Scardino, "Early Detection of Prostate Cancer."

CHAPTER 7: RISK FACTORS AND PREVENTION

1. Bianco, F. J. Jr., M. W. Kattan, and P. T. Scardino. "PSA Velocity and Prostate Cancer." *N Engl J Med* 351, no. 17 (2004): 1800-1802.

2. Reddy, S., M. Shapiro, R. Morton, Jr., and O. W. Brawley. "Prostate Cancer in Black and White Americans." *Cancer Metastasis Rev* 22, no. 1 (2003): 83–6.

3. Carter, H. B., and D. S. Coffey. "The Prostate—An Increasing Medical Problem." *Prostate* 16, no. 1 (1990): 39–48.

4. Tominaga, S. "Cancer Incidence in Japanese in Japan, Hawaii, and Western United States." *National Cancer Institute Monographs* 69 (1985): 83–92.

5. Calle, E. E., C. Rodriguez, K. Walker-Thurmond, and M. J. Thun. "Overweight, Obesity, and Mortality from Cancer in a Prospectively Studied Cohort of U.S. Adults." *N Engl J Med* 348, no. 17 (2003): 1625–38.

6. Bishop, D. T., A. W. Meikle, M. L. Slattery, J. D. Stringham, M. H. Ford, and D. W. West. "The Effect of Nutritional Factors on Sex Hormone Levels in Male Twins." *Genet Epidemiol* 5, no. 1 (1988): 43–59.

7. Stanford, J. L., E. A. Noonan, L. Iwasaki, S. Kolb, R. B. Chadwick, Z. Feng, and E. A. Ostrander. "A Polymorphism in the Cyp17 Gene and Risk of Prostate Cancer." *Cancer Epidemiol Biomarkers Prev* 11, no. 3 (2002): 243–7.

8. Zeegers, M. P., A. Jellema, and H. Ostrer. "Empiric Risk of Prostate Carcinoma for Relatives of Patients with Prostate Carcinoma: A Meta-Analysis." *Cancer* 97, no. 8 (2003): 1894–903.

9. Lichtenstein, P., N. V. Holm, P. K. Verkasalo, A. Iliadou, J. Kaprio, M. Koskenvuo, E. Pukkala, A. Skytthe, and K. Hemminki. "Environmental and Heritable Factors in the Causation of Cancer—Analyses of Cohorts of Twins from Sweden, Denmark, and Finland." *N Engl J Med* 343, no. 2 (2000): 78–85.

10. Xu, J., E. M. Gillanders, S. D. Isaacs, B. L. Chang, K. E. Wiley, S. L. Zheng, M. Jones, D. Gildea, E. Riedesel, J. Albertus, D. Freas-Lutz, C. Markey, D. A. Meyers, P. C. Walsh, J. M. Trent, and W. B. Isaacs. "Genome-Wide Scan for Prostate Cancer Susceptibility Genes in the Johns Hopkins Hereditary Prostate Cancer Families." *Prostate* 57, no. 4 (2003): 320–5.

11. Leitzmann, M. F., E. A. Platz, M. J. Stampfer, W. C. Willett, and E. Giovannucci. "Ejaculation Frequency and Subsequent Risk of Prostate Cancer" *JAMA* 291, no. 13 (2004): 1578–86.

12. Goldstein, I. "Bicycle Riding and Perineal Injuries." *Family Urology* 9, no. 1 (2004): Available at: http://www.impotence.org/hottopics/bicycle.asp. Last accessed on 10/07/2004.

13. De Marzo, A. M., T. L. DeWeese, E. A. Platz, A. K. Meeker, M. Nakayama, J. I. Epstein, W. B. Isaacs, and W. G. Nelson. "Pathological and Molecular Mechanisms of Prostate Carcinogenesis: Implications for Diagnosis, Detection, Prevention, and Treatment." *J Cell Biochem* 91, no. 3 (2004): 459–77.

14. Verougstraete, V., D. Lison, and P. Hotz. "Cadmium, Lung and Prostate Cancer: A Systematic Review of Recent Epidemiological Data." *J Toxicol Environ Health B Crit Rev* 6, no. 3 (2003): 227–55.

15. *Veterans and Agent Orange: Health Effects of Herbicides Used in Vietnam: Update 1998. Institute of Medicine.* Washington, DC: National Academy Press, 1998.

16. Hickson, R. C., K. L. Ball, and M. T. Falduto. "Adverse Effects of Anabolic Steroids." *Med Toxicol Adverse Drug Exp* 4, no. 4 (1989): 254–71.

17. Moyad, M. A. *The ABCs of Nutrition and Supplements for Prostate Cancer.* Chelsea, Mich.: Sleeping Bear Press, 2000.

18. Thompson, I. M., P. J. Goodman, C. M. Tangen, M. S. Lucia, G. J. Miller, L. G. Ford, M. M. Lieber, R. D. Cespedes, J. N. Atkins, S. M. Lippman, S. M. Carlin, A. Ryan, C. M. Szczepanek, J. J. Crowley, and C. A. Coltman, Jr. "The Influence of Finasteride on the Development of Prostate Cancer." *N Engl J Med* 349, no. 3 (2003): 215–24.

19. Scardino, P. T. "The Prevention of Prostate Cancer—The Dilemma Continues." *N Engl J Med* 349, no. 3 (2003): 297–9.

20. Studies reevaluating the prostate cancer prevention trial will be published in 2005.

21. Moyad; and Thompson et al.
22. Cassileth, B. R. *The Alternative Medicine Handbook.* New York: W. W. Norton & Co., 1998; and http://www.mskcc.org/aboutherbs.
23. http://www.mskcc.org/aboutherbs.

CHAPTER 8: DETECTING PROSTATE CANCER
WITH PSA AND OTHER TESTS

1. Han, M., P. H. Gann, and W. J. Catalona. "Prostate-Specific Antigen and Screening for Prostate Cancer." *Med Clin North Am* 88, no. 2 (2004): 245–65, ix.
2. Woolf, S. H. "Screening for Prostate Cancer with Prostate-Specific Antigen. An Examination of the Evidence." *N Engl J Med* 333, no. 21 (1995): 1401–5; and McGregor, M., J. A. Hanley, J. F. Boivin, and R. G. McLean. "Screening for Prostate Cancer: Estimating the Magnitude of Overdetection." *CMAJ* 159, no. 11 (1998): 1368–72.
3. Brawley, O. W. "Prostate Cancer Screening: Clinical Applications and Challenges." *Urol Oncol* 22, no. 4 (2004): 353–7; and Chan, E. C., S. W. Vernon, F. T. O'Donnell, C. Ahn, A. Greisinger, and D. W. Aga. "Informed Consent for Cancer Screening with Prostate-Specific Antigen: How Well Are Men Getting the Message?" *Am J Public Health* 93, no. 5 (2003): 779–85.
4. Ferrini, R., and S. H. Woolf. "Screening for Prostate Cancer in American Men." http://www.acpm.org/prostate.htm, 10/07/2004.
5. "American Urological Society. Prostate Screening." In http://www.auanet.org, 10/07/2004; and "American Cancer Society. Prostate Cancer Screening." In http://search.cancer.org/search?client=amcancer&site=amcancer&output=xml_no_dtd&proxystylesheet=amcancer&restrict=cancer&q=prostate+cancer+screening, 10/07/2004.
6. "American Healthcare Research and Quality. Prostate Cancer Screening." In http://www.ahrq.gov/query/query.idq?CiRestriction=prostate+cancer+screening&CiScope=%2F&CiMaxRecordsPerPage=10&TemplateName=query&CiSort=rank%5Bd%5D&HTMLQueryForm=query.htm: 10/07/2004.
7. Lilja, H. "Biology of Prostate-Specific Antigen." *Urology* 62, no. 5 Suppl 1 (2003): 27–33.
8. Han et al.; and Gretzer, M. B., and A. W. Partin. "PSA Markers in Prostate Cancer Detection." *Urol Clin North Am* 30, no. 4 (2003): 677–86.
9. Crawford, E. D., S. Leewansangtong, S. Goktas, K. Holthaus, and M. Baier. "Efficiency of Prostate-Specific Antigen and Digital Rectal Examination in Screening, Using 4.0 Ng/Ml and Age-Specific Reference Range as a Cutoff for Abnormal Values." *Prostate* 38, no. 4 (1999): 296–302.
10. Catalona, W. J., J. P. Richie, F. R. Ahmann, M. A. Hudson, P. T. Scardino, R. C. Flanigan, J. B. deKernion, T. L. Ratliff, L. R. Kavoussi, B. L. Dalkin, et al. "Comparison of Digital Rectal Examination and Serum Prostate Specific Antigen in the Early Detection of Prostate Cancer: Results of a Multicenter Clinical Trial of 6,630 Men." *J Urol* 151, no. 5 (1994): 1283–90.
11. Lilja; and Gretzer et al.
12. Catalona et al.
13. Andriole, G. L., H. A. Guess, J. I. Epstein, H. Wise, D. Kadmon, E. D. Crawford, P. Hudson, C. L. Jackson, N. A. Romas, L. Patterson, T. J. Cook, and J. Waldstreicher. "Treatment with Finasteride Preserves Usefulness of Prostate-Specific Antigen in the Detection of Prostate Cancer: Results of a Randomized, Double-Blind, Placebo-Controlled Clinical Trial. Pless Study Group. Proscar Long-Term Efficacy and Safety Study." *Urology* 52, no. 2 (1998): 195–201; discussion 01–2.
14. Crawford, E. D., M. J. Schutz, S. Clejan, J. Drago, M. I. Resnick, G. W. Chodak, L. G. Gomella, M. Austenfeld, N. N. Stone, and B. J. Miles. "The Effect of Digital Rectal Examination on Prostate-Specific Antigen Levels." *JAMA* 267, no. 16 (1992): 2227–8.

15. Catalona et al.

16. Eastham, J. A., E. Riedel, P. T. Scardino, M. Shike, M. Fleisher, A. Schatzkin, E. Lanza, L. Latkany, and C. B. Begg. "Variation of Serum Prostate-Specific Antigen Levels: An Evaluation of Year-to-Year Fluctuations." *JAMA* 289, no. 20 (2003): 2695–700.

17. Stamey, T. A., M. Caldwell, J. E. McNeal, R. Nolley, M. Hemenez, and J. Downs. "The Prostate Specific Antigen Era in the United States Is Over for Prostate Cancer: What Happened in the Last 20 Years?" *J Urol* 172, no. 4, Pt 1 of 2 (2004): 1297–301.

18. Gann, P. H., C. H. Hennekens, and M. J. Stampfer. "A Prospective Evaluation of Plasma Prostate-Specific Antigen for Detection of Prostatic Cancer." *JAMA* 273, no. 4 (1995): 289–94.

19. Carter, H. B., J. D. Pearson, E. J. Metter, L. J. Brant, D. W. Chan, R. Andres, J. L. Fozard, and P. C. Walsh. "Longitudinal Evaluation of Prostate-Specific Antigen Levels in Men with and without Prostate Disease." *JAMA* 267, no. 16 (1992): 2215–20.

20. D'Amico, A. V., M. H. Chen, K. A. Roehl, and W. J. Catalona. "Preoperative PSA Velocity and the Risk of Death from Prostate Cancer After Radical Prostatectomy." *N Engl J Med* 351, no. 2 (2004): 125–35.

21. Bianco, F. J. "Letter Response to A. V. D'Amico: Preoperative PSA Velocity and Risk of Death from Prostate Cancer After Radical Prostatectomy." *N Engl J Med* in press (2004).

22. Catalona, W. J., A. W. Partin, K. M. Slawin, M. K. Brawer, R. C. Flanigan, A. Patel, J. P. Richie, J. B. deKernion, P. C. Walsh, P. T. Scardino, P. H. Lange, E. N. Subong, R. E. Parson, G. H. Gasior, K. G. Loveland, and P. C. Southwick. "Use of the Percentage of Free Prostate-Specific Antigen to Enhance Differentiation of Prostate Cancer from Benign Prostatic Disease: A Prospective Multicenter Clinical Trial." *JAMA* 279, no. 19 (1998): 1542–7.

23. Benson, M. C., I. S. Whang, A. Pantuck, K. Ring, S. A. Kaplan, C. A. Olsson, and W. H. Cooner. "Prostate Specific Antigen Density: A Means of Distinguishing Benign Prostatic Hypertrophy and Prostate Cancer." *J Urol* 147, no. 3 Pt 2 (1992): 815–6.

24. Lilja.

CHAPTER 9: BIOPSY

1. Eastham, J. A., E. Riedel, P. T. Scardino, M. Shike, M. Fleisher, A. Schatzkin, E. Lanza, L. Latkany, and C. B. Begg. "Variation of Serum Prostate-Specific Antigen Levels: An Evaluation of Year-to-Year Fluctuations." *JAMA* 289, no. 20 (2003): 2695–700.

2. Partin, A. W., H. B. Carter, D. W. Chan, J. I. Epstein, J. E. Oesterling, R. C. Rock, J. P. Weber, and P. C. Walsh. "Prostate Specific Antigen in the Staging of Localized Prostate Cancer: Influence of Tumor Differentiation, Tumor Volume and Benign Hyperplasia." *J Urol* 143, no. 4 (1990): 747–52.

3. Catalona, W. J., J. P. Richie, F. R. Ahmann, M. A. Hudson, P. T. Scardino, R. C. Flanigan, J. B. deKernion, T. L. Ratliff, L. R. Kavoussi, B. L. Dalkin, et al. "Comparison of Digital Rectal Examination and Serum Prostate Specific Antigen in the Early Detection of Prostate Cancer: Results of a Multicenter Clinical Trial of 6,630 Men." *J Urol* 151, no. 5 (1994): 1283–90.

4. Watanabe, H. "History of Ultrasound in Nephrourology." *Ultrasound Med Biol* 27, no. 4 (2001): 447–53.

5. Ragde, H., H. C. Aldape, and C. M. Bagley, Jr. "Ultrasound-Guided Prostate Biopsy. Biopsy Gun Superior to Aspiration." *Urology* 32, no. 6 (1988): 503–6.

6. Gore, J. L., S. F. Shariat, B. J. Miles, D. Kadmon, N. Jiang, T. M. Wheeler, and K. M. Slawin. "Optimal Combinations of Systematic Sextant and Laterally Directed Biopsies for the Detection of Prostate Cancer." *J Urol* 165, no. 5 (2001): 1554–9.

7. Carey, J. M., and H. J. Korman. "Transrectal Ultrasound Guided Biopsy of the Prostate. Do Enemas Decrease Clinically Significant Complications?" *J Urol* 166, no. 1 (2001): 82–5.

8. Rodriguez, L. V., and M. K. Terris. "Risks and Complications of Transrectal Ultrasound Guided Prostate Needle Biopsy: A Prospective Study and Review of the Literature." *J Urol* 160, no. 6 Pt 1 (1998): 2115–20.

9. AAOS. "Antibiotic Prophylaxis for Urological Patients with Total Joint Replacements." In http://www.aaos.org/wordhtml/papers/advistmt/1023.htm: 10/08/2004.

10. Obek, C., B. Ozkan, B. Tunc, G. Can, V. Yalcin, and V. Solok. "Comparison of 3 Different Methods of Anesthesia Before Transrectal Prostate Biopsy: A Prospective Randomized Trial." *J Urol* 172, no. 2 (2004): 502–5.

11. Rodriguez et al.

12. Roehl, K. A., J. A. Antenor, and W. J. Catalona. "Serial Biopsy Results in Prostate Cancer Screening Study." *J Urol* 167, no. 6 (2002): 2435–9.

13. Beyersdorff, D., M. Taupitz, B. Winkelmann, T. Fischer, S. Lenk, S. A. Loening, and B. Hamm. "Patients with a History of Elevated Prostate-Specific Antigen Levels and Negative Transrectal US-Guided Quadrant or Sextant Biopsy Results: Value of MR Imaging." *Radiology* 224, no. 3 (2002): 701–6.

14. Frauscher, F., A. Klauser, H. Volgger, E. J. Halpern, L. Pallwein, H. Steiner, A. Schuster, W. Horninger, H. Rogatsch, and G. Bartsch. "Comparison of Contrast Enhanced Color Doppler Targeted Biopsy with Conventional Systematic Biopsy: Impact on Prostate Cancer Detection." *J Urol* 167, no. 4 (2002): 1648–52.

15. Bastacky, S. S., P. C. Walsh, and J. I. Epstein. "Needle Biopsy Associated Tumor Tracking of Adenocarcinoma of the Prostate." *J Urol* 145, no. 5 (1991): 1003–7.

16. Bostwick, D. G., and J. Qian. "High-Grade Prostatic Intraepithelial Neoplasia." *Mod Pathol* 17, no. 3 (2004): 360–79.

17. NCI. "Cancer Facts: Tumor Grade: Questions and Answers." In http://cis.nci.nih.gov/fact/5_9.htm: 10/08/2004.

18. Humphrey, P. A. "Gleason Grading and Prognostic Factors in Carcinoma of the Prostate." *Mod Pathol* 17, no. 3 (2004): 292–306.

19. Epstein, J. I., and S. R. Potter. "The Pathological Interpretation and Significance of Prostate Needle Biopsy Findings: Implications and Current Controversies." *J Urol* 166, no. 2 (2001): 402–10.

20. Herman, C. M., M. W. Kattan, M. Ohori, P. T. Scardino, and T. M. Wheeler. "Primary Gleason Pattern as a Predictor of Disease Progression in Gleason Score 7 Prostate Cancer: A Multivariate Analysis of 823 Men Treated with Radical Prostatectomy." *Am J Surg Pathol* 25, no. 5 (2001): 657–60.

21. Stamey, T. A., C. M. Yemoto, J. E. McNeal, B. M. Sigal, and I. M. Johnstone. "Prostate Cancer Is Highly Predictable: A Prognostic Equation Based on All Morphological Variables in Radical Prostatectomy Specimens." *J Urol* 163, no. 4 (2000): 1155–60.

22. King, C. R., J. E. McNeal, H. Gill, and J. C. Presti, Jr. "Extended Prostate Biopsy Scheme Improves Reliability of Gleason Grading: Implications for Radiotherapy Patients." *Int J Radiat Oncol Biol Phys* 59, no. 2 (2004): 386–91.

23. O'Malley, K. J., C. R. Pound, P. C. Walsh, J. I. Epstein, and A. W. Partin. "Influence of Biopsy Perineural Invasion on Long-Term Biochemical Disease-Free Survival After Radical Prostatectomy." *Urology* 59, no. 1 (2002): 85–90.

24. Patel, M. I., D. T. DeConcini, E. Lopez-Corona, M. Ohori, T. Wheeler, and P. T. Scardino. "An Analysis of Men with Clinically Localized Prostate Cancer Who Deferred Definitive Therapy." *J Urol* 171, no. 4 (2004): 1520–4.

25. Hansson, J., and P. A. Abrahamsson. "Neuroendocrine Pathogenesis in Adenocarcinoma of the Prostate." *Ann Oncol* 12 Suppl 2 (2001): S145–52.

26. Bock, B. J., and D. G. Bostwick. "Does Prostatic Ductal Adenocarcinoma Exist?" *Am J Surg Pathol* 23, no. 7 (1999): 781–5.

27. Bostwick et al.

28. Lopez-Corona, E., M. Ohori, P. T. Scardino, V. E. Reuter, M. Gonen, and M. W. Kattan. "A Nomogram for Predicting a Positive Repeat Prostate Biopsy in Patients with a Previous Negative Biopsy Session." *J Urol* 170, no. 4 Pt 1 (2003): 1184–8; discussion 88.

29. Epstein et al.

30. Ylikoski, A., K. Pettersson, J. Nurmi, K. Irjala, M. Karp, H. Lilja, T. Lovgren, and M. Nurmi. "Simultaneous Quantification of Prostate-Specific Antigen and Human Glandular Kallikrein 2 MRNA in Blood Samples from Patients with Prostate Cancer and Benign Disease." *Clin Chem* 48, no. 8 (2002): 1265–71.

CHAPTER 10: UNDERSTANDING YOUR CANCER

1. NCI. "Search Results for Prostate Cancer Survivors." In http://www.cancer.gov/search/results.aspx: 10/08/2004.

2. Gretzer, M. B., and A. W. Partin. "PSA Markers in Prostate Cancer Detection." *Urol Clin North Am* 30, no. 4 (2003): 677–86.

3. Stamey, T. A., M. Caldwell, J. E. McNeal, R. Nolley, M. Hemenez, and J. Downs. "The Prostate Specific Antigen Era in the United States Is Over for Prostate Cancer: What Happened in the Last 20 Years?" *J Urol* 172, no. 4, Pt 1 of 2 (2004): 1297–301.

4. Shinohara, K., T. M. Wheeler, and P. T. Scardino. "The Appearance of Prostate Cancer on Transrectal Ultrasonography: Correlation of Imaging and Pathological Examinations." *J Urol* 142, no. 1 (1989): 76–82.

5. Frauscher, F., A. Klauser, H. Volgger, E. J. Halpern, L. Pallwein, H. Steiner, A. Schuster, W. Horninger, H. Rogatsch, and G. Bartsch. "Comparison of Contrast Enhanced Color Doppler Targeted Biopsy with Conventional Systematic Biopsy: Impact on Prostate Cancer Detection." *J Urol* 167, no. 4 (2002): 1648–52.

6. Mullerad, M., H. Hricak, L. Wang, H. N. Chen, M. W. Kattan, and P. T. Scardino. "Prostate Cancer: Detection of Extracapsular Extension by Genitourinary and General Body Radiologists at MR Imaging." *Radiology* 232, no. 1 (2004): 140–6.

7. Singh, H., E. I. Canto, S. F. Shariat, D. Kadmon, B. J. Miles, T. M. Wheeler, and K. M. Slawin. "Six Additional Systematic Lateral Cores Enhance Sextant Biopsy Prediction of Pathological Features at Radical Prostatectomy." *J Urol* 171, no. 1 (2004): 204–9.

8. Greene, F. L., D. L. Page, I. D. Fleming, A. Fritz, C. M. Balch, D. G. Haller, and M. Morrow. *AJCC Cancer Staging Manual.* 6th ed. New York: Springer-Verlag, 2002.

9. Partin, A. W., L. A. Mangold, D. M. Lamm, P. C. Walsh, J. I. Epstein, and J. D. Pearson. "Contemporary Update of Prostate Cancer Staging Nomograms (Partin Tables) for the New Millennium." *Urology* 58, no. 6 (2001): 843–8.

10. Kattan, M. W., A. M. Stapleton, T. M. Wheeler, and P. T. Scardino. "Evaluation of a Nomogram Used to Predict the Pathologic Stage of Clinically Localized Prostate Carcinoma." *Cancer* 79, no. 3 (1997): 528–37.

11. Gretzer et al.

12. D'Amico, A. V., M. H. Chen, K. A. Roehl, and W. J. Catalona. "Preoperative PSA Velocity and the Risk of Death from Prostate Cancer After Radical Prostatectomy." *N Engl J Med* 351, no. 2 (2004): 125–35; and Bianco, F. J. "Letter Response to A. V. D'Amico: Preoperative PSA Velocity and Risk of Death from Prostate Cancer After Radical Prostatectomy." *N Engl J Med* in press (2004).

13. Carter, H. B., J. D. Pearson, E. J. Metter, L. J. Brant, D. W. Chan, R. Andres, J. L. Fozard, and P. C. Walsh. "Longitudinal Evaluation of Prostate-Specific Antigen Levels in Men with and without Prostate Disease." *JAMA* 267, no. 16 (1992): 2215–20; and Ulmert, D., C. Becker, T. Bjork, J. A. Malmo, G. Berglund, and H. Lilja. "Rates of Change in Levels of HK2, Free and Total PSA up to 20 Years Before Diagnosis of Prostate Cancer." *J Urol* 169, no. 4 (2003): 384.

14. Eastham, J. A., E. Riedel, P. T. Scardino, M. Shike, M. Fleisher, A. Schatzkin, E. Lanza, L. Latkany, and C. B. Begg. "Variation of Serum Prostate-Specific Antigen Levels: An Evaluation of Year-to-Year Fluctuations." *JAMA* 289, no. 20 (2003): 2695–700.

15. Kikuchi, E., P. T. Scardino, T. M. Wheeler, K. M. Slawin, and M. Ohori. "Is Tumor Volume an Independent Prognostic Factor in Clinically Localized Prostate Cancer?" *J Urol* 172, no. 2 (2004): 508–11.

16. Partin, A. W., H. B. Carter, D. W. Chan, J. I. Epstein, J. E. Oesterling, R. C. Rock, J. P. Weber, and P. C. Walsh. "Prostate Specific Antigen in the Staging of Localized Prostate Cancer: Influence of Tumor Differentiation, Tumor Volume and Benign Hyperplasia." *J Urol* 143, no. 4 (1990): 747–52.

17. Aihara, M., R. M. Lebovitz, T. M. Wheeler, B. M. Kinner, M. Ohori, and P. T. Scardino. "Prostate Specific Antigen and Gleason Grade: An Immunohistochemical Study of Prostate Cancer." *J Urol* 151, no. 6 (1994): 1558–64.

18. NCCN. "Guidelines on Bone Scans: Search Results." In http://www.nccn.org/cgi-bin/perlfect/search/search.pl?p=1&lang=en&include=&exclude=&penalty=0&mode=all&q=guidelines+on+bone+scans&submit.x=25&submit.y=13: 10/08/2004.

19. Di Blasio, C. J., A. C. Rhee, D. Cho, P. T. Scardino, and M. W. Kattan. "Predicting Clinical End Points: Treatment Nomograms in Prostate Cancer." *Semin Oncol* 30, no. 5 (2003): 567–86.

20. Huncharek, M., and J. Muscat. "Serum Prostate-Specific Antigen as a Predictor of Radiographic Staging Studies in Newly Diagnosed Prostate Cancer." *Cancer Invest* 13, no. 1 (1005): 31–5.

21. Ibid.

22. D'Amico, A. V., R. Whittington, S. B. Malkowicz, D. Schultz, K. Blank, G. A. Broderick, J. E. Tomaszewski, A. A. Renshaw, I. Kaplan, C. J. Beard, and A. Wein. "Biochemical Outcome After Radical Prostatectomy, External Beam Radiation Therapy, or Interstitial Radiation Therapy for Clinically Localized Prostate Cancer." *JAMA* 280, no. 11 (1998): 969–74.

23. Kattan, M. W. "Nomograms Are Superior to Staging and Risk Grouping Systems for Identifying High-Risk Patients: Preoperative Application in Prostate Cancer." *Curr Opin Urol* 13, no. 2 (2003): 111–6; and Eastham, J. A., M. W. Kattan, and P. T. Scardino. "Nomograms as Predictive Models." *Semin Urol Oncol* 20, no. 2 (2002): 108–15.

CHAPTER 11: UNDERSTANDING YOURSELF

1. Roth, A. J., B. Rosenfeld, A. B. Kornblith, C. Gibson, H. I. Scher, T. Curley-Smart, J. C. Holland, and W. Breitbart. "The Memorial Anxiety Scale for Prostate Cancer: Validation of a New Scale to Measure Anxiety in Men with Prostate Cancer." *Cancer* 97, no. 11 (2003): 2910–8.

2. "NCCN Practice Guidelines for the Management of Psychosocial Distress. National Comprehensive Cancer Network." *Oncology (Huntingt)* 13, no. 5A (1999): 113–47.

3. USTOO "Prostate Cancer Education and Support." In http://www.ustoo.com/: 10/08/2004.

4. Ross, P. L., B. Littenberg, P. Fearn, P. T. Scardino, P. I. Karakiewicz, and M. W. Kattan. "Paper Standard Gamble: A Paper-Based Measure of Standard Gamble Utility for Current Health." *Int J Technol Assess Health Care* 19, no. 1 (2003): 135–47.

CHAPTER 12: DECIDING HOW TO TREAT
LOCALIZED PROSTATE CANCER

1. Fleming, C., J. H. Wasson, P. C. Albertsen, M. J. Barry, and J. E. Wennberg. "A Decision Analysis of Alternative Treatment Strategies for Clinically Localized Prostate Cancer. Prostate Patient Outcomes Research Team." *JAMA* 269, no. 20 (1993): 2650–8; and CHE. "Centre for Health Evidence: How to Use a Clinical Decision Analysis." In http://www.cche.net/usersguides/decision.asp: 10/08/2004.

2. Albertsen, P. C., D. G. Fryback, B. E. Storer, T. F. Kolon, and J. Fine. "Long-Term Survival Among Men with Conservatively Treated Localized Prostate Cancer." *JAMA* 274, no. 8 (1995): 626–31; and Johansson, J. E., O. Andren, S. O. Andersson, P. W. Dickman, L. Holmberg, A. Magnuson, and H. O. Adami. "Natural History of Early, Localized Prostate Cancer." *JAMA* 291, no. 22 (2004): 2713–9.

3. Holmberg, Lars, A. Bill-Axelson, Fred Helgesen, J. Salo, P. Folmerz, M. Haggman, Swen-Olof Andersson, A. Spangberg, J. E. Johansson, and Bo Johan Norlen. "A Randomized Trial Comparing Radical Prostatectomy with Watchful Waiting in Early Prostate Cancer." *N Engl J Med* 347, no. 11 (2002): 781–89.

4. D'Amico, A. V., R. Whittington, S. B. Malkowicz, D. Schultz, K. Blank, G. A. Broderick, J. E. Tomaszewski, A. A. Renshaw, I. Kaplan, C. J. Beard, and A. Wein. "Biochemical Outcome After Radical Prostatectomy, External Beam Radiation Therapy, or Interstitial Radiation Therapy for Clinically Localized Prostate Cancer." *JAMA* 280, no. 11 (1998): 969–74.

5. CDC. "Department of Health and Human Resources. CDC. Search Results for Life Expectancy Tables." In http://www.CDC.gov/search.do?action=search&queryText=life+expectancy+tables&x=14&y=10: 10/08/2004.

6. de Groot, V., H. Beckerman, G. J. Lankhorst, and L. M. Bouter. "How to Measure Comorbidity. A Critical Review of Available Methods." *J Clin Epidemiol* 56, no. 3 (2003): 221–9.

7. Eastham, J. A., and P. T. Scardino. "Radical Prostatectomy." In *Campbell's Urology* 8th edition. Edited by P. C. Walsh, A. B. Retik, E. D. Vaughan, Jr. and A. J. Wein, Philadelphia: W. B. Saunders, Co., 2002.

8. Shipley, W. U., P. T. Scardino, D. S. Kaufman, and M. W. Kattan. "Advising Patients with Early Prostatic Cancer on Their Treatment Decision." In *The Comprehensive Textbook of Genitourinary Oncology,* ed. N. J. Vogelzang, P. T. Scardino, W. U. Shipley, and C. S. Coffey. Philadelphia: Lippincott Williams & Wilkins, 2004.

9. Kattan, M. W., A. M. Stapleton, T. M. Wheeler, and P. T. Scardino. "Evaluation of a Nomogram Used to Predict the Pathologic Stage of Clinically Localized Prostate Carcinoma." *Cancer* 79, no. 3 (1997): 528–37.

10. Memorial Sloan-Kettering Cancer Center. "Nomograms." Available at http://www.mskcc.org/mskcc/html/5794.cfm: 10/08/2004.

11. Kattan, M. W., M. J. Zelefsky, P. A. Kupelian, P. T. Scardino, Z. Fuks, and S. A. Leibel. "Pretreatment Nomogram for Predicting the Outcome of Three-Dimensional Conformal Radiotherapy in Prostate Cancer." *J Clin Oncol* 18, no. 19 (2000): 3352–9.

12. Kattan, M. W., J. A. Eastham, A. M. Stapleton, T. M. Wheeler, and P. T. Scardino. "A Preoperative Nomogram for Disease Recurrence Following Radical Prostatectomy for Prostate Cancer." *J Natl Cancer Inst* 90, no. 10 (1998): 766–71.

13. Kattan, M. W. "Nomograms Are Superior to Staging and Risk Grouping Systems for Identifying High-Risk Patients: Preoperative Application in Prostate Cancer." *Curr Opin Urol* 13, no. 2 (2003): 111–6.

14. Begg, C. B., E. R. Riedel, P. B. Bach, M. W. Kattan, D. Schrag, J. L. Warren, and P. T. Scardino. "Variations in Morbidity After Radical Prostatectomy." *N Engl J Med* 346, no. 15 (2002): 1138–44.

CHAPTER 13: WATCHFUL WAITING

1. Scardino, P. T., R. Weaver, and M. A. Hudson. "Early Detection of Prostate Cancer." *Human Pathology* 23, no. 3 (1992): 211–22.

2. Parker, C. "Active Surveillance: Towards a New Paradigm in the Management of Early Prostate Cancer." *Lancet Oncol* 5, no. 2 (2004): 101–6.

3. Johansson, J. E., L. Holmberg, S. Johansson, R. Bergstrom, and H. O. Adami. "Fifteen-Year Survival in Prostate Cancer. A Prospective, Population-Based Study in Sweden [see comments] [published erratum appears in *JAMA* 278, no. 3 (July 16,1997): 206." *JAMA* 277, no. 6 (1997): 467–71.

4. Holmberg, L., A. Bill-Axelson, F. Helgesen, J. O. Salo, P. Folmerz, M. Haggman, S. O. Andersson, A. Spangberg, C. Busch, S. Nordling, J. Palmgren, H. O. Adami, J. E. Johansson, and B. J. Norlen. "A Randomized Trial Comparing Radical Prostatectomy with Watchful Waiting in Early Prostate Cancer." *N Engl J Med* 347, no. 11 (2002): 781–9.

5. Schmid, H. P., J. E. McNeal, and T. A. Stamey. "Observations on the Doubling Time of Prostate Cancer. The Use of Serial Prostate-Specific Antigen in Patients with Untreated Disease as a Measure of Increasing Cancer Volume." *Cancer* 71, no. 6 (1993): 2031–40.

6. Patel, M. I., D. T. DeConcini, E. Lopez-Corona, M. Ohori, T. Wheeler, and P. T. Scardino. "An Analysis of Men with Clinically Localized Prostate Cancer Who Deferred Definitive Therapy." *J Urol* 171, no. 4 (2004): 1520–4.

7. Epstein, J. I., P. C. Walsh, M. Carmichael, and C. B. Brendler. "Pathologic and Clinical Findings to Predict Tumor Extent of Nonpalpable (Stage T1c) Prostate Cancer." *JAMA* 271, no. 5 (1994): 368–74; and Ohori, M., T. M. Wheeler, J. K. Dunn, T. A. Stamey, and P. T. Scardino. "The Pathological Features and Prognosis of Prostate Cancer Detectable with Current Diagnostic Tests." *J Urol* 152, no. 5 Pt 2 (1994): 1714–20.

8. Ohori et al. "The Pathological Features and Prognosis of Prostate Cancer Detectable with Current Diagnostic Tests."

9. Ohori, M., T. M. Wheeler, N. Maru, A. Erbersdobler, M. Graefen, H. Huland, H. Koh, S. F. Shariat, K. M. Slawin, J. A. Eastham, P. T. Scardino, and M. W. Kattan. "Counseling Men with Prostate Cancer (PCA): A Nomogram for Predicting the Presence of Indolent (Small, Well-Moderately Differentiated, Confined) Tumors." *J Urol* 169, no. 4 (2003): 425–6.

10. CDC. "Department of Health and Human Resources. CDC. Search Results for Life Expectancy Tables." In http://www.CDC.gov/search.do?action=search&queryText=life+expectancy+tables&x=14&y=10: 10/08/2004.

11. Patel et al.; and Carter, H. B., P. C. Walsh, P. Landis, and J. I. Epstein. "Expectant Management of Nonpalpable Prostate Cancer with Curative Intent: Preliminary Results." *J Urol* 167, no. 3 (2002): 1231–4.

12. Eastham, J. A., E. Riedel, P. T. Scardino, M. Shike, M. Fleisher, A. Schatzkin, E. Lanza, L. Latkany, and C. B. Begg. "Variation of Serum Prostate-Specific Antigen Levels: An Evaluation of Year-to-Year Fluctuations." *JAMA* 289, no. 20 (2003): 2695–700.

13. Schmid et al.

14. Ross, P. L., S. Mahmud, A. J. Stephenson, L. Souhami, S. Tanguay, and A. G. Aprikian. "Variations in PSA Doubling Time in Patients with Prostate Cancer on 'Watchful Waiting': Value of Short-Term PSADT Determinations." *Urology* 64, no. 2 (2004): 323–8.

15. Patel et al.

16. Ibid.

17. Ibid.

18. Johansson, J. E., O. Andren, S. O. Andersson, P. W. Dickman, L. Holmberg, A. Magnuson, and

H. O. Adami. "Natural History of Early, Localized Prostate Cancer." *JAMA* 291, no. 22 (2004): 2713–9.

19. Schatzkin, A., E. Lanza, D. Corle, P. Lance, F. Iber, B. Caan, M. Shike, J. Weissfeld, R. Burt, M. R. Cooper, J. W. Kikendall, J. Cahill, L. Freedman, J. Marshall, R. E. Schoen, and M. Slattery. "Lack of Effect of a Low-Fat, High-Fiber Diet on the Recurrence of Colorectal Adenomas." *N Engl J Med* 342, no. 16 (2000): 1149-55; and Shike, M., L. Latkany, E. Riedel, M. Fleisher, A. Schatzkin, E. Lanza, D. Corle, and C. B. Begg. "Lack of Effect of a Low-Fat, High-Fruit, -Vegetable, and -Fiber Diet on Serum Prostate-Specific Antigen of Men without Prostate Cancer: Results from a Randomized Trial." *J Clin Oncol* 20, no. 17 (2002): 3592–8.

20. Patel et al.

21. Johansson et al. "Natural History of Early, Localized Prostate Cancer."

22. Carter et al.; and Ross et al.

CHAPTER 14: SURGERY

1. Stamey, T. A., F. S. Freiha, J. E. McNeal, E. A. Redwine, A. S. Whittemore, and H. P. Schmid. "Localized Prostate Cancer. Relationship of Tumor Volume to Clinical Significance for Treatment of Prostate Cancer." *Cancer* 71, Suppl 3 (1993): 933–8.

2. Kikuchi, E., P. T. Scardino, T. M. Wheeler, K. M. Slawin, and M. Ohori. "Is Tumor Volume an Independent Prognostic Factor in Clinically Localized Prostate Cancer?" *J Urol* 172, no. 2 (2004): 508–11.

3. Greene, D. R., S. R. Taylor, T. M. Wheeler, and P. T. Scardino. "DNA Ploidy by Image-Analysis of Individual Foci of Prostate-Cancer—A Preliminary Report." *Cancer Research* 51, no. 15 (1991): 4084–9.

4. Watanabe, H. "History of Ultrasound in Nephrourology." *Ultrasound Med Biol* 27, no. 4 (2001): 447–53.

5. Young, H. H. "The Early Diagnosis and Cure of Carcinoma of the Prostate: Being a Study of 40 Cases and Presentation of a Radical Operation Which Was Carried Out in Four Cases." *Johns Hopkins Hosp Bull* 16 (1905): 315.

6. Walsh, P. C., and P. J. Donker. "Impotence Following Radical Prostatectomy: Insight into Etiology and Prevention." *J Urol* 128, no. 3 (1982): 492–7.

7. Walsh, P. C. "Radical Prostatectomy for Localized Prostate Cancer Provides Durable Cancer Control with Excellent Quality of Life: A Structured Debate." *J Urol* 163, no. 6 (2000): 1802–7; and Rabbani, F., A. M. Stapleton, M. W. Kattan, T. M. Wheeler, and P. T. Scardino. "Factors Predicting Recovery of Erections After Radical Prostatectomy." *J Urol* 164, no. 6 (2000): 1929–34.

8. Eastham, J. A., and P. T. Scardino. "Radical Prostatectomy for Clinical Stage T1 and T2 Prostate Cancer." In *The Comprehensive Textbook of Genitourinary Oncology,* ed. Vogelzang, N. J., P. T. Scardino, W. U. Shipley, and D. S. Coffey, 722–38. Philadelphia: Lippincott Williams & Wilkins, 2000.

9. Scardino P. T., Kim E. D. "Rationale for and Results of Nerve Grafting During Radical Prostatectomy." *Urology* 57, no. 6 (2001): 1016–9; and Eastham, J. A., and P. T. Scardino. "Update on Nerve Grafting During Radical Prostatectomy." *AUA News* 8 (2003): 40–41.

10. Kim, E. D., P. T. Scardino, D. Kadmon, K. Slawin, and R. K. Nath. "Interposition Sural Nerve Grafting During Radical Retropubic Prostatectomy." *Urology* 57, no. 2 (2001): 211–6.

11. Kim, E. D., R. Nath, K. M. Slawin, D. Kadmon, B. J. Miles, and P. T. Scardino. "Bilateral Nerve Grafting During Radical Retropubic Prostatectomy: Extended Follow-Up." *J Urol* 168, no. 1 (2002): 376–77.

12. Rabbani, F. "Recovery of Potency After Cavernous Nerve Graft Reconstruction at Radical Prostatectomy: The MSKCC Experience." Paper presented at the 101st Annual Meeting of the New York Section American Urological Association, Athens and Crete, October 11–18, 2003.

13. Kim, E. D., P. T. Scardino, O. Hampel, N. L. Mills, T. M. Wheeler, and R. K. Nath. "Interposition of Sural Nerve Restores Function of Cavernous Nerves Resected During Radical Prostatectomy." *J Urol* 161, no. 1 (1999): 188–92.

14. Scardino and Kim.

15. Eastham and Scardino. "Radical Prostatectomy for Clinical Stage T1 and T2 Prostate Cancer."

16. Ohori, M., and P. T. Scardino. "Localized Prostate Cancer." *Curr Probl Surg* 39, no. 9 (2002): 833–957.

17. Stanford, J. L., Z. Feng, A. S. Hamilton, F. D. Gilliland, R. A. Stephenson, J. W. Eley, P. C. Albertsen, L. C. Harlan, and A. L. Potosky. "Urinary and Sexual Function After Radical Prostatectomy for Clinically Localized Prostate Cancer: The Prostate Cancer Outcomes Study." *JAMA* 283, no. 3 (2000): 354–60.

18. Begg, C. B., E. R. Riedel, P. B. Bach, M. W. Kattan, D. Schrag, J. L. Warren, and P. T. Scardino. "Variations in Morbidity After Radical Prostatectomy." *N Engl J Med* 346, no. 15 (2002): 1138–44; and Wei, J. T., R. L. Dunn, H. M. Sandler, P. W. McLaughlin, J. E. Montie, M. S. Litwin, L. Nyquist, and M. G. Sanda. "Comprehensive Comparison of Health-Related Quality of Life After Contemporary Therapies for Localized Prostate Cancer." *J Clin Oncol* 20, no. 2 (2002): 557–66.

19. Fromont, G., B. Guillonneau, P. Validire, and G. Vallancien. "Laparoscopic Radical Prostatectomy. Preliminary Pathologic Evaluation." *Urology* 60, no. 4 (2002): 661–5.

20. Su, L. M., R. E. Link, S. B. Bhayani, W. Sullivan, and C. P. Pavlovich. "Nerve-Sparing Laparoscopic Radical Prostatectomy: Replicating the Open Surgical Technique." *Urology* 64, no. 1 (2004): 123–7.

21. Bishoff, J. T., A. Reyes, I. M. Thompson, M. J. Harris, S. R. St. Clair, L. Gomella, and C. A. Butzin. "Pelvic Lymphadenectomy Can Be Omitted in Selected Patients with Carcinoma of the Prostate: Development of a System of Patient Selection." *Urology* 45, no. 2 (1995): 270–4.

22. Touijer, A. K., and B. Guillonneau. "Laparoscopic Radical Prostatectomy." *Urol Oncol* 22, no. 2 (2004): 133–8.

23. Hull, G. W., F. Rabbani, F. Abbas, T. M. Wheeler, M. W. Kattan, and P. T. Scardino. "Cancer Control with Radical Prostatectomy Alone in 1,000 Consecutive Patients." *J Urol* 167, no. 2 Pt 1 (2002): 528–34.

24. Eastham, J. A., and P. T. Scardino. "Radical Prostatectomy." In *Campbell's Urology,* 8th edition, ed. Walsh, P. C. Philadelphia: Saunders, 2002. 3080–3106.

25. Bianco, F. J., Jr., D. P. Wood, Jr., M. L. Cher, I. J. Powell, J. W. Souza, and J. E. Pontes. "Ten-Year Survival After Radical Prostatectomy: Specimen Gleason Score Is the Predictor in Organ-Confined Prostate Cancer." *Clin Prostate Cancer* 1, no. 4 (2003): 242–7.

26. Eastham, J. A., J. R. Goad, E. Rogers, M. Ohori, M. W. Kattan, T. B. Boone, and P. T. Scardino. "Risk Factors for Urinary Incontinence After Radical Prostatectomy." *J Urol* 156, no. 5, (1996): 1707–13.

27. Rabbani et al.

28. Goad, J. R., and P. T. Scardino. "Modifications in the Technique of Radical Retropubic Prostatectomy to Minimize Blood Loss." *Atlas Urol Clin North Am* 2, no. 2 (1994): 65–80.

29. Rosenblum, N., M. A. Levine, T. Handler, and H. Lepor. "The Role of Preoperative Epoetin Alfa in Men Undergoing Radical Retropubic Prostatectomy." *J Urol* 163, no. 3 (2000): 829–33.

30. Catalona, W. J., and D. S. Smith. "Cancer Recurrence and Survival Rates After Anatomic

Radical Retropubic Prostatectomy for Prostate Cancer: Intermediate-Term Results." *J Urol* 160, no. 6 Pt 2 (1998): 2428–34; and Dillioglugil, O., B. D. Leibman, N. S. Leibman, M. W. Kattan, A. L. Rosas, and P. T. Scardino. "Risk Factors for Complications and Morbidity After Radical Retropubic Prostatectomy." *J Urol* 157, no. 5 (1997): 1760–7.

31. Begg et al.
32. Ibid.
33. Eastham and Goad et al.
34. Wille, S., A. Sobottka, A. Heidenreich, and R. Hofmann. "Pelvic Floor Exercises, Electrical Stimulation and Biofeedback After Radical Prostatectomy: Results of a Prospective Randomized Trial." *J Urol* 170, no. 2 Pt 1 (2003): 490–3.
35. Eastham and Goad, et al.
36. Rabbani et al.
37. Ibid.
38. Begg et al.; and Wei et al.
39. Eastham, J. A., M. W. Kattan, E. Riedel, C. B. Begg, T. M. Wheeler, C. Gerigk, M. Gonen, V. Reuter, and P. T. Scardino. "Variations Among Individual Surgeons in the Rate of Positive Surgical Margins in Radical Prostatectomy Specimens." *J Urol* 170, no. 6, Pt 1 (2003): 2292–5.
40. America's Top Doctors, www.castleconnolly.com. Accessed 10/16/2004.
41. Begg et al.
42. Eastham and Goad et al.
43. Ang-Lee, M. K., J. Moss, and C. S. Yuan. "Herbal Medicines and Perioperative Care." *JAMA* 286, no. 2 (2001): 208–16.
44. Kamat, A. M., K. Babaian, M. R. Cheung, Y. Naya, S. H. Huang, D. Kuban, and R. J. Babaian. "Identification of Factors Predicting Response to Adjuvant Radiation Therapy in Patients with Positive Margins After Radical Prostatectomy." *J Urol* 170, no. 5 (2003): 1860–3.
45. Zelefsky, M. J., E. Aschkenasy, S. Kelsen, and S. A. Leibel. "Tolerance and Early Outcome Results of Postprostatectomy Three-Dimensional Conformal Radiotherapy." *Int J Radiat Oncol Biol Phys* 39, no. 2 (1997): 327–33.
46. Burnett, A. L. "Neuroprotection and Nerve Grafts in the Treatment of Neurogenic Erectile Dysfunction." *J Urol* 170, no. 2, Pt 2 (2003): S31–4; discussion S34.

CHAPTER 15: RADIATION THERAPY

1. Garcia-Barros, M., F. Paris, C. Cordon-Cardo, D. Lyden, S. Rafii, A. Haimovitz-Friedman, Z. Fuks, and R. Kolesnick. "Tumor Response to Radiotherapy Regulated by Endothelial Cell Apoptosis." *Science* 300, no. 5622 (2003): 1155–9; and Kolesnick, R., and Z. Fuks. "Radiation and Ceramide-Induced Apoptosis." *Oncogene* 22, no. 37 (2003): 5897–906.
2. Hanks, G. E., A. L. Hanlon, B. Epstein, and E. M. Horwitz. "Dose Response in Prostate Cancer with 8–12 Years' Follow-Up." *Int J Radiat Oncol Biol Phys* 54, no. 2 (2002): 427–35.
3. History of Radiation. At http://www.Physics.Isu.Edu/Radinf/Hist.Htm. Last accessed on 10/16/2004.
4. Barringer, B. "Radium in the Treatment of Carcinoma of the Bladder and Prostate." *JAMA* 68 (1917): 1227–30.
5. Bagshaw, M. A. "Definitive Radiotherapy in Carcinoma of the Prostate." *JAMA* 210, no. 2 (1969): 326–7.
6. Sogani, P. C., W. F. Whitmore, Jr., B. S. Hilaris, and M. A. Batata. "Experience with Interstitial Implantation of Iodine 125 in the Treatment of Prostatic Carcinoma." *Scand J Urol Nephrol Suppl* 55 (1980): 205–11.

7. Gottesman, J. E., D. G. Tesh, and W. D. Weissman. "Failure of Open Radioactive 125 Iodine Implantation to Control Localized Prostate Cancer: A Study of 41 Patients." *J Urol* 146, no. 5 (1991): 1317–9; discussion 19–20.

8. Hanks.

9. Bagshaw, M. A., G. R. Ray, and R. S. Cox. "Radiotherapy of Prostatic Carcinoma: Long- or Short-Term Efficacy (Stanford University Experience)." *Urology* 25, Suppl 2 (1985): 17–23.

10. Zelefsky, M. J., Z. Fuks, M. Hunt, H. J. Lee, D. Lombardi, C. C. Ling, V. E. Reuter, E. S. Venkatraman, and S. A. Leibel. "High Dose Radiation Delivered by Intensity Modulated Conformal Radiotherapy Improves the Outcome of Localized Prostate Cancer." *J Urol* 166, no. 3 (2001): 876–81.

11. Ibid.

12. Shipley, W. U., L. J. Verhey, J. E. Munzenrider, H. D. Suit, D. Phil, M. M. Urie, P. L. McManus, R. H. Young, J. W. Shipley, A. L. Zietman, P. J. Biggs, N. M. Heney, and M. Goitein. "Advanced Prostate Cancer: The Results of a Randomized Comparative Trial of High Dose Irradiation Boosting with Conformal Protons Compared with Conventional Dose Irradiation Using Photons Alone." *Int J Radiat Oncol Biol Phys* 32, no.1 (1995): 3–12.

13. Lindsley, K. L., P. Cho, K. J. Stelzer, W. J. Koh, M. Austin-Seymour, K. J. Russell, G. E. Laramore, and T. W. Griffin. "Fast Neutrons in Prostatic Adenocarcinomas: Worldwide Clinical Experience." *Recent Results Cancer Res* 150 (1998): 125–36.

14. Rosser, C. J., D. A. Kuban, L. B. Levy, R. Chichakli, A. Pollack, A. K. Lee, and L. L. Pisters. "Prostate Specific Antigen Bounce Phenomenon After External Beam Radiation for Clinically Localized Prostate Cancer." *J Urol* 168, no. 5 (2002): 2001–5.

15. Ibid.

16. Sandler, H. M., P. W. McLaughlin, R. K. Ten Haken, H. Addison, J. Forman, and A. Lichter. "Three Dimensional Conformal Radiotherapy for the Treatment of Prostate Cancer: Low Risk of Chronic Rectal Morbidity Observed in a Large Series of Patients." *Int J Radiat Oncol Biol Phys* 33, no. 4 (1995): 797–801.

17. Zelefsky et al. "High Dose Radiation Delivered by Intensity Modulated Conformal Radiotherapy Improves the Outcome of Localized Prostate Cancer."

18. Zelefsky, M. J., D. Cowen, Z. Fuks, M. Shike, C. Burman, A. Jackson, E. S. Venkatraman, and S. A. Leibel. "Long Term Tolerance of High Dose Three-Dimensions Conformal Radiotherapy in Patients with Localized Prostate Carcinoma." *Cancer* 85, no. 11 (1999): 2460–8.

19. Ellis, R. J., and E. Kim. "Brachytherapy: Update and Results." *Curr Urol Rep* 4, no. 3 (2003): 233–9.

20. Stromberg, J. S., A. A. Martinez, E. M. Horwitz, G. S. Gustafson, J. A. Gonzalez, W. F. Spencer, D. S. Brabbins, C. F. Dmuchowski, J. B. Hollander, and F. A. Vicini. "Conformal High Dose Rate Iridium-192 Boost Brachytherapy in Locally Advanced Prostate Cancer: Superior Prostate-Specific Antigen Response Compared with External Beam Treatment." *Cancer J Sci Am* 3, no. 6 (1997): 346–52.

21. Mallick, S., R. Azzouzi, L. Cormier, D. Peiffert, and P. H. Mangin. "Urinary Morbidity After 125i Brachytherapy of the Prostate." *BJU Int* 92, no. 6 (2003): 555–8.

22. Rosser et al.

23. "Consensus Statement: Guidelines for PSA Following Radiation Therapy. American Society for Therapeutic Radiology and Oncology Consensus Panel." *Int J Radiat Oncol Biol Phys* 37, no. 5 (1997): 1035–41.

24. Merrick, G. S., W. M. Butler, K. E. Wallner, and R. W. Galbreath. "Effect of Transurethral Resection on Urinary Quality of Life After Permanent Prostate Brachytherapy." *Int J Radiat Oncol Biol Phys* 58, no. 1 (2004): 81–8.

25. Raina, R., A. Agarwal, K. K. Goyal, C. Jackson, J. Ulchaker, K. Angermeier, E. Klein,

J. Ciezki, and C. D. Zippe. "Long-Term Potency After Iodine-125 Radiotherapy for Prostate Cancer and Role of Sildenafil Citrate." *Urology* 62, no. 6 (2003): 1103–8.

26. Zelefsky, M. J., Y. Yamada, G. Cohen, E. S. Venkatraman, A. Y. Fung, E. Furhang, D. Silvern, and M. Zaider. "Postimplantation Dosimetric Analysis of Permanent Transperineal Prostate Implantation: Improved Dose Distributions with an Intraoperative Computer-Optimized Conformal Planning Technique." *Int J Radiat Oncol Biol Phys* 48, no. 2 (2000): 601–8.

27. Ragde, H., J. C. Blasko, P. D. Grimm, G. M. Kenny, J. E. Sylvester, D. C. Hoak, K. Landin, and W. Cavanagh. "Interstitial Iodine-125 Radiation without Adjuvant Therapy in the Treatment of Clinically Localized Prostate Carcinoma." *Cancer* 80, no. 3 (1997): 442–53.

28. Bolla, M. "Combination of Radiotherapy and Hormonotherapy in Locally Advanced Cancers of the Prostate." *Cancer Radiother* 1, no. 5 (1997): 439–42.

29. Bolla, M., L. Collette, L. Blank, P. Warde, J. B. Dubois, R. O. Mirimanoff, G. Storme, J. Bernier, A. Kuten, C. Sternberg, J. Mattelaer, J. Lopez Torecilla, J. R. Pfeffer, C. Lino Cutajar, A. Zurlo, and M. Pierart. "Long-Term Results with Immediate Androgen Suppression and External Irradiation in Patients with Locally Advanced Prostate Cancer (an EORTC Study): A Phase III Randomised Trial." *Lancet* 360, no. 9327 (2002): 103–6; and Pilepich, M. V., K. Winter, C. Lawton, R. E. Krisch, H. Wolkov, B. Movsas, E. Hug, S. Asbell, and D. Grignon. "Androgen Suppression Adjuvant to Radiotherapy in Carcinoma of the Prostate. Long-Term Results of Phase III RTOG Study 85-31." *Int J Radiat Oncol Biol Phys* 57, Suppl 2 (2003): S172–3.

30. Higano, C. S. "Side Effects of Androgen Deprivation Therapy: Monitoring and Minimizing Toxicity." *Urology* 61, no. 2 Suppl 1 (2003): 32–8.

31. Zelefsky, M. J., Z. Fuks, and S. A. Leibel. "Intensity-Modulated Radiation Therapy for Prostate Cancer." *Semin Radiat Oncol* 12, no. 3 (2002): 229–37.

32. Zelefsky et al. "High Dose Radiation Delivered by Intensity Modulated Conformal Radiotherapy Improves the Outcome of Localized Prostate Cancer."

CHAPTER 16: OTHER LOCAL THERAPIES

1. Robinson, J. W., S. Moritz, and T. Fung. "Meta-Analysis of Rates of Erectile Function After Treatment of Localized Prostate Carcinoma." *Int J Radiat Oncol Biol Phys* 54, no. 4 (2002): 1063–8.

2. Anastasiadis, A. G., R. Sachdev, L. Salomon, M. A. Ghafar, B. C. Stisser, R. Shabsigh, and A. E. Katz. "Comparison of Health-Related Quality of Life and Prostate-Associated Symptoms After Primary and Salvage Cryotherapy for Prostate Cancer." *J Cancer Res Clin Oncol* 129, no. 12 (2003): 676–82.

3. Blana, A., B. Walter, S. Rogenhofer, and W. F. Wieland. "High-Intensity Focused Ultrasound for the Treatment of Localized Prostate Cancer: 5-Year Experience." *Urology* 63, no. 2 (2004): 297–300.

4. Muschter, R. "Photodynamic Therapy: A New Approach to Prostate Cancer." *Curr Urol Rep* 4, no. 3 (2003): 221–8.

5. Shalev, M., D. Kadmon, B. S. Teh, E. B. Butler, E. Aguilar-Cordova, T. C. Thompson, J. R. Herman, H. L. Adler, P. T. Scardino, and B. J. Miles. "Suicide Gene Therapy Toxicity After Multiple and Repeat Injections in Patients with Localized Prostate Cancer." *J Urol* 163, no. 6 (2000): 1747–50; and Herman, J. R., H. L. Adler, E. Aguilar-Cordova, A. Rojas-Martinez, S. Woo, T. L. Timme, T. M. Wheeler, T. C. Thompson, and P. T. Scardino. "In Situ Gene Therapy for Adenocarcinoma of the Prostate: A Phase I Clinical Trial." *Hum Gene Ther* 10, no. 7 (1999): 1239–49.

CHAPTER 17: URINARY SIDE EFFECTS

1. Steiner, M. S., R. A. Morton, and P. C. Walsh. "Impact of Anatomical Radical Prostatectomy on Urinary Continence." *J Urol* 145, no. 3 (1991): 512–4; discussion 14–5.

2. Lepor, H., L. Kaci, and X. Xue. "Continence Following Radical Retropubic Prostatectomy Using Self-Reporting Instruments." *J Urol* 171, no. 3 (2004): 1212–5.

3. Begg, C. B., E. R. Riedel, P. B. Bach, M. W. Kattan, D. Schrag, J. L. Warren, and P. T. Scardino. "Variations in Morbidity After Radical Prostatectomy." *N Engl J Med* 346, no. 15 (2002): 1138–44.

4. Eastham, J. A., M. W. Kattan, J. R. Goad, E. Rogers, M. Ohori, T. B. Boone, and P. T. Scardino. "Risk Factors for Urinary Incontinence After Radical Prostatectomy." *J Urol* 156 (1996): 1707–13.

5. Begg et al.

6. Terk, M. D., R. G. Stock, and N. N. Stone. "Identification of Patients at Increased Risk for Prolonged Urinary Retention Following Radioactive Seed Implantation of the Prostate." *J Urol* 160, no. 4 (1998): 1379–82.

7. Anastasiadis, A. G., R. Sachdev, L. Salomon, M. A. Ghafar, B. C. Stisser, R. Shabsigh, and A. E. Katz. "Comparison of Health-Related Quality of Life and Prostate-Associated Symptoms After Primary and Salvage Cryotherapy for Prostate Cancer." *J Cancer Res Clin Oncol* 129, no. 12 (2003): 676–82.

8. Kegel, A. "Progressive Exercise in the Functional Restoration of the Perineal Muscles." *American Journal of Obstetrics and Gynecology* 56 (1948): 238–48.

9. Van Kampen, M., W. De Weerdt, H. Van Poppel, D. De Ridder, H. Feys, and L. Baert. "Effect of Pelvic-Floor Re-Education on Duration and Degree of Incontinence After Radical Prostatectomy: A Randomised Controlled Trial." *Lancet* 355, no. 9198 (2000): 98–102.

10. Smith, D. N., R. A. Appell, R. R. Rackley, and J. C. Winters. "Collagen Injection Therapy for Post-Prostatectomy Incontinence." *J Urol* 160, no. 2 (1998): 364–7.

11. Comiter, C. V. "The Male Sling for Stress Urinary Incontinence: A Prospective Study." *J Urol* 167, no. 2 Pt 1 (2002): 597–601.

12. Dalkin, B. L., H. Wessells, and H. Cui. "A National Survey of Urinary and Health Related Quality of Life Outcomes in Men with an Artificial Urinary Sphincter for Post-Radical Prostatectomy Incontinence." *J Urol* 169, no. 1 (2003): 237–9.

CHAPTER 18: SEXUAL SIDE EFFECTS

1. Huggins, C. "Endocrine-Induced Regression of Cancers." *Cancer Res* 27, no. 11 (1967): 1925–30.

2. Sadovsky, R., and J. P. Mulhall. "The Potential Value of Erectile Dysfunction Inquiry and Management." *Int J Clin Pract* 57, no. 7 (2003): 601–8.

3. Bodie, J. A., W. W. Beeman, and M. Monga. "Psychogenic Erectile Dysfunction." *Int J Psychiatry Med* 33, no. 3 (2003): 273–93.

4. Montorsi, P., A. Briganti, A. Salonia, A. Margonato, and F. Montorsi. "Impaired Vascular Reactivity in Patients with Erectile Dysfunction." *J Am Coll Cardiol* 44, no. 6 (2004): 1339–40; author reply 40–1.

5. Foresta, C., N. Caretta, M. Rossato, A. Garolla, and A. Ferlin. "Role of Androgens in Erectile Function." *J Urol* 171, no. 6 Pt 1 (2004): 2358–62, quiz 435.

6. Jackson, G. "Sexual Dysfunction and Diabetes." *Int J Clin Pract* 58, no. 4 (2004): 358–62.

7. Munarriz, R., J. Hwang, I. Goldstein, A. M. Traish, and N. N. Kim. "Cocaine and Ephedrine-Induced Priapism: Case Reports and Investigation of Potential Adrenergic Mechanisms." *Urology* 62, no. 1 (2003): 187–92.

8. Scardino, P. T., and E. D. Kim. "Rationale for and Results of Nerve Grafting During Radical Prostatectomy." *Urology* 57, no. 6 (2001): 1016–9.

9. Montorsi, F., and A. L. Burnett. "Erectile Dysfunction After Radical Prostatectomy." *BJU Int* 93, no. 1 (2004): 1–2.

10. Sethi, A., N. Mohideen, L. Leybovich, and J. Mulhall. "Role of IMRT in Reducing Penile Doses in Dose Escalation for Prostate Cancer." *Int J Radiat Oncol Biol Phys* 55, no. 4 (2003): 970–8.
11. Higano, C. S. "Side Effects of Androgen Deprivation Therapy: Monitoring and Minimizing Toxicity." *Urology* 61, no. 2, Suppl 1 (2003): 32–8.
12. Gresser, U., and C. H. Gleiter. "Erectile Dysfunction: Comparison of Efficacy and Side Effects of the PDE-5 Inhibitors Sildenafil, Vardenafil and Tadalafil—Review of the Literature." *Eur J Med Res* 7, no. 10 (2002): 435–46.
13. Brock, G., L. M. Tu, and O. I. Linet. "Return of Spontaneous Erection During Long-Term Intracavernosal Alprostadil (Caverject) Treatment." *Urology* 57, no. 3 (2001): 536–41.
14. Fulgham, P. F., J. S. Cochran, J. L. Denman, B. A. Feagins, M. B. Gross, K. T. Kadesky, M. C. Kadesky, A. R. Clark, and C. G. Roehrborn. "Disappointing Initial Results with Transurethral Alprostadil for Erectile Dysfunction in a Urology Practice Setting." *J Urol* 160, no. 6 Pt 1 (1998): 2041–6.
15. Mulhall, J. P., A. Ahmed, J. Branch, and M. Parker. "Serial Assessment of Efficacy and Satisfaction Profiles Following Penile Prosthesis Surgery." *J Urol* 169, no. 4 (2003): 1429–33.

CHAPTER 19: BOWEL SIDE EFFECTS

1. Wei, J. T., R. L. Dunn, H. Sandler, W. McLaughlin, J. E. Montie, M. S. Litwin, L. Nyquist, and M. G. Sanda. "Comprehensive Comparison of Health-Related Quality of Life After Contemporary Therapies for Localized Prostate Cancer." *J Clin Oncol* 20, no. 2 (2002): 557–66.
2. Zelefsky, M. J., Z. Fuks, M. Hunt, H. J. Lee, D. Lombardi, C. C. Ling, V. E. Reuter, E. S. Venkatraman, and S. A. Leibel. "High Dose Radiation Delivered by Intensity Modulated Conformal Radiotherapy Improves the Outcome of Localized Prostate Cancer." *J Urol* 166, no. 3 (2001): 876–81.
3. Yeoh, E. E., R. H. Holloway, R. J. Fraser, R. J. Botten, A. C. Di Matteo, J. W. Moore, M. N. Schoeman, and F. D. Bartholomeusz. "Anorectal Dysfunction Increases with Time Following Radiation Therapy for Carcinoma of the Prostate." *Am J Gastroenterol* 99, no. 2 (2004): 361–9.
4. Waterman et al.
5. Menard, C., K. Camphausen, T. Muanza, N. Sears-Crouse, S. Smith, E. Ben-Josef, and C. N. Coleman. "Clinical Trial of Endorectal Amifostine for Radioprotection in Patients with Prostate Cancer: Rationale and Early Results." *Semin Oncol* 30, no. 6 Suppl 18 (2003): 63–7.

CHAPTER 20: RISING PSA AFTER SURGERY
OR RADIATION THERAPY

1. Horwitz, E. M., F. A. Vicini, E. L. Ziaja, C. F. Dmuchowski, J. S. Stromberg, and A. A. Martinez. "The Correlation between the Astro Consensus Panel Definition of Biochemical Failure and Clinical Outcome for Patients with Prostate Cancer Treated with External Beam Irradiation. American Society of Therapeutic Radiology and Oncology." *Int J Radiat Oncol Biol Phys* 41, no. 2 (1998): 267–72.
2. Fowler, J. E., Jr., J. Brooks, P. Pandey, and L. E. Seaver. "Variable Histology of Anastomotic Biopsies with Detectable Prostate Specific Antigen After Radical Prostatectomy." *J Urol* 153, no. 3, Pt 2 (1995): 1011–4.
3. Jhaveri, F. M., and E. A. Klein. "How to Explore the Patient with a Rising PSA After Radical Prostatectomy: Defining Local Versus Systemic Failure." *Semin Urol Oncol* 17, no. 3 (1999): 130–4.

446 *Notes*

4. Swindle, P. W., M. W. Kattan, and P. T. Scardino. "Markers and Meaning of Primary Treatment Failure." *Urol Clin North Am* 30, no. 2 (2003): 377–401.

5. D'Amico, A. V., J. W. Moul, P. R. Carroll, L. Sun, D. Lubeck, and M. H. Chen. "Surrogate End Point for Prostate Cancer-Specific Mortality after Radical Prostatectomy or Radiation Therapy." *J Natl Cancer Inst* 95, no. 18 (2003): 1376–83.

6. Swindle et al.

7. Bander, N. H., D. M. Nanus, M. I. Milowsky, L. Kostakoglu, S. Vallabahajosula, and S. J. Goldsmith. "Targeted Systemic Therapy of Prostate Cancer with a Monoclonal Antibody to Prostate-Specific Membrane Antigen." *Semin Oncol* 30, no. 5 (2003): 667–76.

8. Stephenson, A. J., S. F. Shariat, M. J. Zelefsky, M. W. Kattan, E. B. Butler, B. S. Teh, E. A. Klein, P. A. Kupelian, C. G. Roehrborn, D. A. Pistenmaa, H. D. Pacholke, S. L. Liauw, M. S. Katz, S. A. Leibel, P. T. Scardino, and K. M. Slawin. "Salvage Radiotherapy for Recurrent Prostate Cancer after Radical Prostatectomy." *JAMA* 291, no. 11 (2004): 1325-32.

9. Maier, J., J. Forman, S. Tekyi-Mensah, S. Bolton, R. Patel, and J. E. Pontes. "Salvage Radiation for a Rising PSA Following Radical Prostatectomy." *Urol Oncol* 22, no. 1 (2004): 50–6.

10. Coakley, F. V., H. S. Teh, A. Qayyum, M. G. Swanson, Y. Lu, M. R. III, B. Pickett, K. Shinohara, D. B. Vigneron, and J. Kurhanewicz. "Endorectal MR Imaging and MR Spectroscopic Imaging for Locally Recurrent Prostate Cancer After External Beam Radiation Therapy: Preliminary Experience." *Radiology* 223, no. 2 (2004): 441–8.

11. Rosser, C. J., D. A. Kuban, L. B. Levy, R. Chichakli, A. Pollack, A. K. Lee, and L. L. Pisters. "Prostate Specific Antigen Bounce Phenomenon After External Beam Radiation for Clinically Localized Prostate Cancer." *J Urol* 168, no. 5 (2002): 2001–5.

12. Pollack, A., A. L. Hanlon, E. M. Horwitz, S. J. Feigenberg, R. G. Uzzo, and G. E. Hanks. "Prostate Cancer Radiotherapy Dose Response: An Update of the Fox Chase Experience." *J Urol* 171, no. 3 (2004): 1132–6.

13. Eastham, J. A., C. J. DiBlasio, and P. T. Scardino. "Salvage Radical Prostatectomy for Recurrence of Prostate Cancer After Radiation Therapy." *Curr Urol Rep* 4, no. 3 (2003): 211–5.

14. Anastasiadis, A. G., R. Sachdev, L. Salomon, M. A. Ghafar, B. C. Stisser, R. Shabsigh, and A. E. Katz. "Comparison of Health-Related Quality of Life and Prostate-Associated Symptoms After Primary and Salvage Cryotherapy for Prostate Cancer." *J Cancer Res Clin Oncol* 129, no. 12 (2003): 676–82.

15. Tannock, I. F., R. de Wit, W. R. Berry, J. Horti, A. Pluzanska, K. N. Chi, S. Oudard, C. Theodore, N. D. James, I. Turesson, M. A. Rosenthal, and M. A. Eisenberger. "Docetaxel Plus Prednisone or Mitoxantrone Plus Prednisone for Advanced Prostate Cancer." *N Engl J Med* 351, no. 15 (2004): 1502–12.

CHAPTER 21: TREATING METASTATIC PROSTATE CANCER

1. Messing, E. M., J. Manola, M. Sarosdy, G. Wilding, D. E. Crawford, and D. Trump. "Immediate Hormonal Therapy Compared with Observation After Radical Prostatectomy and Pelvic Lymphadenectomy in Men with Node-Positive Prostate Cancer." *N Engl J Med* 341, no. 24 (1999): 1781–8.

2. Schroder, F. H., K. H. Kurth, S. D. Fossa, W. Hoekstra, P. P. Karthaus, M. Debois, and L. Collette. "Early Versus Delayed Endocrine Treatment of Pn1–3 M0 Prostate Cancer without Local Treatment of the Primary Tumor: Results of European Organisation for the Research and Treatment of Cancer 30846—a Phase III Study." *J Urol* 172, no. 3 (2004): 923–7.

3. Albrecht, W., L. Collette, C. Fava, O. B. Kariakine, P. Whelán, U. E. Studer, T. M. De Reijke, P. J. Kil, and L. A. Rea. "Intermittent Maximal Androgen Blockade in Patients with Metastatic Prostate Cancer: An EORTC Feasibility Study." *Eur Urol* 44, no. 5 (2003): 505–11.

4. Chen, C. D., D. S. Welsbie, C. Tran, S. H. Baek, R. Chen, R. Vessella, M. G. Rosenfeld, and C. L. Sawyers. "Molecular Determinants of Resistance to Antiandrogen Therapy." *Nat Med* 10, no. 1 (2004): 33–9.

5. Berry, W., S. Dakhil, M. Modiano, M. Gregurich, and L. Asmar. "Phase III Study of Mitoxantrone plus Low Dose Prednisone versus Low Dose Prednisone Alone in Patients with Asymptomatic Hormone Refractory Prostate Cancer." *J Urol* 168, no. 6 (2002): 2439–43.

6. Petrylak, D. P., C. M. Tangen, M. H. Hussain, P. N. Lara, Jr., J. A. Jones, M. E. Taplin, P. A. Burch, D. Berry, C. Moinpour, M. Kohli, M. C. Benson, E. J. Small, D. Raghavan, and E. D. Crawford. "Docetaxel and Estramustine Compared with Mitoxantrone and Prednisone for Advanced Refractory Prostate Cancer." *N Engl J Med* 351, no. 15 (2004): 1513–20; and Tannock, I. F., R. de Wit, W. R. Berry, J. Horti, A. Pluzanska, K. N. Chi, S. Oudard, C. Theodore, N. D. James, I. Turesson, M. A. Rosenthal, and M. A. Eisenberger. "Docetaxel Plus Prednisone or Mitoxantrone Plus Prednisone for Advanced Prostate Cancer." *N Engl J Med* 351, no. 15 (2004): 1502–12.

7. Morris, M. J., and H. I. Scher. "Clinical Approaches to Osseous Metastases in Prostate Cancer." *Oncologist* 8, no. 2 (2003): 161–73.

8. Cassileth, B. R. *The Alternative Medicine Handbook*. New York: W. W. Norton & Co., 1998.

9. Mercadante, S. "World Health Organization Guidelines: Problem Areas in Cancer Pain Management." *Cancer Control* 6, no. 2 (1999): 191–7.

10. Olson, K. B., and K. J. Pienta. "Pain Management in Patients with Advanced Prostate Cancer." *Oncology (Huntingt)* 13, no. 11 (1999): 1537–49.

GLOSSARY OF TERMS

3-D conformal radiation therapy (3D-CRT): A form of external beam radiation therapy in which the tissue exposed to radiation precisely matches the shape of the organ or tumor being targeted.

5(alpha)-reductase: An enzyme that converts testosterone (T) to dihydrotestosterone (DHT), the male hormone most active in the prostate. (See also **finasteride**.)

active monitoring: A strategy for managing disease in which the patient is regularly examined but not treated until the disease shows signs of worsening. Also called *deferred therapy* and *expectant management*, as opposed to traditional watchful waiting, which meant do nothing.

acute prostatitis: An inflammation or infection in the prostate of sudden onset.

acute urinary retention: A sudden inability to urinate.

adenocarcinoma: A cancer that begins in epithelial cells of glands and glandlike organs. Almost all prostate cancers are adenocarcinomas.

alternative medicine: Approaches outside mainstream medical therapy that are promoted as viable treatment options but are unproven and could be harmful.

androgen: A hormone that stimulates activity of male sex organs or promotes development of male sex characteristics. The principal androgen is testosterone.

androgen deprivation therapy: A treatment for prostate cancer in which surgery or, more commonly, drugs, prevent the body from making or using androgens.

androstenedione (Andro): A steroidal hormone that the body can convert to testosterone. It is naturally produced in testicles, adrenal glands, and ovaries, and has recently been declared a controlled substance by the FDA.

antiandrogens: Medications used to block the effects of male hormones. A form of androgen deprivation therapy.

apoptosis: Programmed cell death, the natural process by which cells self-destruct to make room for new cells. Cancer cells, resistant to this process, are virtually immortal.

artificial sphincter: A surgically implanted device that replaces the urinary sphincter to treat incontinence.

benign: Not malignant, not cancerous, lacks the capacity to spread beyond the organ of origin.

benign prostatic hyperplasia (BPH): Non-cancerous overgrowth of cells within the prostate. As the prostate enlarges, it may block the urinary stream.

biopsy: The process of removing tissue from a patient to check for cancer. Also, a sample of tissue removed as part of this process. A "positive" result means cancer has been detected.

bladder: A muscular organ that stores and periodically empties ("voids") urine.

bladder neck: The opening of the bladder into the urethra. Contains the internal urinary sphincter.

bladder outlet obstruction: A blockage at the point where the bladder drains into the urethra. BPH is a frequent cause.

bone scan: A medical test that uses trace amounts of radioisotopes to detect the spread of cancer to bones.

brachytherapy (seed implants): A form of radiation therapy in which the radioactive material is implanted near or in direct contact with the tissue being treated.

cancer: Any disease in which abnormal cells grow in an uncontrolled manner and have the potential to invade nearby tissue and spread to distant sites (metastasize).

capsule: The soft, fibrous outer layer or "skin" of the prostate.

castration: Blocking the production of testosterone by surgical removal of the testicles (see **orchiectomy**) or with drugs.

cavernous (erectile) nerves: The erectile nerves that run along the left and right side of the prostate to the penis and control erections. Surgery or radiation therapy to treat prostate cancer can damage these nerves.

chemotherapy: Cancer treatment involving one or a combination ("cocktail") of drugs.

chronic prostatitis/chronic pelvic pain syndrome (CP–CPPS): The most common type of prostatitis, defined by symptoms that persist for three months or more with no evidence of bacterial infection of the prostate.

cold spot: In radiation therapy, an area that received a lower-than-intended radiation dose, inadequately treating cancer cells.

comorbidity: A disease or medical condition in addition to the condition under consideration. For example, a urologist discussing a man's prostate cancer would consider his heart disease a comorbidity.

complementary medicine: Supportive measures used in addition to conventional medical treatments to alleviate stress, reduce symptoms, and promote a feeling of well-being, e.g. acupuncture, massage.

constricting ring: A ring or band placed at the base of the penis to help maintain an erection.

conventional radiation therapy: A form of external beam therapy in which the radiation is delivered to a box-shaped area around the target organ.

corpus cavernosum (pl., **corporora cavernosa**): One of two erectile chambers filled with spongy tissues that run the length of the penis. An influx of blood to these chambers is required for penile erection.

corpus spongiosum: A small erectile chamber near the urethra that runs to the head of the penis.

Cowper's glands: A pair of pea-sized glands that lie beneath the prostate gland and produce part of the seminal fluid.

cryotherapy (cryoablation, cryosurgery): A treatment in which prostate tissue is destroyed by freezing.

cystoscope: A slim, lighted instrument that allows a doctor to visually examine the urethra and the bladder internally.

dehydroepiandro sterone (DHEA): A steroidal hormone alleged to reverse many effects of aging, although its effectiveness and safety are doubtful.

digital rectal exam (DRE): A screening test in which the physician inserts a lubricated, gloved finger into the rectum to detect abnormalities in the prostate.

dihydrotestosterone (DHT): A male hormone derived from testosterone that is required for development of the prostate and other secondary male characteristics (including male pattern baldness).

disease state: A distinct stage in the natural history of an illness.

DNA: The molecule that makes up genes and chromosomes and carries all hereditary information.

doubling time: The time required for a tumor to double in size or for the PSA level to double.

dry orgasm: Orgasm without ejaculation.

dysorgasmia: Pain in the penis, scrotum, or perineum during orgasm.

ejaculation: The sudden release of semen through the penis during sexual climax. (The semen is the "ejaculate.")

ejaculatory ducts: Tubes that run from the seminal vesicles and prostate into the urethra near the tip or apex of the prostate.

emission: The discharge of sperm and seminal fluid into the urethra during sexual climax.

endorectal MRI (with spectroscopy): A technique used to visualize the prostate and surrounding tissues using magnetic resonance imaging. A coil placed in the rectum permits greater detail and clarity. Spectroscopy detects chemical signals that distinguish cancer from normal tissue.

epididymis: Long, slender, tightly coiled tubes behind the testes in which sperm mature and are stored.

epithelial cells: Cells that line or cover body organs and protect the underlying tissue (e.g. skin).

erectile dysfunction (ED): A consistent inability to get or maintain an erection satisfactory for sexual intercourse.

erection: A sudden inflow of blood to the penis that causes enlargement and rigidity.

estrogen: A female sex hormone.

expressed prostatic fluid: Liquid removed from the prostate for diagnosis purposes during a digital rectal exam.

external beam therapy: A treatment for cancer that uses high-energy radiation from an energy source outside the body to kill cancer cells.

external urinary sphincter: The muscular structure that constricts the urethra below the prostate, retaining urine until the sphincter is relaxed. During ejaculation, the external sphincter relaxes while the internal sphincter constricts to allow release of semen through the urethra.

extracapsular extension (ECE): Spread of prostate cancer outside the membranous covering (capsule) of the prostate.

fecal incontinence: The inability to control the passage of feces or gas.

finasteride (Proscar, Propecia): See **5 alpha-reductase inhibitors**. Finasteride is approved for use in treating BPH (Proscar) and baldness (Propecia) and may have a role in prostate-cancer prevention.

Foley catheter: A tube inserted through the urethra into the bladder to drain urine.

free PSA (% free PSA, %fPSA): PSA that is not bound to another protein. The ratio of free to total PSA, expressed as a percent, helps to distinguish BPH from prostate cancer.

gene therapy: A process to treat or to prevent disease by inserting genes into cells.

Gleason pattern: The degree of disorganization and cellular abnormalities of prostatic glands expressed on a scale from 1 (nearly normal) to 5 (markedly abnormal). Indicates the aggressiveness of a prostate cancer.

Gleason sum (score): Used to describe the seriousness of prostate cancer; the sum of the most common Gleason pattern and the second most common Gleason pattern in a given cancer.

grade: A description of a cancer based on how abnormal the cancer cells appear under a microscope, ranked as low (nearly normal), intermediate, or high (markedly abnormal).

Gray (Gy): A unit designating a certain amount of radiation absorbed by the body during radiation therapy (formerly known as a **rad**).

half-life: The time required for the radioactivity of a given substance to decrease by half. Also, the time required for half the amount of a substance in the body to be eliminated.

hematospermia: Blood in the semen.

hematuria: Blood in the urine.

high-grade PIN (prostatic intraepithelial neoplasia): Premalignant clusters of abnormal cells that have not invaded through the basement membrane of a gland. High-grade PIN is thought to be a precursor of cancer.

high-intensity focused ultrasound (HIFU): A treatment that destroys prostate cells using heat generated by high-frequency soundwaves.

hormone: A signaling chemical produced in one organ that regulates the function of another.

hormone refractory: Prostate cancer that no longer responds to androgen deprivation therapy.

hormone therapy: See **androgen deprivation therapy.**

hot spot: In radiation therapy, an area that receives a higher-than-intended radiation dose, causing damage.

impotence: See **erectile dysfunction.**

incidental cancer: Small, insignificant cancer found when prostate tissue is removed to treat symptoms of BPH or as part of an operation for bladder cancer.

incontinence: Inability to control the release of urine or feces.

indolent cancer: A tiny cancer that poses no immediate threat to life or health.

infertility: The inability to conceive children.

inflammation: A response of the body to injury or infection.

intensity modulated radiation therapy (IMRT): A form of external radiation in which the dose is highly targeted to the tumor, increasing effectiveness and decreasing side effects.

internal urinary sphincter: Muscular structure of the bladder neck that retains urine in the bladder until it is voluntarily released.

international prostate symptom score (IPSS): A questionnaire used to assess urinary symptoms.

irritative voiding symptoms: Urinary symptoms that result from irritations, e.g. frequency, urgency, blood in the urine, burning.

Kegel (pelvic floor) exercises: Repetitive exercises to strengthen the muscles of the pelvic floor to improve urinary control.

LHRH agonist: Injectable medication that suppresses the body's production of androgens (a form of androgen deprivation therapy).

laparoscopic prostatectomy: Removal of the entire prostate and seminal vesicles through tiny incisions, using a laparoacope.

libido: Sexual desire.

lower urinary tract symptoms (LUTS): Urinary problems, including frequent, slow, or painful urination, nocturia, hesitancy, and dribbling.

magnetic resonance imaging (MRI): A diagnostic tool that uses a powerful magnetic field to generate three-dimensional images of internal organs.

malignant: Cancerous, has the capacity to escape the organ or origin and spread to other sites.

meatus: The opening in the head of the penis.

medical informatics: The development of mathematical models designed to improve communication, understanding, and management of medical information.

minimal peripheral dose (MPD): In brachytherapy, the least amount of radiation exposure to the edges of the prostate that provides an adequate radiation dose throughout the gland.

monoclonal antibodies: Substances produced in the lab to diagnose or treat cancer.

morbidity: Any disease condition. Also, the rate of disease; the number of people sick divided by the population.

mortality: Death. Also, the death rate; the number of deaths from a given cause divided by the population.

myogenic: Caused by or associated with muscle contractions.

nerve graft: Transfer of a segment of a nerve from one site in the body to another to repair a nerve that has been damaged or removed.

nerve sparing: Radical prostatectomy in which the erectile (cavernous) nerves are preserved.

neurogenic: Caused by or originating in the nervous system.

nocturia: Waking at night to urinate.

nocturnal penile tumescence (NPT): Erections that occur during sleep.

nomogram: A mathematical tool for estimating a disease stage or the probability of a medical outcome.

nonsteroidal anti-inflammatory drugs (NSAIDs): A class of substances (e.g. ibuprofen, aspirin) used to relieve pain and suppress inflammation.

obstructive voiding symptoms: Urinary symptoms caused by blockage, e.g. slow stream, hesitancy, intermittency, waking at night to urinate.

open radical prostatectomy: Removal of prostate tissue through an incision in the abdomen.

orchiectomy: Surgical removal of the testes (see **castration**).

organ confined: A cancer that has not escaped the prostate.

outer urinary sphincter: See **external urinary sphincter.**

overflow incontinence: Urinary incontinence that occurs when there is leakage of urine because the bladder is always full.

Partin tables: Staging tables used to predict what the pathologist will find on examining the prostate after it is surgically removed to treat cancer.

pelvic lymph node dissection (PLND): A procedure in which lymph nodes near the site of a malignant tumor are removed and examined for cancer.

penile implant (prothesis): A semi-rigid or inflatable device that is surgically implanted in the penis to enable erections.

penis: The male organ of sexual intercourse and urination.

perineal prostatectomy: Removal of the prostate through an incision between the scrotum and rectum.

perineum: Area between the scrotum and the rectum.

perineural invasion (PNI): The spread of prostate cancer into the sheath surrounding the prostate nerves.

peripheral zone: The part of the prostate beneath the capsule that surrounds the transition zone. Most prostate cancers arise in the peripheral zone.

Peyronie's disease: A condition in which hard areas (fibrous plaques) form in the erectile bodies of the penis, causing the penis to bend and sometimes feel painful during erections.

photodynamic therapy: An experimental treatment for prostate cancer in which a light source inserted into the prostate activates the therapeutic drug.

positive surgical margin: The presence of cancer at the edge of tissue removed during surgery. Suggests that some of the cancer likely remains in the body.

priapism: A dangerous erection that lasts four hours or more.

proctitis: Inflammation of the mucous membranes that line the rectum; sometimes follows radiation therapy.

prostadynia: Pain in the prostate.

prostaglandin: Potent hormone-like substance that can trigger inflammation, pain, and various other processes.

ProstaScint: A test for prostate cancer metastases using a monoclonal antibody.

prostate-specific antigen (PSA): A protein, produced in the prostate, normally present in high levels in the semen. Elevated PSA levels in the blood may indicate a problem in the prostate.

prostatectomy: Surgical removal of prostate tissue.

prostatism: Urinary symptoms associated with prostate enlargement.

prostatitis: Inflammation or infection of the prostate.

proton beam radiation: A form of external radiation that uses protons instead of gamma rays.

PSA density (PSAD): The ratio of PSA level to prostate size.

PSA doubling time (PSA velocity): How quickly the PSA level rises (the rate of rise, measured in nanograms per milliliter per year). The time required for a man's PSA level to double.

PSA nadir: The lowest PSA level after treatment for prostate cancer.

psychogenic: Caused by or related to stress.

rad: A unit that describes radiation dosage. See **Gray.**

radiation cystitis: Inflammation of the urinary bladder caused by exposure to radiation.

radiation proctitis: Inflammation of the rectum caused by radiation exposure.

radical prostatectomy: Surgery that completely removes the prostate and seminal vesicles.

radiofrequency ablation (RFA): A treatment that uses heat to kill tissue.

rectum: The lowest part of the large intestine, connecting to the anus.

retrograde ejaculation: The release of semen into the bladder instead of out through the penis.

salvage radiation: Radiation therapy to treat a cancer that has recurred after surgery or another initial treatment.

salvage radical prostatectomy: Removal of the entire prostate, performed to treat prostate cancer that has recurred after radiation or other primary therapy.

seed implants: See **brachytherapy.**

semen: The thick fluid released from the penis during orgasm containing sperm.

seminal vesicle: One of two glands, connected to the base (top) of the prostate behind the bladder, which secretes a component of seminal fluid.

seminal vesicle invasion (SVI): Speed of prostate cancer into the seminal vesicles.

simple prostatectomy: A surgical procedure to remove prostate tissue to treat the urinary symptoms of BPH.

sling procedure: A treatment for urinary incontinence in which a piece of synthetic material is attached to the pelvis to compress the urethra.

stage: Describes the size and location of a cancer and how large and extensive a cancer is.

stress incontinence (stress urinary incontinence, SUI): Leakage of urine from an increase in pressure on the abdomen, as from coughing, straining, or sudden movement.

stricture: A narrowing of the urethra caused by scarring.

surgical margin: The outer surface of the tissue that is surgically removed.

tenesmus: An urgent desire to empty the bowel, resulting in passage of mucus but little fecal matter.

testis (testicle): One of the two male reproductive glands that produce sperm and testosterone.

testosterone: The principal male hormone. See **androgen.**

thermal therapy: Using heat to destroy tissue.

TNM staging: A system for expressing the size and degree of spread of a cancer by separately describing the extent of tumor as its original location (T), whether and to what extent the cancer has spread to nearby lymph nodes (N), and whether and to what extent the cancer has metastasized to distant sites (M).

total (complete) androgen blockade: Therapy that completely blocks the effects of testosterone.

transition zone: The part of the prostate immediately surrounding the urethra. The transition zone is the site of benign prostate hyperplasia (BPH). Prostate cancers can arise in this zone as well.

transrectal ultrasound (TRUS): Imaging technique in which the prostate is examined through an ultrasound probe inserted in the rectum.

transurethral resection of the prostate (TURP): Removal of excess prostate tissue by chipping away with a special instrument. The most common surgical treatment for symptoms of BPH.

ureter: A tube that carries urine from a kidney to the bladder.

urethra: The tube that carries urine from the bladder to the outside of the body.

urethral stricture: See **stricture.**

urge incontinence: Involves a strong, sudden need to urinate immediately.

urinary flow rate: The speed of the stream during urination.

urinary tract: The organs that produce and eliminate urine: the kidneys, ureters, bladder, and urethra.

urodynamic testing: A set of medical tests to measure urinary flow, bladder capacity, and bladder function, used to determine the cause of urinary symptoms.

urology: The field of medicine concerned with the function and disorders of the male genitals and the male and female urinary system.

vacuum erection device (VED): Induces an erection by creating a vacuum around the penis. A constricting ring maintains the erection.

vas deferens: Ducts that carry sperm from the testicles to the prostate.

watchful waiting: An approach to managing prostate cancer. Traditionally, watchful waiting meant to make no attempt to cure or regularly monitor the cancer. Today, the term is often used to mean the deferral of treatment, though patients are actively, regularly monitored and treated when the cancer shows signs of worsening.

GLOSSARY OF MEDICATIONS

5 alpha-reductase inhibitors: Drugs (e.g. finasteride or dutasteride) used to treat BPH symptoms by shrinking the prostate. These drugs block the conversion of testosterone (T) to dihydrotestosterone (DHT), the male hormone that stimulates prostate growth.

alfuzosin (Uroxatral): See **alpha blockers.**

alpha blockers: A group of drugs (e.g. doxazosin, terazosin, tamsulosin, and alfuzosin) used to treat urinary symptoms in men. Alpha blockers, originally developed to treat high blood pressure, work by blocking the effects of adrenaline, allowing the muscles of the prostate and bladder neck to relax.

alprostadil: A drug used to treat erectile dysfunction, supplied as a suppository (MUSE) or in a syringe for injection (Caverject. Also one component of injectible "Trimix"). Alprostadil increases blood flow to the penis, producing an erection.

aminoglutethimide: See **antiandrogens.** A second-line hormonal agent, used for hormone refractory prostate cancer, works by blocking the production of androgens by the adrenal gland. Must be given in combination with steroid hormones (e.g. corticosteroids), which are essential to life but are also blocked by the drug.

ansamycins: A group of experimental drugs being tested as chemotherapeutic agents for prostate cancer.

antiandrogens: A group of drugs (e.g. bicalutamide, flutamide, and nilutamide) used in hormone therapy that block the stimulatory effects of male hormones on prostate-cancer cells.

antibiotics: Drugs that kill microorganisms, especially bacteria. Antibiotics can cure both acute and chronic bacterial prostatitis. They are often tried, with limited success, to treat chronic prostatitis/chronic pelvic pain syndrome.

anticholinergics: A group of drugs (e.g. oxybutinin, tolterodine, and banthine) used to relax the bladder and relieve bladder spasms.

Aredia (pamidronate): See **bisphosphonates.**

Avodart (dutasteride): See **5 alpha-reductase inhibitors** and **dutasteride.**

bicalutamide (Casodex): See **antiandrogens.** Bicalutamide, taken by mouth, is the most widely prescribed antiandrogen. The dose is lower when bicalutamide is used with LHRH agonists than alone.

bisphosphonates: A group of drugs (e.g. pamidronate, sodium dodronate, zoledronic acid, and etidronate) used to reduce bone mass loss caused by hormone therapy or by metastases of cancer to bone.

bone protective agent: See **bisphosphonates.**

Bonefos (sodium clodronate): See **bisphosphonates.**

buprenorphine: See **opioids.**

carboplatin: See **chemotherapeutic drugs.** Carboplatin is an intravenous chemotherapeutic drug with less effect on kidney function than its cousin, cisplatinum, but also less effect on cancer.

Cardura (doxazosin): See **alpha blockers.**

Casodex (bicalutamide): See **bicalutamide.**

Caverject (alprostadil): An injectable medication for erectile dysfunction. Caverjet consists of a syringe filled with alprostadil, which can produce an erection by increasing blood flow to the penis.

Celebrex (celecoxib): See **celecoxib.**

celecoxib (Celebrex): See **COX-2 inhibitors.**

chemotherapeutic drugs: A group of drugs that kill cancer cells and other rapidly dividing cells in the body. These drugs typically have more side effects (e.g. hair loss, nausea, diarrhea, loss of appetite, mouth ulcers) than biologic or immunologic agents.

Cialis (tadalafil): See **PDE-5 inhibitors.** Tadalafil is sometimes called the "weekend drug" because its effects last longer than sildenafil or vardalafil.

Cipro (ciprofloxacin): See **ciprofloxacin.**

ciprofloxacin (Cipro): An antibiotic that is especially effective for urinary tract infections and to prevent infection from prostate biopsies.

codeine: See **opioids.** Codeine, taken by mouth, is an effective medicine for pain after prostate surgery.

Colace (docusate): See **stool softeners.**

complete (total) androgen blockade: Hormone therapy that combines an LHRH agonist and an antiandrogen to stop production of male hormones by the testicles and block the effects of the small amount of androgens produced by the adrenal gland.

Contigen (bovine collagen): Bulking agent that is injected into the urinary sphincter to treat incontinence.

corticosteroids: Hormones (or drugs that have similar hormonal effects) produced by the adrenal gland that reduce inflammation and bleeding from radiation proctitis and prevent nausea and vomiting from chemotherapy.

Coumadin (warfarin): Taken by mouth, this drug prevents clotting of blood by reducing the amount of vitamin K produced by the liver.

COX-2 inhibitors: A group of drugs (e.g. celecoxib and rofecoxib) used to relieve the pain and inflammation of prostatitis and other conditions; thought to have fewer side effects than aspirin or NSAIDs, such as ibuprofen, though the COX-2 inhibitor Vioxx was recently taken off the market when it was found to increase the risk of heart attack and stroke.

DES (diethylstilbestrol): A female hormone taken by mouth which stops the production of male hormone by the testicles by blocking the necessary signals from the brain (LHRH).

Detrol (tolterodine): See **anticholinergics.**

Didronel (etidronate): See **bisphosphonates.**

Ditropan (oxybutynin): See **anticholinergics.**

docetaxel (Taxotere): A chemotherapeutic agent used to treat cancer. The combination of docetaxel with other agents has been shown to prolong life in men with hormone refractory prostate cancer.

doxazosin (Cardura): See **alpha blockers.**

Dulcolax (bisacodyl): A mild laxative, used to relieve constipation; can be taken by mouth or as a rectal suppository.

Durasphere: Bulking agent that is injected into the urinary sphincter as a treatment for incontinence.

dutasteride (Avodart): See **5 alpha-reductase inhibitors**. Dutasteride differs from finasteride in blocking both type I and II reductase enzyme, but it is not clear that this distinction makes any difference in how well it works.

Eligard (leuprolide): See **LHRH agonists.**

Elmiron (pentosan polysulfate): A drug used to treat bladder pain caused by interstitial cystitis. Elmiron has also been tested as a treatment for chronic prostatitis/chronic pelvic pain syndrome.

estramustine: A **chemotherapeutic drug** that combines the effect of an estrogen (female hormone) and a chemotherapeutic agent that kills cancer cells directly, designed especially to treat prostate cancer.

estrogen: Female hormone. Estrogen has been used to treat prostate cancer by inhibiting the production of hormone-stimulating substances (LHRH) in the brain, thus blocking the production of testosterone by the testicles.

etidronate (Didronel): See **bisphosphonates.**

Eulexin (flutamide): See **antiandrogens.**

fentanyl: See **opioids.** Fentanyl provides powerful quick but short-lasting pain relief and is often used in epidural anesthesia or as a skin patch for postoperative pain.

finasteride (Proscar, Propecia): See **5 alpha-reductase inhibitors.** Finasteride is approved for use in treating BPH (Proscar) and baldness (Propecia) and may have a role in prostate-cancer prevention.

Flomax (tamsulosin): See **tamulosin**.

flutamide (Eulexin): See **antiandrogens**.

ganciclovir: Antiviral drug used in an experimental gene therapy for prostate cancer.

gentamicin: See **antibiotics**. Given by injection, gentamicin is one of the most effective antibiotics for urinary infections and prevention of infection after prostate biopsy.

goserelin (Zoladex): See **LHRH agonists**.

heparin: See **blood thinners**.

hydrocodone: See **opioids**.

hydrocortisone: See **corticosteroids**.

hydromorphone: See **opioids**.

Hytrin (terazosin): See **alpha blockers**.

Imodium (loperamide): A drug used to treat diarrhea.

ketoconazole (Nizoral): See **antiandrogens**.

ketorolac (Toradol): A powerful anti-inflammatory drug and pain reliever sometimes used to reduce pain after surgery.

leuprolide (Lupron, Eligard): See **LHRH agonists**.

Levaquin (levofloxacin): See **antibiotics**.

Levitra (vardenafil): See **PDE-5 inhibitors**.

levofloxacin (Levaquin) See **antibiotics**.

LHRH agonists: A group of drugs used in hormone therapy that shut down testosterone production by the testicles.

lidocaine: A local anesthetic sometimes used before a prostate biopsy.

loperamide (Imodium): A drug used to treat diarrhea.

Lupron (leuprolide): See **LHRH agonists**.

methadone: See **opioids**.

mitoxantrone (Novantrone): See **chemotherapeutic drugs**.

monoclonal antibodies: A group of substances produced in the laboratory that track and bind to cancer cells. Monoclonal antibodies have been studied as a means of diagnosing and treating prostate cancer.

morphine: See **opioids**.

MUSE (Medical Urethral System for Erection): A treatment for erectile dysfunction consisting of a suppository containing alprostadil that is inserted into the urethra. Alprostadil increases blood flow to the penis, which enables an erection.

neuroprotective agents: A group of drugs that protect nerves from damage.

Nilandron (nilutamide): See **antiandrogens**.

nilutamide (Nilandron): See **antiandrogens**.

nitrates: Drugs used medically to treat chest pain (e.g. nitroglycerin) and recreationally (e.g. "poppers"). Nitrates can interact dangerously with PDE-5 inhibitors.

nitroglycerin: A drug used to treat chest pain (angina).

Nizoral (ketoconazole): See **antiandrogens**.

non-opioid drugs: A group of drugs used to relieve mild to moderate pain (e.g. aspirin, acetaminophin, NSAIDs), which are not addictive.

nonsteroidal anti-inflammatory drugs (NSAIDs): A class of substances (e.g. ibuprofen, aspirin) used to relieve pain and suppress inflammation.

Novantrone (mitoxantrone): See **chemotherapeutic drugs**.

opioids: A group of drugs used to relieve moderate to severe pain. Examples include codeine, tramadol, morphine, methadone, hydrocodone, and buprenorphine.

oxybutynin (Ditropan): See **anticholinergics**.

pamidronate (Aredia): See **bisphosphonates**.

PDE-5 inhibitors: A group of drugs (e.g. sildenafil, vardenafil, tadalafil) used to treat erectile dysfunction by relaxing smooth muscles and increasing blood flow to the penis.

pentosan polysulfate (Elmiron): Prescription drug approved for treating bladder pain caused by interstitial cystitis. Pentosan polysulfate has also been tested as a treatment for chronic prostatitis/chronic pelvic pain syndrome.

Percocet: A combination of the opioid pain reliever hydrocodone and the milder pain reliever acetaminophen. Percocet is often used for relief of pain after surgery.

Prednisone: See **corticosteroids**.

Propecia (finasteride): See **5 alpha-reductase inhibitors**.

Proscar (finasteride): See **5 alpha-reductase inhibitors**.

sildenafil (Viagra): See **PDE-5 inhibitors**.

sodium clodronate (Bonefos): See **bisphosphonates**.

spironolactone (Aldactone): A diuretic used to reduce the swelling and weight gain from fluid retention after surgery.

steroid foam: Medication used to treat rectal irritation, bleeding, and diarrhea.

stool softeners: Drugs that relieve constipation by causing the stool to contain more moisture, making it easier to pass.

tadalafil (Cialis): See **PDE-5 inhibitors**.

tamsulosin (Flomax): See **alpha blockers**. Tamulosin inhibits the specific type of receptor that constricts the bladder neck and the prostate and may have fewer side effects than doxazosin or terazosin.

Taxotere (docetaxel): See **docetaxel**.

terazosin (Hytrin): See **alpha blockers**.

tobramycin: See **antibiotics**.

tolterodine tartrate (Detrol LA): See **anticholinergics**.

Toradol (ketorolac): See **anti-inflammatory drugs**.

total androgen blockade: See **complete (total) androgen blockade**.

tramadol: See **opioids**.

Trimix: Injectable mixture of alprostadil, papaverine, and phentolamine used to treat erectile dysfunction by expanding blood vessels and increasing blood flow to the penis. Trimix is not commercially available and must be compounded by a pharmacy.

UroXatral (alfuzosin): See **alpha blockers**.

Vaccine: Any preparation designed to prevent or treat disease by stimulating the immune system.

vardenafil (Levitra): See **PDE-5 inhibitors**.

Viagra (sildenafil): See **PDE-5 inhibitors**.

Vicodin: A combination of the opioid pain reliever hydrocodone and the milder pain reliever acetaminophen. Vicodin is often used for relief of pain after surgery.

Vioxx (rofecoxib): See **COX-2 inhibitors**.

warfarin (Coumadin): A blood thinner used to prevent clotting.

Zoladex (goserelin): See **LHRH agonists**.

zoledronic acid (Zometa): See **bisphosphonates**.

Zometa (zoledronic acid): See **bisphosphonates**.

RESOURCES

Countless resources are available to men with prostate diseases and their loved ones. Here is a representative sample of some of the best Web sites, organizations, and suggested additional readings. Listings are alphabetical by category.

AGING

Rowe, J. W., and R. I. Kan. *Successful Aging*. New York, Dell Publishing; Division of Random House (1998).
Based on the findings of the MacArthur Foundation Study of Successful Aging, this book details lifestyle factors that can improve quality of life as we age.

Vaillant, George E. *Aging Well: Surprising Guideposts to a Happier Life from the Landmark Harvard Study of Adult Development*. Boston: Little Brown (2002).
This report, based on a fifty-year study of people from highly diverse cultural backgrounds, identifies the apparent keys to successful aging.

ALTERNATIVE AND COMPLEMENTARY MEDICINES

Cassileth, B. R. *The Alternative Medicine Handbook*. New York: W. W. Norton & Co. (1998).
A guide to helpful and harmful alternatives to mainstream medical treatments by a leading expert in the field.

Cassileth, B. R., Lucarelli. *Herb-Drug Interactions in Oncology* (CD). Hamilton: BC Decker, Inc. (2003).
Scientifically based information for cancer patients and physicians on the values and dangers of herbs and remedies.

MEMORIAL SLOAN-KETTERING CANCER CENTER

www.mskcc.org/mskcc/html/11570.cfm
1-212-639-2000
Comprehensive information about herbs, botanicals, and other products, as well as a link to the hospital's integrative medicine services and research on alternative healing practices.

Moyad, M. A. *ABC's of Nutrition and Supplements for Prostate Cancer*. Chelsea, Mich.: Sleeping Bear Press (2000).
Practical advice for prostate-cancer patients on nutrients and supplements from a leading expert.

NATIONAL CENTER FOR COMPLEMENTARY
  AND ALTERNATIVE MEDICINE
www.nccam.nih.gov
1-888-644-6226
An organization of the National Institutes of Health (NIH) that investigates complementary and alternative healing practices in the context of rigorous science. Focuses include research, training, outreach, and integration of proven complementary and alternative practices with conventional medicine.

BENIGN PROSTATIC HYPERPLASIA (BPH)

AMERICAN UROLOGY ASSOCIATION
www.urologyhealth.org
The patient Web site of this organization has information on the causes, diagnosis, and treatment of BPH. (The site also offers information on prostate cancer and prostatitis.)

NATIONAL GUIDELINE CLEARINGHOUSE: GUIDELINES FOR
  THE DIAGNOSIS AND TREATMENT OF BPH
www.guideline.gov/summary/summary.aspx?doc_id=3740&nbr=2966&string=BPH,
or go to www.guideline.gov and type "BPH" in the search bar
info@guideline.gov
2003 guidelines for the diagnosis and treatment of BPH from the American Urological Association.

NATIONAL KIDNEY AND UROLOGIC DISEASE
  INFORMATION CLEARINGHOUSE
www.kidney.niddk.nih.gov/kudiseases/pubs/prostateenlargement
1-800-891-5390
Information about BPH, including clinical trials.

CANCER

AMERICAN CANCER SOCIETY
www.cancer.org
1-800-ACS-2345
Information from the leading private cancer organization in the United States.

INFORMÁCION EN ESPAÑOL DE LA NCI
www.nci.nih.gov/espanol
1-800-4-CANCER
Comprehensive information about cancer in Spanish from the National Cancer Institute.

MEMORIAL SLOAN-KETTERING CANCER CENTER
www.mskcc.org
1-212-639-2000; 1-800-525-2225
Comprehensive information about all aspects of cancer prevention, diagnosis, and treatment from the world's oldest medical center dedicated to cancer care.

NATIONAL CANCER INSTITUTE (NCI)
www.nci.nih.gov
1-800-4-CANCER
A thorough discussion of cancer screening, diagnosis, and treatment from the government's National Institutes of Health.

NCI LIST OF DESIGNATED CANCER CENTERS
http://www3.cancer.gov/cancercenters/centerslist.html

PEOPLE LIVING W/CANCER
www.oncology.com/plwc
1-703-797-1914
The patient information Web site of the American Society of Clinical Oncology (ASCO) provides oncologist-approved information on more than fifty types of cancer and their treatments, clinical trials, coping, and side effects. Additional resources include a Find on Oncologist database, live chats, message boards, a drug database, and links to patient-support organizations. The site is designed to help people with cancer make informed health-care decisions.

UNDERSTANDING CANCER
www.cancer.gov/cancertopics
1-800-4-CANCER
Comprehensive information about cancer types, diagnosis, treatments, and clinical trials.

CHEMOTHERAPY

AMERICAN CANCER SOCIETY (ACS)
www.cancer.org/docroot/MBC/MBC_2X_ChemotherapyEffects.asp?sitearea=MBC
1-800-ACS-2345
A comprehensive discussion of chemotherapy, including possible side effects and means to deal with them.

NATIONAL CANCER INSTITUTE (NCI)
www.nci.nih.gov/cancerinfo/chemotherapy-and-you
1-800-4-CANCER
Information about chemotherapy from the National Cancer Institute, including how it works, what to expect during treatment, nutritional needs during therapy, and possible means of financing.

CLINICAL TRIALS

CLINIC TRIALS.GOV
www.clinicaltrials.gov/
1-800-4-CANCER
Information about federally and privately supported clinical trials of new diagnostic tools and treatments for various medical conditions, including all prostate diseases.

PHYSICIAN DATA QUERY (PDQ)
http://www.cancer.gov/cancertopics/pdq
An NCI database that contains the latest information about cancer treatment, screening, prevention, genetics, supportive care, and complementary and alternative medicine, plus clinical trials.

DRUG INFORMATION

MEDLINEPLUS
www.nlm.nih.gov/medlineplus/druginformation.html
custserv@nlm.nih.gov
Information on prescription and nonprescription drugs.

ERECTILE DYSFUNCTION

WWW.IMPOTENCE.ORG
www.impotence.org
1-410-689-3990
Comprehensive information about erectile dysfunction from the Sexual Function Health Council of the American Foundation for Urologic Disease, Inc. (AFUD).

Lue, Tom F. *Contemporary Diagnosis and Management of Male Erectile Dysfunction.* Newtown, Pa.: Handbooks in Health Care (2000).
Written by a prominent urologist, this book offers an in-depth look at the causes and treatments for ED.

NATIONAL KIDNEY AND UROLOGIC DISEASE
  INFORMATION CLEARINGHOUSE
www.kidney.niddk.nih.gov/kudiseases/pubs/impotence/index.htm
1-800-891-5390
Information about erectile dysfunction from the NIH includes access to a search of the recent medical literature, clinical trials, and resources (*en español también*).

Ridwan, Shabsigh, MD, and Louis Ignarro, Phd. *Back to Great Sex: Overcome ED and Reclaim Lost Intimacy.* New York: Kensington Books (2002).
Reassuring, scientifically based information on overcoming erectile dysfunction.

FREE AND SUBSIDIZED SERVICES FOR PATIENTS

ANGELFLIGHT AMERICA
www.angelflightamerica.org
1-800-446-1231
Provides long-distance transportation in private planes free of charge for patients and their families traveling for essential medical treatment.

CANCER CARE
www.cancercare.org
1-800-813-HOPE
One of the oldest private, not-for-profit organizations in the United States. Provides advice and support services free of charge for cancer patients, including counseling, education, information, and referrals, as well as financial assistance.

HELPINGPATIENTS.ORG
www.helpingpatients.org
This site, from the Pharmaceutical Research & Manufacturers of America, allows patients and doctors to determine whether the patient is eligible to receive medications free of charge because of financial need.

NATIONAL ASSOCIATION OF HOSPITAL
  HOSPITALITY HOUSES, INC.
www.nahhh.org
1-800-542-9730
Provides lodging and support services to patients and their families who are receiving medical treatment far from their home communities.

NATIONAL PATIENT AIR TRANSPORT HELPLINE
www.patienttravel.org
1-800-296-1217
Provides information and referrals for charitable medical transportation for patients and their families.

GENERAL MEDICAL

AMERICAN BOARD OF MEDICAL SPECIALTIES
www.abms.org
1-866-ASK-ABMS
A nonprofit organization of twenty-four specialty societies that list board-certified medical specialists who have completed approved training programs and successfully passed a specialty examination in their fields.

MEDLINEPLUS
www.nlm.nih.gov/medlineplus/healthtopics.html
custserv@nlm.nih.gov
Health information from the National Library of Medicine, including a searchable database of health topics, drug information, a medical encyclopedia and dictionary, health news, and a directory of specialists and hospitals.

NIH SENIORHEALTH
www.nihseniorhealth.gov
custserv@nlm.nih.gov
Health information from the National Institutes of Health; can be viewed in large type and will read text aloud.

HORMONE THERAPY

www.casodex.com
Information from AstraZeneca about bicalutamide (Casodex).

www.lupron.com
Information on (leuprolide acetate) Lupron from TAP Pharmaceuticals.

www.zoladex.com
Information about goserelin acetate (Zoladex) from AstraZeneca.

HOSPICE AND OTHER END-OF-LIFE RESOURCES

Hospice Services provide comprehensive support services to terminally ill patients and their families.

HOSPICE FOUNDATION OF AMERICA
www.hospicefoundation.org
1-305-981-2522

HOSPICE NET
www.hospicenet.org
Suite 51
401 Bowling Avenue
Nashville, Tenn. 37205-5124

NATIONAL HOSPICE AND PALLIATIVE CARE ORGANIZATION
www.nhpco.org
1-703-837-1500

INCONTINENCE, BOWEL AND URINARY

INCONTINENCE.ORG
www.incontinence.org
Information about urinary incontinence sponsored by the Bladder Advisory Council of the American
Foundation for Urologic Disease, Inc. (AFUD).

There are many additional online sources for mens' incontinence supplies. You can also purchase pads
specially designed for men at many drugstores and supermarkets.

INCONTINENCE SUPPLIES

At Home Medical
www.athomemedical.com
1-800-526-5895

UroMed
www.umed.com
1-800-403-9189

Direct Medical
directmedicalinc.com/pad.html
1-800-659-8037

NATIONAL KIDNEY AND UROLOGIC DISEASE
    INFORMATION CLEARINGHOUSE
www.kidney.niddk.nih.gov/kudiseases/pubs/uimen/index.htm
www.digestive.niddk.nih.gov/ddiseases/pubs/fecalincontinence/index.htm.
1-800-891-5390
A comprehensive source of information about urinary and fecal incontinence.

PROSTATE CANCER

AMERICAN UROLOGICAL ASSOCIATION PATIENT SITE
    (SEE BPH ABOVE)
www.urologyhealth.org

CANADIAN PROSTATE CANCER NETWORK
www.cpcn.org
1-705-652-9200
The national association of prostate-cancer support groups in Canada.

Campbell, Meredith F., Patrick C. Walsh, and Alan B. Retik. *Campbell's Urology.* 4 volumes. Philadelphia: Saunders (2000).
The definitive textbook of urology, updated every three to five years. Detailed descriptions of the current medical understanding and treatment of BPH, prostatitis, and prostate cancer, with sections on normal anatomy and physiology, and urinary and sexual function and dysfunction.

DEPARTMENT OF DEFENSE CONGRESSIONALLY DIRECTED MEDICAL RESEARCH PROGRAMS
www.cdmrp.army.mil/pcrp
1-301-619-7071
The U.S. Department of Defense is the second largest source of funding for medical research in prostate cancer, after the National Cancer Institute. This site provides information about research grants and research projects.

MEMORIAL SLOAN-KETTERING CANCER CENTER
www.mskcc.org/mskcc/html/403.cfm
For information about prostate cancer.

NATIONAL CANCER INSTITUTE: PROSTATE CANCER
www.cancer.gov/cancerinfo/types/prostate
1-800-4-CANCER
Comprehensive information from the U.S. government's National Institutes of Health about prostate cancer, including support groups and resources, clinical trials, complementary and alternative medicine, statistics, diagnosis and treatment, access to PDQ (a listing of approved clinical trials), and a list of the major research centers for prostate cancer in the United States.

NATIONAL COMPREHENSIVE CANCER NETWORK
www.nccn.org
1-215-690-0300
The National Comprehensive Cancer Network (NCCN), an alliance of nineteen of the world's leading cancer centers, provides detailed guidelines for the diagnosis and treatment of cancer to help patients and health professionals make informed decisions. For prostate-cancer guidelines, go to www.nccn.org/patient_gls/_english/_prostate/index.htm.

NATIONAL GUIDELINE CLEARINGHOUSE: GUIDELINES FOR THE DIAGNOSIS AND TREATMENT OF PROSTATE CANCER
www.guideline.gov/search/searchresults.aspx?=3&txtsearch=prostate+cancer&num=20, or go to www.guideline.gov and type "prostate cancer" in the search bar.
A wide variety of guidelines for screening, diagnosis, and treatment of prostate cancer.

NATIONAL PROSTATE CANCER COALITION
www.4npcc.org
Information on research and treatment for prostate cancer.

Nomograms: computer-based tools to predict clinical stage and treatment results

www.nomograms.org

This URL takes you to a page on the Memorial Sloan-Kettering Cancer Center Web site that allows you to calculate the probability of success with various treatments for prostate cancer, depending upon the characteristics of your disease (stage, grade, PSA, etc.). Use online or download the software to your computer or PDA.

Ohori, Mak, and P. T. Scardino. "Localized Prostate Cancer" *Current Problems in Surgery* 39 (2002): 833–960.
Comp Textbk GU Oncology, 3rd ed. (2005).
The most comprehensive medical textbook of genitourinary oncology, including prostate cancer, written by international authorities in urology, medical oncology, and radiation therapy. Every aspect of prostate cancer is covered in detail.

Phoenix 5

www.phoenix5.org

A patient-to-patient site with a particularly good online glossary (www.phoenix5.org/glossary/glossary.html) and abundant links to other patient-oriented resources.

Prostate Cancer Foundation

www.prostatecancerfoundation.org

1-800-757-CURE

The world's largest source of philanthropic funding for prostate-cancer research. Also disseminates information to promote public awareness.

Resources in Languages other than English

www.cancerindex.org/clinks13.htm

A site with links to cancer resources in many languages.

Us Too! Prostate Cancer Education and Support

www.ustoo.com

1-630-795-1002; Fax: 1-630-795-1602

PCa Support Hotline: 1-800-80-UsTOO, 1-800-808-7866

The oldest patient support group for men with prostate cancer and their partners, with chapters across the United States and Canada.

Virgil's Prostate Online

www.prostate-online.com/index.html

One man's dedicated effort to provide patient-friendly information about prostate cancer.

Walsh, P. C., and J. F. Worthington. *Dr. Patrick Walsh's Guide to Surviving Prostate Cancer.* New York: Warner Books (2001).

PROSTATE CANCER PERSONAL ACCOUNTS

Howe, Desiree Lyon. *His Prostate and Me: A Couple Deals with Prostate Cancer.* Houston: Winedale Publishing (2002).

Korda, M. *Man to Man: Surviving Prostate Cancer.* New York: Vintage Books (1997).

Martin, W. C. *My Prostate and Me: Dealing with Prostate Cancer.* New York: Cadell & Davies (1994).

PROSTATITIS

AMERICAN UROLOGICAL ASSOCIATION PATIENT SITE
(SEE BPH ABOVE)
www.urologyhealth.org

NATIONAL GUIDELINE CLEARINGHOUSE: GUIDELINES FOR THE DIAGNOSIS AND TREATMENT OF PROSTATITIS
www.guideline.gov/summary/summary.aspx?doc_id=3041&nbr=2267&string=prostatitis,
or go to www.guideline.gov and type "prostatitis" in the search bar.
Prostatitis guidelines from the Association of Genitourinary Medicine in London.

NATIONAL KIDNEY AND UROLOGIC DISEASE
INFORMATION CLEARINGHOUSE
www.kidney.niddk.nih.gov/kudiseases/pubs/prostatitis
1-800-891-5390
Information about prostatitis from the NIH; includes access to a search of the recent medical literature.

INDEX

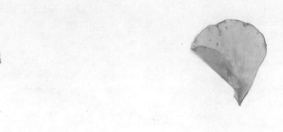